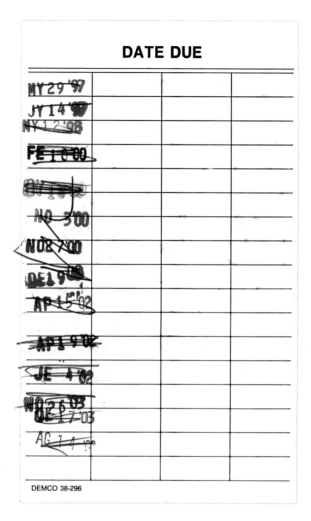

DATE DUE

MY 29 '97			
JY 14 '97			
MY 12 '98			
FE 1 6 00			
NO 3 00			
NO 27 00			
DE 19 00			
AP 15 '02			
AP 19 02			
JE 4 '02			
NO 26 03			
DE 17 03			
AG 14			

DEMCO 38-296

PREVENTING HIV Transmission

The Role of Sterile Needles and Bleach

Jacques Normand, David Vlahov, and Lincoln E. Moses, editors

Panel on Needle Exchange and Bleach Distribution Programs

Commission on Behavioral and Social Sciences and Education

National Research Council

and

Institute of Medicine

NATIONAL ACADEMY PRESS
Washington, D.C. 1995

Preventing HIV transmission

iis report was approved by the Governing Board
ibers are drawn from the councils of the National
/ of Engineering, and the Institute of Medicine.
The members of the committee responsible for the report were chosen for their special competences
and with regard for appropriate balance.

This report has been reviewed by a group other than the authors according to procedures
approved by a Report Review Committee consisting of members of the National Academy of
Sciences, the National Academy of Engineering, and the Institute of Medicine.

This project was sponsored by the National Institute on Drug Abuse.

Library of Congress Cataloging-in-Publication Data

Preventing HIV transmission : the role of sterile needles and bleach /
    Jacques Normand, David Vlahow, and Lincoln E. Moses, editors.
        p. cm.
        "Panel on Needle Exchange and Bleach Distribution Programs,
    Commission on Behavioral and Social Sciences and Education, National
    Research Council and Institute of Medicine."
        ISBN 0-309-05296-3
        1. Needle exchange programs—United States. 2. Chlorine and
    derivatives as disinfectants. 3. AIDS (Disease)—United States—
    Prevention. I. Vlahov, David. II. Moses, Lincoln E.
    III. National Research Council (U.S.). Panel on Needle Exchange and
    Bleach Distribution Programs. IV. Institute of Medicine (U.S.)
        [DNLM: 1. HIV Infections—prevention & control. 2. Needle-
    Exchange Programs. 3. Disinfectants—supply & distribution.
    4. Substance Abuse, Intravenous—complications. 5. Health Policy—
    United States. WC 503.6 P944 1995]
    RA644.A25P754   1995
    616.97'9205—dc20
    DNLM/DLC
    for Library of Congress   95-35458
                                                                              CIP

W. WAYNE WIEBEL, AIDS Outreach Intervention Project *and* School of Public Health, Epidemiology and Biostatistics, University of Illinois at Chicago

DAVID R. WILLIAMS, Department of Sociology and Institute for Social Research, University of Michigan, Ann Arbor

ALEXANDRA K. WIGDOR, *Division Director*
JACQUES NORMAND, *Study Director*
SUSAN R. McCUTCHEN, *Senior Project Assistant*

Contents

PREFACE   xi

ACKNOWLEDGMENTS   xv

EXECUTIVE SUMMARY   1
    The Problem, 1
    The Panel's Charge, 3
    Scientific Assessment of Program Effectiveness, 3
    Community and Legal Factors, 5
    Recommended Course of Action, 6

INTRODUCTION   9
    Dimensions of the Problem, 9
    Responses to the Epidemic, 11
    The Charge to the Panel, 12
    The Panel's Report, 14

PART 1
DIMENSIONS OF THE PROBLEM

1   THE EPIDEMIOLOGY OF HIV AND AIDS   23
    Biological Mechanisms of Transmission, 24
    Injection Drug Use Transmission, 24

v

Sexual Transmission, 28
Perinatal Transmission, 29
Conclusion, 30
Epidemiologic Data, 31
HIV and AIDS Surveillance, 31
Mode of Acquisition of Infection, 32
HIV and AIDS Among Injection Drug Users, 37
Surveillance, 37
Sexual Transmission Among Injection Drug Users, 40
Perinatal Transmission from Injection Drug Users, 43
Summary, 44
Conclusions, 45
Recommendations, 45

2   THE EPIDEMIOLOGY OF INJECTION DRUG USE   57
Estimates of Injection Drug Users, 58
Geographic Variations, 59
National Surveys of Drug Abuse, 60
Characteristics of Injection Drug Users, 64
A National Profile, 64
Local Drug Use Trends and Patterns, 66
Summary, 69
Recommendation, 69

3   NEEDLE EXCHANGE AND BLEACH DISTRIBUTION
PROGRAMS IN THE UNITED STATES   74
Introduction, 74
Needle Exchange Programs, 75
Legal Issues, 75
Program Operations, 77
Characteristics of Program Participants, 83
Cost and Cost-Effectiveness, 86
Organizational Characteristics, 89
Comparisons Across Programs, 93
Bleach Distribution Programs, 95
Characteristics of Program Participants, 96
Outreach Strategies, 97
Conclusions, 99

4   COMMUNITY VIEWS   103
Moral/Ethical Arguments, 105
Public Opinion Polls, 106
African American Views, 107

Latino/Hispanic Views, 120
Law Enforcement Views, 121
Health Professional Views, 123
    Pharmacists, 123
    Treatment Service Providers, 126
Summary, 133
Conclusions, 133

5   THE LEGAL ENVIRONMENT   143
U.S. Drug Control Policy, 143
    Legislative/Statutory Environment, 145
    Judicial Rulings, 147
Do Paraphernalia and Prescription Laws Contribute to
    HIV Transmission?, 149
    Needle Scarcity and Sharing, 150
    Changes in the Laws in Connecticut, 152
Should the Laws Be Changed?, 155
    Changing the Laws, 156
    Consequences, 157
Conclusions, 158
Recommendations, 158

PART 2
THE IMPACT OF NEEDLE EXCHANGE AND
BLEACH DISTRIBUTION PROGRAMS

6   THE EFFECTIVENESS OF BLEACH AS A DISINFECTANT
    OF INJECTION DRUG EQUIPMENT   167
Transmission of HIV Among Injection Drug Users, 168
Bleach as a Disinfectant, 169
    Definition of Terms, 169
    The Role of Cleaning in Disinfection, 170
    Susceptibility of HIV to Disinfection, 172
Bleach Distribution Programs, 175
    Program Evaluation, 177
    The Chicago Experience, 180
    Limitations of Bleach Disinfection, 186
    Impact of Bleach Disinfection on HIV Transmission, 187
Summary, 190
    Conclusions, 191
    Recommendations, 192

7 THE EFFECTS OF NEEDLE EXCHANGE PROGRAMS 198
    Potential Outcomes, 199
        Possible Positive Outcomes, 199
        Possible Negative Outcomes, 199 *opposing*
    The Panel's Approach to the Evidence, 200
        The Traditional Approach: Considering the Preponderance
            of the Evidence, 200
        An Alternative Approach: Looking at the Patterns of Evidence, 201
        The Panel's Synthesis, 204
    U.S. General Accounting Office Review, 205
        Procedure, 205
        Results, 206
    University of California Report, 208
        Procedure, 208
        Results, 210
        Possible Positive Outcomes, 211
        Possible Negative Outcomes, 214
        Summary, 216
    Evidence from Recent Studies, 217
        Possible Positive Outcomes, 217
        Possible Negative Outcomes, 224
    The New Haven Studies, 226
        Program Implementation, 228
        Estimated Effects on HIV Incidence, 229
        Assessment of the Models, 230
        New Initiates to Injection Drug Use, 231
        Enrollment in Drug Treatment, 232
        Alternative Explanations, 232
        Summary, 233
    The Tacoma Studies, 234
        The Program, 235
        HIV Seroprevalence Studies, 240
        Hepatitis Surveillance and Case Reporting, 240
        Hepatitis B and C Case-Control Study, 242
        Interview Studies with Injection Drug Users, 243
        Potential Alternative Explanations, 244
        Program Effects on New Initiates to Drug Use or Abuse, 248
    Summary, 250
        Conclusions, 251
        Recommendations, 252

8 DIRECTIONS FOR FUTURE RESEARCH 263
    Research on Program Effectiveness, 264

good

Needle Exchange Evaluation, 264
Program Characteristics, 267
Research on Bleach Efficacy in Disinfection, 270
Epidemiologic Research, 270
Research on Community Issues, 272
Other Future Research Issues, 273
Deregulation of Syringe Sale and Possession, 273
Incarcerated Populations, 274
Randomized Trial of Needle Exchange Programs, 274
Broader Issues, 275
Conclusion, 276

APPENDIXES

A   DESCRIPTION AND REVIEW OF RESEARCH PROJECTS
IN THREE CITIES   281
San Francisco, 281
Review, 283
Montréal, 285
Needle Exchange Evaluation Project, 285
Epidemiologic Study, 289
Chicago, 293
Demand for Free Needles and Their Effect on Injecting Frequency
and Needle Use, 293
Effects of Exchange Use on HIV Risk Behavior and Incidence, 302
Conclusion, 304

B   PROFESSIONAL ASSOCIATION POSITIONS ON NEEDLE
EXCHANGE AND BLEACH DISTRIBUTION PROGRAMS   307

C   BIOGRAPHICAL SKETCHES   313

INDEX   321

The National Academy of Sciences is a private, nonprofit, self-perpetuating society of distinguished scholars engaged in scientific and engineering research, dedicated to the furtherance of science and technology and to their use for the general welfare. Upon the authority of the charter granted to it by the Congress in 1863, the Academy has a mandate that requires it to advise the federal government on scientific and technical matters. Dr. Bruce M. Alberts is president of the National Academy of Sciences.

The National Academy of Engineering was established in 1964, under the charter of the National Academy of Sciences, as a parallel organization of outstanding engineers. It is autonomous in its administration and in the selection of its members, sharing with the National Academy of Sciences the responsibility for advising the federal government. The National Academy of Engineering also sponsors engineering programs aimed at meeting national needs, encourages education and research, and recognizes the superior achievement of engineers. Dr. Harold Liebowitz is president of the National Academy of Engineering.

The Institute of Medicine was established in 1970 by the National Academy of Sciences to secure the services of eminent members of appropriate professions in the examination of policy matters pertaining to the health of the public. The Institute acts under the responsibility given to the National Academy of Sciences by its congressional charter to be an adviser to the federal government and, upon its own initiative, to identify issues of medical care, research, and education. Dr. Kenneth I. Shine is president of the Institute of Medicine.

The National Research Council was organized by the National Academy of Sciences in 1916 to associate the broad community of science and technology with the Academy's purposes of furthering knowledge and advising the federal government. Functioning in accordance with general policies determined by the Academy, the Council has become the principal operating agency of both the National Academy of Sciences and the National Academy of Engineering in providing services to the government, the public, and the scientific and engineering communities. The Council is administered jointly by both Academies and the Institute of Medicine. Dr. Bruce M. Alberts and Dr. Harold Liebowitz are chairman and vice chairman, respectively, of the National Research Council.

Preface

The July 1992 ADAMHA Reorganization Act mandated that the Secretary of Health and Human Services, acting through the Director of the National Institute on Drug Abuse, request the National Academy of Sciences to conduct a study on the impact of needle exchange and bleach distribution programs on drug use behavior and the spread of the human immunodeficiency virus (HIV). In response to that legislative directive, in May 1993 the National Research Council (NRC) and the Institute of Medicine (IOM) of the National Academy of Sciences organized the Panel on Needle Exchange and Bleach Distribution Programs within the Commission on Behavioral and Social Sciences and Education.

The panel's overall charge was to determine the effectiveness of needle exchange and bleach distribution programs. More specifically, the panel was asked to gather and analyze the relevant research regarding the effect of such programs on rates of drug use, the behavior of injection drug users, and the spread of AIDS and other diseases, such as hepatitis, among injection drug users and their sexual partners. In addition, the panel was asked to examine related issues of importance to the research and service communities, such as the characteristics associated with effective exchange programs, and to provide recommendations for future research directions and methods applicable to the evaluation of needle exchange and bleach programs. In the latter task, the panel was asked to identify the relevant evaluation hypotheses and delineate the most appropriate methodologies for testing such hypotheses. The panel was authorized, but not committed, to assess the potential risks and benefits associated with the implementation of such programs if it judged the data adequate to make such an assessment. The panel first met in June 1993 and over two years worked to come to grips with the range of conceptual, methodological, and ideological issues associated with these controversial AIDS prevention programs.

From the outset we recognized the importance, whenever there is a proposal to institute, cancel, or substantially modify a public health policy, of taking both ethical and empirical concerns into account. The wisdom of a public policy depends not only on its consistency with social consensus, but also on pragmatic consequences. With this base, the panel attempted to distill the essence of the ongoing and sometimes acrimonious debate on whether the federal government should provide financial assistance for implementing needle exchange and bleach distribution programs.

Prohibitions, even those that are legally sound and represent well-intentioned efforts to limit the purchase or possession of equipment used to inject drugs, may be found to be ethically problematic. Furthermore, they may not be wise or proper when empirical judgments are warranted to accurately assess the effect of prevention programs on public health. The degree to which institutionalized needle exchange programs are considered ethical is based on measuring to whom they may be offensive and to what degree, whether drug abusers are encouraged to enter drug treatment programs, whether systematic harm is suffered by people of a particular social status, and whether a meaningful impact on reducing HIV transmission is made.

It became apparent early in our work that several concerned constituencies held strong and varied views about the soundness of integrating these types of health promotion and disease prevention programs as part of the nation's public health efforts to reduce the spread of HIV infection. Hence, we proceeded to educate ourselves as fully as possible and carefully consider the broad range of views involved.

The panel held several meetings and two workshops to which representatives of various community groups and researchers were asked to present their views on key issues. In its effort to gather and analyze the relevant scientific evidence, the panel invited both U.S. and foreign experts to participate in a two-day workshop (September 1993) devoted to the presentation and discussion of recent research on and experience with needle exchange and bleach distribution programs. A second workshop (January 1994) was designed to elicit the views of representatives of many of the communities with a stake in the outcome of the needle exchange and bleach distribution debate who have been actively engaged in the ongoing discussions.

As the panel was concluding its deliberations, the Assistant Secretary for Health made public statements that a number of unpublished needle exchange evaluation reports had raised doubts in his mind about the effectiveness of these programs. The panel deemed these statements to be significant in the public debate, therefore necessitating appropriate consideration in order for the panel to be fully responsive to its charge. We therefore reviewed the unpublished studies—by investigators in Chicago, Montréal, and San Francisco—that had raised concerns. As unpublished findings, these studies, though clearly salient, lack the authority provided by the peer review and publication process. For this reason, in the report we give special attention (in an appendix) to scrutinizing and describing in detail their results, as well as appraising their probative value.

This report is the collective product of a panel whose members represent a balance in both expertise and points of view. Its contents reflect the careful deliberations and final consensus of the members. The panel is particularly indebted to two members, David Cordray and Don Des Jarlais, whose contributions of time, energy, and expertise to the crafting of the report were indeed extraordinary. The committee also benefited from the quality and dedication of the NRC and IOM staff. These included Eugenia Grohman, Michael Stoto, and Alexandra Wigdor, who provided constructive advice and guidance throughout the project. Christine McShane contributed significantly to the presentation of the panel's views through both substantive and technical editorial work. Her contributions to the language and structure of the report go far beyond what her title of editor might imply. Special thanks are due to Susan McCutchen, who coordinated all of our meetings, planned the workshop sessions, updated successive drafts of the report and prepared it for production, kept track of the work flow, and generally kept our work team organized. Her commitment and support at every stage of the panel's work was indispensible to the project. We are appreciative of and grateful for the efforts of these talented people.

> Lincoln E. Moses, *Chair*
> Jacques Normand, *Study Director*
> David Vlahov, *Member*
> Panel on Needle Exchange and
>   Bleach Distribution Programs

Acknowledgments

During the course of this study, the panel and staff have been assisted by many researchers and other individuals working in the field who took time to share their insights and expertise. Without this generous assistance, the panel would not have been able to complete its task.

At the panel's September 1993 workshop in Baltimore, Maryland, a number of people made presentations on current research in needle exchange and bleach distribution: Benjamin Bowser (California State University), Alice Gleghorn (The Johns Hopkins University), Lawrence Gostin (Georgetown University), Samuel Groseclose (Centers for Disease Control and Prevention), Holly Hagan (Seattle-King County Health Department), Catherine Hankins (Montréal General Hospital), Noreen Harris (Seattle-King County Department of Public Health [deceased]), James G. Kahn (University of California at San Francisco), Edward Kaplan (Yale School of Management), Peter Lurie (University of California at San Francisco), Linda Martin (Centers for Disease Control and Prevention), Rose Martinez (U.S. General Accounting Office), Clyde McCoy (University of Miami), Margaret Millson (University of Toronto), Sheigla Murphy (Institute for Scientific Analysis), Ted Myers (University of Toronto), Kathy Oliver (Outside In, Portland), Denise Paone (Beth Israel Medical Center), Paul Shapshak (University of Miami), Linda Valleroy (Centers for Disease Control and Prevention), Anneke van den Hoek (Municipal Health Service Amsterdam), John Watters (University of California at San Francisco), and Alex Wodak (St. Vincent's Hospital, Darlinghurst, New South Wales). Robert Booth (University of Colorado), T. Stephen Jones (Centers for Disease Control and Prevention),

Andrew Moss (University of California), Lane Porter (consultant), and Peter Selwyn (Yale University) served as discussants.

At an informal workshop held in January 1994, briefings on relevant community issues were provided by Russell Coon (National Association of Chain Drug Stores [*affiliation* American Drug Stores]), George Doane (law enforcement community [*affiliation* Bureau of Narcotic Enforcement]), Sairus Faruque (Latino community [*affiliation* Association for Drug Abuse Prevention and Treatment]), Gilbert Gallegos (law enforcement community [*affiliation* Fraternal Order of Police]), Wilbert Jordan (African American community [*affiliation* Los Angeles County AIDS Program]), Cleo Malone (African American community, California Coalition of Clergy and Congress of National Black Churches [*affiliation* Palavra Tree]), Suzi Rodriguez (Chicano/Mexican community [*affiliation* Los Angeles County Substance Abuse Task Force]), and Rose Sparks (American Pharmaceutical Association [*affiliation* South Coast Medical Center]).

Many people assisted the panel in its deliberations by providing commissioned papers and/or data in specific research areas: Philip Alcabes (Yale University), Michael Aldrich (California AIDS Intervention Training Center), Walter Bond (Centers for Disease Control and Prevention), Barry Brown (University of North Carolina at Wilmington), Julie Bruneau (Hôpital St.-Luc, Montréal), Mary Ann Chiasson (New York City Department of Health), Richard Clayton (University of Kentucky), Sandra Crouse Quinn (Westat, Inc.), Dominick DePhilippis (University of Pennsylvania), Meg Doherty (The Johns Hopkins University), Martin Favero (Centers for Disease Control and Prevention), Blanche Frank (New York State Office of Alcoholism and Substance Abuse Services), Samuel Friedman (National Development and Research Institutes), Joseph Gfroerer (Substance Abuse and Mental Health Services Administration), Alice Gleghorn (The Johns Hopkins University), Janet Greenblatt (Substance Abuse and Mental Health Services Administration), Holly Hagan (Seattle-King County Health Department), Diana Hartel (Montefiore Medical Center), T. Stephen Jones (Centers for Disease Control and Prevention), Benny Jose (National Development and Research Institutes), Mark Kleiman (Harvard University), Thomas Lampinen (University of Washington), Carl Leukefeld (University of Kentucky), Jerry Mandel (La Familia Unida AIDS Outreach Project), Linda Martin (Centers for Disease Control and Prevention), David Metzger (University of Pennsylvania), Lynne Mofenson (National Institutes of Health), James Murray (University of Illinois at Chicago), John Newmeyer (Haight Ashbury Free Medical Clinics), Mary Utne O'Brien (University of Illinois at Chicago), Lawrence Ouellet (University of Illinois at Chicago), Denise Paone (Beth Israel Medical Center), Jenny Rudolph (BOTEC Analysis Corporation), Peter Selwyn (Yale University), Stephen Thomas (Emory University), Thomas Ward (National Development and Research Institutes), and Norman Williams (New York State Office of Alcoholism and Substance Abuse Services). In addition, researchers Antonio Jimenez, Wendell Johnson, and Afsaneh Rahimian, together with outreach workers Hermando Lira, Ed Mulligan, and Larry Smith, are some of the many intervention staff at field stations in Chicago, Illinois, who provided the panel with invaluable insight into working with drug users and abusers on the street.

The panel and staff would like to acknowledge project staff of the National Institute on Drug Abuse, the project's sponsoring agency, for their assistance in making our work run smoothly. Our project officers were especially helpful: Peter Hartsock provided guidance and technical support throughout the project; Sander Genser offered guidance, particularly in the early stages of the panel's deliberations; Richard Needle served as a project officer as well; and Carol Cushing provided advice and assisted in the administration of the contract. T. Stephen Jones, of the Centers for Disease Control and Prevention, assisted the panel through briefings and providing data during the course of the study. Ripley Forbes, of the House Subcommittee on Health and Environment, briefed the panel in the early stages of its deliberations and helped members focus on the task at hand from the legislative perspective.

The panel extends its sincere thanks and appreciation to all those who have assisted us in our work.

Lincoln E. Moses, *Chair*
Jacques Normand, *Study Director*
David Vlahov, *Member*
Panel on Needle Exchange and Bleach
Distribution Programs

Executive Summary

THE PROBLEM

HIV (human immunodeficiency virus) infection and injection drug use are major public health problems in the United States today. The focus of this study lies at the interface of these two critical threats to public health. The epidemiologic data indicate that the HIV epidemic in this country is now clearly driven by infections occurring in the population of injection drug users, their sexual partners, and their offspring. The proportion of new AIDS cases attributed to the exposure category labeled *men who have sex with men* has declined steadily over the past 13 years (from 74 percent in 1981 to 47 percent in 1993). At the same time, the proportion of cases attributed to *injection drug use* has steadily increased during the same period (from 12 percent in 1981 to 28 percent in 1993). These trends in AIDS cases reflect the rising injection drug use related infections of several years ago. By now, the spread of HIV among injection drug users, their sexual partners, and their offspring accounts for a major proportion of new HIV infections in the United States and the continuing expansion of the AIDS epidemic.

Note: Documentation for the material in this Executive Summary appears in the body of the report. Moreover, it should be noted that this summary focuses on the core conclusions and recommendations of the report. Additional conclusions and recommendations appear at the end of individual chapters.

1

The main factor associated with HIV infection among injection drug users is the practice of sharing injection equipment. This multiperson use of syringes is particularly dangerous because residual blood retained in the syringe from one person can be unintentionally and, even with rinsing, inconspicuously passed along to the next person using the syringe. This sharing behavior is in part a consequence of the restricted availability of sterile needles and syringes. An injection drug user infected with HIV can cause a cascade of new infections in many other individuals, not only through sharing of injection equipment, but also through sexual and perinatal transmission.

Needle exchange programs, in which used needles are exchanged for new, sterile ones, are one level of response to this crisis in some communities. They have been implemented in many countries (including France, the Netherlands, Great Britain, Australia, and Canada) as part of a more comprehensive public health effort to reduce the spread of HIV and other bloodborne infections among drug users, their sexual partners, and the general population. In the United States, approximately 75 needle exchange programs have been initiated in 55 cities, although many are small and the programs have not been endorsed by the federal government as a viable intervention for the prevention of AIDS. Obstacles to this approach include legal, economic, and behavioral factors.

For injection drug users who cannot or will not stop injecting drugs, the once-only use of sterile needles and syringes remains the safest, most effective approach for limiting HIV transmission. However, with significant legal impediments to syringe availability, bleach distribution programs were conceived as a means for injection drug users to disinfect needles and syringes between use. If properly used, bleach is effective in the disinfection of HIV and other pathogens—but the effectiveness of bleach as used by injection drug users under street conditions has not been optimal.

The use of federal funds to support needle exchange programs has been specifically prohibited or restricted by the language contained in a series of statutes enacted by Congress since 1988. The ban on federal support remains in effect ". . . unless the Surgeon General of the United States determines that such programs are effective in preventing the spread of HIV and do not encourage the use of illegal drugs." This current prohibition applies regardless of whether the programs operating in individual states are legally authorized. As a result, needle exchange programs in communities across the country cannot use federal funds to support services involving the provision of sterile needles, but are limited in their funding to state, municipal, and private sources.

THE PANEL'S CHARGE

At the request of Congress, the Panel on Needle Exchange and Bleach Distribution Programs was established by the National Research Council/ Institute of Medicine, with support from the National Institute on Drug Abuse. The panel was asked to undertake a study to determine the effectiveness of needle exchange and bleach distribution programs. The panel's charge is as follows:

The panel will gather and analyze the relevant research regarding the effect of such programs on rates of drug use, the behavior of drug users, and the spread of AIDS and other diseases, such as hepatitis, among intravenous drug users and their partners. In addition, the panel will examine closely related issues of importance to the research and service communities, such as the characteristics associated with effective exchange programs, and will provide recommendations for future research directions and methods applicable to the evaluation of syringe exchange and bleach programs. In the latter task, the study will identify the relevant evaluation hypotheses and delineate the most appropriate methodologies for testing such hypotheses. The panel is authorized, but not committed, to assess the potential risks and benefits associated with the implementation of such programs if it judges the data adequate to make such an assessment.

SCIENTIFIC ASSESSMENT OF PROGRAM EFFECTIVENESS

To examine the context that frames needle exchange and bleach distribution programs, the panel assessed a wide range of studies concerning the magnitude and severity of injection drug use; HIV infection among injection drug users and their partners; and the effects of needle exchange and bleach distribution programs on drug use, HIV risk behaviors, and the spread of HIV/AIDS.

The studies that examine needle exchange and bleach distribution programs have various limitations, including inadequate samples, sample attrition, improper controls, problematic measures, and incomplete analyses. Nevertheless, *the limitations of individual studies do not necessarily preclude us from being able to reach scientifically valid conclusions based on the entire body of literature available.* The situation resembles the exploration of the relationship between cigarette smoking and lung cancer; virtually every individual study was vulnerable to some particular objection, yet collectively those studies justified a compelling conclusion.

It was essential for the panel first to distinguish between studies of high quality and those of lesser quality, and then to weigh the credibility of the findings according to their completeness and soundness. *Using this approach, the panel based its conclusions on the pattern of evidence provided by a set of high-quality studies, rather than relying on the preponderance of evidence across less scientifically sound studies.*

Needle Exchange

On the basis of its review of the scientific evidence, the panel concludes:

• Needle exchange programs increase the availability of sterile injection equipment. For the participants in a needle exchange program, the fraction of needles in circulation that are contaminated is lowered by this increased availability. This amounts to a reduction in an important risk factor for HIV transmission.
• The lower the fraction of needles in circulation that are contaminated, the lower the risk of new HIV infections.

The act of giving a needle to an injection drug user has a powerful symbolism that has sparked fears about the potential negative effects of needle exchange programs. However:

• There is no credible evidence to date that drug use is increased among participants as a result of programs that provide legal access to sterile equipment.
• The available scientific literature provides evidence based on self-reports that needle exchange programs do not increase the frequency of injection among program participants and do not increase the number of new initiates to injection drug use.
• The available scientific literature provides evidence that needle exchange programs have public support, depending on locality, and that public support tends to increase over time.

Needle exchange programs should be regarded as an effective component of a comprehensive strategy to prevent infectious disease.

Bleach Distribution

Although HIV has been shown to be susceptible to inactivation by bleach under idealized conditions in the laboratory, epidemiologic studies have not demonstrated a significant protective effect against HIV infection for injection drug users who report consistent use of bleach to decontaminate needles and syringes previously used by others (see Chapter 6). Consequently, substantial uncertainty now exists among public health officials, laboratory scientists, community outreach workers, and injection drug users concerning the value of bleach disinfection as a public health intervention. Additional investigation into optimizing disinfection methods is clearly necessary.

The panel concludes:

• Bleach, *if used according to the recommendations of the Centers for Disease Control and Prevention, the National Institute on Drug Abuse, and the Center for Substance Abuse Treatment* (see Chapter 6 for a detailed discussion of these recommendations), is likely to be an effective HIV prevention strategy for injection drug users who share needles and syringes.

• Concerted efforts are essential to increase the awareness of injection drug users of the importance of disinfecting shared injection equipment and the importance of following the appropriate procedures.

Bleach use is clearly an intervention to be used when injection drug users have no safer alternatives.

• Health research funding agencies (e.g., the National Institutes of Health, the Centers for Disease Control and Prevention, and the Agency for Health Care Policy and Research) should support research directed toward identifying the simplest to use and most effective disinfection strategies, employing agents that are readily available to injection drug users.

COMMUNITY AND LEGAL FACTORS

In policy decisions about needle exchange and bleach distribution programs, the scientific evidence on whether the behaviors of injection drug users change and the rates at which new infections are reduced are but one dimension of an immensely complex issue. These AIDS prevention programs, in different environments, face various levels of community support, different levels of HIV prevalence[1] in the local population of injection drug users, and operate within different legal environments. And so the scientific issues cannot be viewed in isolation but must be considered along with these other factors.

A range of views about needle exchange programs has been expressed by various groups, including racial and ethnic minority representatives, law enforcement officials, pharmacists, and drug treatment providers. Specific community concerns range from fears that such programs will worsen already severe drug abuse problems and elevate extant high levels of crime to concerns that such programs promote immoral activities. Although there is much variety among the views of different groups, all share the concern that handing out sterile injection equipment or bleach bottles to injection drug users does not address the underlying problems associated with drug abuse.

The high levels of concern about potential negative effects of needle exchange and bleach distribution programs cannot be ignored, despite the paucity of evidence supporting them. Furthermore, the long-term effects of these programs on the level of illicit drug use in communities are not yet known. Communities experiencing high levels of drug use and addiction, AIDS, crime, and poverty may well resent the institution of needle exchange and bleach distribution programs, seeing them as a wholly inadequate response to the underlying problems associated with drug abuse and perceiving that they do more harm than good. The panel urges that local community members (e.g., police, church, treatment providers, pharmacists, local public health authorities) should be involved in determining whether such programs should be implemented locally and how they should be institutionalized.

The legal environment is another, very different factor impinging on needle exchange and bleach distribution programs. On the basis of its review of the legal circumstances in which these programs operate, the panel concludes:

• Any marked increase in the supply of sterile needles to injection drug users above current levels through pharmacy sales is likely to call for new measures to ensure the safe disposal of used needles. Whereas this problem has been solved in other countries (e.g., Australia provides special containers in public places that allow for proper disposal of used syringes, as well as individual returnable containers for used syringes), it is important to design good solutions to the disposal issue in the United States now.

• Laws that make it a criminal offense to possess injection equipment (paraphernalia laws) were designed to decrease the prevalence of injection drug abuse, but they also inhibit users from carrying their own supply of needles and thus unwittingly contribute to the sharing of contaminated ones.

• Laws requiring a prescription for the purchase of new needles and syringes (prescription laws) constrain the availability of sterile injection equipment and thus promote the sharing of contaminated equipment.

RECOMMENDED COURSE OF ACTION

The panel concludes that well-implemented needle exchange programs can be effective in preventing the spread of HIV and do not increase the use of illegal drugs. Hence, we recommend that:

• **The Surgeon General make the determination called for in P.L. 102-394, section 514, 1993, necessary to rescind the present prohibition against applying any federal funds to support needle exchange programs.**

Observe that the panel does not recommend a mandated national program of needle exchange and bleach distribution programs. As documented in this report, regional variations in the prevalence of HIV infection, the extent and kind of drug use, the presence of other AIDS programs, operational characteristics of existing needle exchange programs, and the attitudes and needs of local communities all influence the potential effects of needle exchange programs and militate against such a mandate. The recommendation is to *allow communities that desire such programs to institute them*, using resources at their disposal and unencumbered by the specific funding handicap that is now in place.

The panel further recommends that:

• A better monitoring system should be established for assessing long-term societal changes in drug use at the community level due to needle exchange programs.

• The Assistant Secretary for Health should charge appropriate agencies (i.e., the National Institutes of Health and the Centers for Disease Control and Prevention), in consultation with academic departments of epidemiology, to develop more effective surveillance of drug use, particularly for local areas. The data collected should move beyond gross prevalence estimation of drug use and toward detailed information about users. This should include data on behavioral dynamics (e.g., pattern of drug use, sharing of drugs and drug paraphernalia, social context of drug use) by drugs of choice, routes of administration for each, and the flow of injection drug users into and out of drug treatment programs.

• Given the serious public health threat associated with HIV infection among injection drug users, their sexual partners, and offspring, the Assistant Secretary for Health should ensure that AIDS prevention efforts targeted to injection drug users are expanded specifically to include behavioral interventions in order to limit the further spread of HIV infection.

• The Assistant Secretary for Health should cause the disposal issue to be studied and appropriate means of needle disposal to be developed. A task force should be appointed and should include health safety specialists, infectious disease specialists, injection drug use researchers, and community representatives/civic leaders.

• Legislative bodies should remove legal sanctions for the possession of injection paraphernalia.

• Appropriate legislative bodies should repeal laws in the nine states that require a prescription in order to purchase injection equipment.

These recommendations must be viewed in the overall context of the drug epidemic. Comprehensive responses to this threat to public health are critical: most critical is the expansion of drug treatment to make it more available. Needle exchange programs report increased referrals to drug abuse treatment and, in the few studies that examined this issue, no increase in the number of dirty needles discarded in public places (e.g., parks, streets, alleys). Needle exchange programs should promote HIV prevention not only by providing sterile equipment, but also by means of education, drug treatment referral, and materials, including bleach, alcohol pads, and condoms. Moreover, needle exchange and bleach distribution programs should make special efforts to reach and retain hard-to-reach subgroups of injection drug users, such as young injection drug users and women.

Incremental funds for needle exchange programs and other AIDS prevention strategies should be appropriated but should not be taken from resources now supporting drug treatment programs. Such a diversion of funds would be unwise because drug treatment programs have been shown to be effective in treating the underlying disorder of drug abuse and can be effective in curtailing HIV risk behaviors. Moreover, for many program participants, needle exchange and bleach distribution programs have been found to serve as a bridge to drug treatment for many needle exchange program participants. Indeed, the appropriate legislative bodies should enact legislation (and should appropriate monies) to increase drug treatment capacity. In this context, both needle exchange and bleach distribution programs should be regarded as strategies for public health promotion and disease prevention.

NOTE

1. *Prevalence* denotes the proportion of a population that is currently (or at a specified point in time) infected. *Incidence* denotes the rate of occurrence of new cases of infection per unit of time.

Introduction

The critical role of injection drug use in the spread of the human immu-nodeficiency virus (HIV) in this country is manifest. Early in the epidemic, it was implicated as a primary mode of transmission (Masur et al., 1981; Centers for Disease Control, 1982). The observed clustering of reported cases of acquired immune deficiency syndrome (AIDS) in specific popula-tions (e.g., homosexual men, injection drug users, recipients of blood and blood products) was one of the original pieces of evidence that indicated the possibility that an infectious agent was the underlying cause of the disease (Friedland and Klein, 1987).

DIMENSIONS OF THE PROBLEM

Although no changes in the primary routes of transmission (sexual con-tact, injection drug use, blood/blood products, perinatal) have been ob-served over the years, the proportion of cases by exposure mode and the distribution of new cases across demographic characteristics (e.g., sex, ethnicity/ race, geographic location) have changed drastically over the last 13 years. As we discuss in this report, the proportion of AIDS cases attributed to the exposure category labeled *men who have sex with men* by the Centers for Disease Control and Prevention (CDC) has declined steadily over the past 13 years (from 74 percent in 1981 to 47 percent in 1993), while the propor-tion of cases attributed to *injection drug use* has steadily increased during that period (from 12 percent in 1981 to 28 percent in 1993). The proportion

9

of heterosexual cases has also increased over the years (from 1 percent in 1981 to 9 percent in 1993), and women are disproportionately affected in this latter category (of all new AIDS cases reported in 1993, heterosexual contact accounted for 4 percent of AIDS cases among men and 37 percent among women). Injection drug use has been tied to the majority of AIDS cases among heterosexuals and is a major risk factor associated with pediatric cases. Furthermore, the rate of AIDS cases linked to injection drug use is disproportionately high for African Americans and Hispanics.

Injection drug users represent a sizable population. Estimates of current injection drug users in the United States range from 1.1 to 1.9 million people (Turner et al., 1989; Office of Technology Assessment, 1990; Research Triangle Institute, 1989; Valdiserri et al., 1993), and more than 3.2 million people have injected drugs at some point in their lives (National Institute on Drug Abuse, 1991). There is of course substantial variation across the country in the number of injectors within specific geographic areas. For example, typically high rates of injection drug use are observed in the Northeast, Miami, and Puerto Rico; moderate rates in the West; and low rates in the Midwest.

The experiences of several large urban areas have shown how infection among injection drug users can explode rapidly after the introduction of the virus into that population. For example, within two years the HIV prevalence[1] rates in Edinburgh, Scotland, soared from 5 percent in 1983 to 57 percent in 1985 (Robertson et al., 1986); the rates in Bangkok, Thailand, increased from 1 to 43 percent in one year (Berkelman et al., 1989); and by 1985, seroprevalence estimate rates as high as 69 percent were reported in Milan, Italy (Titti et al., 1987; Angarano et al., 1985). Similarly in the United States, the virus spread rapidly in New York City in the early 1980s, with seroprevalence stabilizing at between 55 and 60 percent in 1984 through 1987 (Des Jarlais et al., 1989). The main factor associated with the accelerated increase in HIV infection among injection drug users is the widespread sharing of needles or syringes, which is in part a consequence of the restricted availability of sterile injection equipment. Moreover, it is a matter of concern that epidemiologic data indicate that, given the large number of injection drug users and their comparatively high incidence of HIV, the basic elements necessary for the rapid diffusion of the virus are apparent. That is, communities of injection drug users with high levels of both HIV infection and risk behaviors (i.e., involving drugs and sex) can serve as a bridge across distinct populations and efficiently impact the infection rate of other groups for which the HIV prevalence rates are currently relatively low. The epidemiologic data do indicate that the HIV epidemic in this country is now clearly driven by infections occurring in the population of injection drug users, their sexual partners, and their offspring.

RESPONSES TO THE EPIDEMIC

The magnitude of the epidemic and the severity of the health consequences posed by HIV infection within the population of injection drug users, their sexual partners, and their offspring are not at issue. What is being strenuously debated in the United States is whether certain AIDS prevention programs, directed at this highly vulnerable population, should be implemented with the assistance of the federal government.

Needle exchange programs, in which used needles are exchanged for new, sterile ones, are widely used in many industrialized countries (e.g., France, the Netherlands, Great Britain, Australia, Canada) as part of public health efforts to reduce the spread of HIV and other blood-borne infections among drug users, their sexual partners, and the general population.

In the United States, although approximately 75 needle exchange programs have been initiated in 55 cities, many are small and the programs have not yet been endorsed by the federal government as a viable intervention for AIDS prevention. The debate in the U.S. Congress has been intense between members who are particularly interested in AIDS prevention initiatives and members who are concerned that the use of federal funds to implement needle exchange programs would have the unintended effect of increasing injection drug use in those communities already plagued by drug abuse. To date, the impasse between these two camps has blocked any use of federal funds for needle exchange program services.

Indeed, the use of appropriated funds by the Department of Health and Human Services to support needle exchange programs has been specifically prohibited or restricted by the language contained in a series of statutes[2] enacted by Congress since 1988. The U.S. General Accounting Office (1993) recently analyzed the legal authority applicable to the federal support of research and services related to needle exchange. It concluded, primarily on the basis of language contained in section 514 of the "General Provisions" of the 1993 *Departments of Labor, Health and Human Services, and Education, and Related Agencies Appropriation Act*, that, although the Department of Health and Human Services is restricted from using certain funds to support the funding of needle exchange programs directly, it does have the authority to conduct demonstration and research projects that involve the provision of needles. Nevertheless, the ban on federal support for needle exchange program services still remains in effect: " . . . unless the Surgeon General of the United States determines that such programs are effective in preventing the spread of HIV and do not encourage the use of illegal drugs" (U.S. Congress, 1992a). This current prohibition applies regardless of the legal standing of the programs operating in individual states. As a result, needle exchange programs across the country cannot use federal funds to support services involving the provision of needles, but must rely on funding from state, municipal, and private sources.

THE CHARGE TO THE PANEL

This unresolved debate led Congress to request, through the ADAMHA Reorganization Act (U.S. Congress, 1992b) that the National Academy of Sciences undertake a study to determine the effectiveness of needle exchange and bleach distribution programs on the spread of HIV in order to allow the Surgeon General to determine whether federal funds can be used to carry out such programs (P.L. 102-394, Section 514). More specifically, the mandate called for the study to make determinations of the following:

"1. The extent to which the programs promote, directly or indirectly, the abuse of drugs through providing information or devices (or both) regarding the manner in which the adverse health consequences of such abuse can be minimized."

"2. In the case of individuals participating in the programs, the number of individuals who have engaged in the abuse of drugs prior to admission to the programs and the number of individuals who have not engaged in such abuse prior to such admission."

"3. The extent to which participation in the programs has altered any behaviors constituting a substantial risk of contracting acquired immune deficiency syndrome or hepatitis, or of transmitting either of the diseases."

"4. The number of programs that provide referrals for the treatment of such abuse and the number of programs that do not provide such referrals."

"5. The extent to which programs safely dispose of used hypodermic syringes and needles."

In response to this request of Congress, the National Research Council/ Institute of Medicine established the Panel on Needle Exchange and Bleach Distribution Programs and outlined its charge as follows:

The panel will gather and analyze the relevant research regarding the effect of such programs on rates of drug use, the behavior of drug users, and the spread of AIDS and other diseases, such as hepatitis, among intravenous drug users and their partners. In addition, the panel will examine closely related issues of importance to the research and service communities, such as the characteristics associated with effective exchange programs, and will provide recommendations for future research directions and methods applicable to the evaluation of syringe exchange and bleach programs. In the latter task, the study will identify the relevant evalu-

ation hypotheses and delineate the most appropriate methodologies for testing such hypotheses. The panel is authorized, but not committed, to assess the potential risks and benefits associated with the implementation of such programs if it judges the data adequate to make such an assessment.

The charge gives special attention to the first three of the five tasks specified in the congressional mandate. The panel addressed tasks 4 and 5 as specified in the mandate by relying primarily on the research findings of two large-scale studies, undertaken with support from the federal government, that devoted a substantial amount of attention to these issues (U.S. General Accounting Office, 1993; Lurie et al., 1993).

The panel's charge refers to both *needle exchange* and *bleach distribution programs*, and a brief characterization of these programs will shed some light on the panel's scope of work. Diverse AIDS prevention programs have been implemented in attempts to reduce the spread of HIV among injection drug users, their sexual partners, and their offspring. These include, but are not limited to, educational, testing and counseling, needle exchange, and bleach distribution programs. A review of the services and devices delivered by needle exchange and bleach distribution programs (see Chapter 3) makes it clear that these programs do have many common elements and are not mutually exclusive. That is, the majority of the needle exchange programs distribute bleach, educational material, and condoms and make referrals to drug treatment and other services. Bleach programs typically dispense bleach, condoms, and educational materials and provide treatment and other referrals (e.g., primary care, public services). Both types of AIDS prevention programs attempt to prevent the transmission of the virus through the use of infected equipment and sexual risk behaviors. Both types of programs adopt multiple strategies in an attempt to reduce high-risk behaviors (e.g., injection and sexual behaviors). The primary distinguishing characteristic between them is that needle exchange programs provide as one of their main services the exchange of sterile needles for the return of used ones, whereas bleach distribution programs provide a readily available disinfectant (i.e., household bleach) to clean needles not meant to be reused.

A recent public health bulletin (Centers for Disease Control and Prevention, 1993), which was issued jointly by the National Institute on Drug Abuse of the National Institutes of Health, the Center for Substance Abuse Treatment of the Substance Abuse and Mental Health Services Administration, and the Centers for Disease Control and Prevention, makes it clear that the use of bleach can play a role in reducing risk of HIV transmission, but it does not always sterilize the injection equipment. Specifically, the bulletin states that sterile, never-used needles and syringes are safer than bleach-disinfected, previously used needles and syringes, which in turn are safer than used needles and syringes that have not been disinfected with bleach. The bulletin also emphasizes that those individuals who continue to inject drugs should be made aware of the limitations associated with using bleach and encouraged to always use sterile injection equipment and warned to never reuse or share needles, syringes, and other injection equipment. Given that disposable needles and syringes are not intended for reuse (their design does not easily allow for efficient disinfection), some have argued that preventive interventions should have as a goal to get every injection drug user to comply with the same standards that are upheld for patient care by the health care delivery system and the medical profession—that is, a new needle and syringe for every injection (Jones, 1994).

THE PANEL'S REPORT

Information Sources

To carry out its charge, the panel undertook a variety of approaches to collect and analyze research data and other pertinent information. In addition to literature searches, panel assessments of evaluation studies, and briefings by technical experts at the panel's scheduled meetings, two informational workshops were convened. The first was designed to examine the impact of needle exchange and bleach distribution programs on drug-use behavior and the spread of HIV infection. The primary purpose of the workshop was to assist the panel in gathering and analyzing the relevant research regarding the effect of needle exchange and bleach distribution programs on rates of drug use, the behavior of drug users, and the spread of AIDS and other diseases, such as hepatitis, among intravenous drug users and their partners. A number of speakers, discussants, and participants were invited on the basis of their demonstrated expertise in the relevant research areas (National Research Council/Institute of Medicine, 1994).

The second workshop brought together community leaders to present their communities' views on and reactions to needle exchange and bleach distribution programs. The intent was to provide panel members with this important input to consider in their deliberations and to encourage a useful discussion of the issues involved in program implementation and the delivery of prevention services.

Approach

This report examines a wide range of studies concerning the magnitude and severity of injection drug use, HIV infection among injection drug users and their partners, the effects of needle exchange and bleach distribution programs on drug use, HIV risk behaviors, and the spread of HIV/ AIDS. These include epidemiologic studies of injection drug use and HIV/ AIDS, laboratory experiments and field studies on the efficacy and effectiveness of bleach in decontaminating injection equipment, and ethnographic accounts as well as empirical evaluations of needle exchange and bleach distribution programs.

The studies that examine needle exchange and bleach distribution programs have a variety of limitations, including inadequate samples, sample attrition, improper controls, problematic measures, and incomplete analyses. *Nevertheless, the limitations of individual studies do not necessarily preclude us from being able to reach scientifically valid conclusions based on the body of literature available on the issues of interest.* The strategy adopted by the panel in reviewing the literature on this topic was to first distinguish between high-quality and lesser-quality studies and to weigh the credibility of the findings according to their completeness and soundness. Using this approach, the panel bases its conclusions on the *pattern of evidence* provided by a set of high-quality studies, rather than relying on the preponderance of evidence across less scientifically sound studies (see Chapter 7). Furthermore, the panel examined whether the results of a number of less rigorous studies conformed with the results of the most rigorous studies. In some areas, however, this was not possible, and consequently the panel's efforts to answer certain questions were hampered by the lack of research.

Acknowledging the methodological limitations of certain individual studies, the panel also recognizes that most of them have been subject to a number of the mechanisms used by the scientific community to ensure the scientific adequacy of research—including the peer review process used in scientific and professional journals, scientific advisory panels and review groups, and external reviews of research—prior to their execution and/or publication. The majority of the studies reviewed in this report have satisfied these scientific criteria. Nonetheless, as is the case with many socially controversial programs (such as those involving sexual behavioral research, teenage pregnancy, contraception), the research findings we discuss have been the topic of heated debates among health policy decision makers who support or oppose such programs (Hartsock, 1993; Des Jarlais and Friedman, 1993; Office of National Drug Control Policy, 1992; Ginzburg, 1993; Kaplan, 1993). *After examining the relevant research, one important conclusion the panel reached is that the body of evidence is sufficient to allow informed scientific judgments to be formulated about the impact of these programs on issues of public health.*

A point worth noting here is that, amidst the controversy, there are some issues on which both proponents and opponents seem to agree. Although the debate is heated, individuals on both sides of the issue would concur that treatment is an efficient approach to dealing with injection drug use. Ultimately, both proponents and opponents would agree that, in dealing with current injection drug users, complete cessation of injection drug use would eliminate needles and syringes as a major route of transmission. Consequently, enrolling injection drug users in drug abuse treatment programs is viewed by both opponents and proponents as a highly desirable goal for countering the spread of HIV. The controversy emerges when attempting to determine the best strategy for achieving such a goal.

Organization

This report is organized into two parts. Part 1: Dimensions of the Problem begins with a summary of current information about the epidemiology of HIV/AIDS in Chapter 1. It is followed by the presentation of data on the epidemiology of injection drug use in Chapter 2. Chapter 3 describes the characteristics of needle exchange and bleach distribution programs, highlighting the many variations in organizational structure, context, and services, as well as the dynamic nature of the programs.

Chapter 4 summarizes the views of various communities on needle exchange programs. We discuss input from diverse communities, including law enforcement, health professionals, and ethnic groups. In this chapter, the panel briefly addresses moral and ethical issues as they relate to the implementation of needle exchange and bleach distribution programs and their potential adverse effect on illicit drug use. The panel discusses concerns that arise as a consequence of implementing prevention programs that attempt to contain the propagation of a deadly disease linked to illicit drug-use behavior with a focus toward the preservation of human life. However, the panel elected not to elaborate on whether the illicit use of drugs is in itself moral or ethical.

Part 2: Impact of Needle Exchange and Bleach Distribution Programs addresses the critical issues concerning the impact of needle exchange and bleach distribution programs. Chapter 5 examines the impact of paraphernalia and prescription laws on sharing behavior and HIV transmission. Chapter 6 reviews laboratory research on the efficacy of bleach as a disinfectant, and the limitations associated with that research literature are highlighted. This chapter also summarizes field studies that have assessed how effectively injection drug users in real-life settings comply with current recommended standards of bleach disinfection. Finally, this chapter summarizes the findings of evaluation studies that have assessed the impact of bleach distribution programs.

Chapter 7 addresses the effectiveness of needle exchange programs in preventing the transmission of HIV and other diseases, as well as the impact of these HIV/AIDS prevention programs on drug-use behaviors. We note that the conclusions and recommendations in this chapter are based not only on the findings presented in this chapter, but also on the findings and conclusions presented in the earlier chapters. This presentation reflects the cumulative development of the panel's understanding about the issues inherent in the establishment of needle exchange and bleach distribution programs and, ultimately, their anticipated effects, based on the pattern of evidence the panel discerned from its collection of descriptive and analytic materials, community views, and reviews of pertinent studies.

Chapter 8 identifies issues that need to be studied further.

The report includes three appendixes. Appendix A is a detailed description and review of some unpublished research findings, which came to the panel's attention as we were completing our review of the available evidence on needle exchange and bleach distribution programs (see the Preface). These studies are significant because their results appear to conflict with the findings of the body of literature reviewed in this report and have the potential of being misinterpreted. Appendix B presents a detailed summary of the views of various professional associations on needle exchange and bleach distribution programs. Appendix C gives biographical information about panel members and the study director.

NOTES

1. *Prevalence* denotes the proportion of a population that is currently (or at a specified point in time) infected. *Incidence* denotes the rate of occurrence of new cases of infection per unit of time.

2. These statutes include the Comprehensive Alcohol Abuse, Drug Abuse, and Mental Health Amendments Act of 1988, the Health Omnibus Programs Extension of 1988, the Ryan White Comprehensive AIDS Resources Emergency Act of 1990, and the Departments of Labor, Health and Human Services, and Education, and Related Agencies Appropriations Acts of 1990 and 1991.

REFERENCES

Angarano, G., G. Pastore, L. Monno, T. Santantonio, N. Luchena, and O. Schiraldi
 1985 Rapid spread of HTLV-III infection among drug addicts in Italy. *Lancet* 2(8467):1302.
Berkelman, R.L., W.L. Heyward, J.K. Stehr-Green, and J.W. Curran
 1989 Epidemiology of human immunodeficiency virus infection and acquired immunodeficiency syndrome. *American Journal of Medicine* 86:761-770.
Centers for Disease Control
 1982 *Pneumocystis* pneumonia. *Morbidity and Mortality Weekly Report* 30:250-252.
Centers for Disease Control and Prevention, Centers for Substance Abuse Treatment, National Institute on Drug Abuse
 1993 *HIV/AIDS Prevention Bulletin* April 19.
Des Jarlais, D.C., S.R. Friedman, D. Novick, J.L. Sotheran, P. Thomas, et al.
 1989 HIV-1 infection among intravenous drug users in Manhattan, from 1977 through 1987. *Journal of the American Medical Association* 261:1008-1012.

Des Jarlais, D.C., and S.R. Friedman
1993   Missing the point: Science and politics in the American debate on syringe exchanges. *Pediatric AIDS and HIV Infection: Fetus to Adolescent* 4(2):61-65.

Friedland, G.H., and R.S. Klein
1987   Transmission of the human immunodeficiency virus. *New England Journal of Medicine* 347(18):1125-1135.

Ginzburg, H.M.
1993   Federal response to needle-exchange programs: Part II: A. Science vs. politics. *Pediatric AIDS and HIV Infection: Fetus to Adolescent* 4(2):88-91.

Hartsock, P.I.
1993   National Institute on Drug Abuse (NIDA) needle exchange research: Maintaining rigorous science. Pp. 414-420 in *Epidemiologic Trends in Drug Abuse, Volume II: Proceedings.* Rockville, MD: National Institute on Drug Abuse.

Jones, T.S.
1994   Update on Upcoming Research Activities Pertaining to Needle Exchange and Bleach Distribution. Presentation at the September meeting of the Panel on Needle Exchange and Bleach Distribution Programs, Woods Hole, MA.

Kaplan, E.H.
1993   Federal response to needle-exchange programs: Part II: B. Needle-exchange research: The New Haven experience. *Pediatric AIDS and HIV Infection: Fetus to Adolescent* 4(2):92-96.

Lurie, P., A.L. Reingold, B. Bowser, D. Chen, J. Foley, J. Guydish, J.G. Kahn, S. Lane, and J. Sorensen
1993   *The Public Health Impact of Needle Exchange Programs in the United States and Abroad, Volume 1.* San Francisco: University of California.

Masur, H., M. Michelis, J. Greene, et al.
1981   An outbreak of community-acquired *Pneumocystis carinii* pneumonia: Initial manifestation of cellular immune dysfunction. *New England Journal of Medicine* 305(24):1431-1438.

National Institute on Drug Abuse
1991   National Household Survey on Drug Abuse: Population Estimates 1991. Rockville, MD: National Institute on Drug Abuse.

National Research Council/Institute of Medicine
1994   *Proceedings, Workshop on Needle Exchange and Bleach Distribution Programs.* Panel on Needle Exchange and Bleach Distribution Programs. Washington, DC: National Academy Press.

Office of National Drug Control Policy
1992   Needle exchange programs: Are they effective? *ONDCP Bulletin No. 7.* Washington, DC: Executive Office of the President.

Office of Technology Assessment
1990   *The Effectiveness of Drug Abuse Treatment: Implications for Controlling AIDS/ HIV Infection.* (Report Number 052-003-0120-3). Washington, DC: U.S. Government Printing Office.

Research Triangle Institute
1989   Estimation of the Size of Population Groups at Increased Risk of HIV Infection and AIDS in the United States (derived from pre-existing data). Research Triangle Institute, Research Triangle Park, NC.

Robertson, J.R., A.B.V. Bucknall, P.D. Welsby, J.J. Roberts, J.M. Inglis, J.F. Peutherer, and R.P. Brettle
1986   Epidemic of AIDS-related virus (HTLV-III/LAV) infection among intravenous drug users. *British Medical Journal* 292(6519):527-529.

Titti, F., A. Lazzarin, P. Costigliola, C. Oliva, L. Nicoletti, C. Negri, E. Ricchi, G. Donati, C. Uberti-Foppa, M.C. Re, et al.

1987   Human immunodeficiency virus (HIV) seropositivity in intravenous (i.v.) drug abusers in three cities of Italy: Possible natural history of HIV infection in i.v. drug addicts in Italy. *Journal of Medicine and Virology* 23(3):241-248.

Turner, C.F., H.G. Miller, and L.E. Moses, eds.

1989   *AIDS, Sexual Behavior, and Intravenous Drug Use.* Committee on AIDS Research and the Behavioral, Social, and Statistical Sciences. Washington, DC: National Academy Press.

U.S. Congress

1992a   Departments of Labor, Health and Human Services, and Education, and Related Agencies Appropriations Act, 1993, October 6. Public Law 102-394, 106 Stat. 1827, Section 514.

1992b   ADAMHA Reorganization Act, July 10. Public Law 102-321, 106 Stat. 439, Section 706.

U.S. General Accounting Office

1993   *Needle Exchange Programs: Research Suggests Promise as an AIDS Prevention Strategy.* Report Number GAO/HRD-93-60. Washington, DC: U.S. Government Printing Office.

Valdiserri, R.O., T.S. Jones, G.R. West, C.H. Campbell, and P.I. Thompson

1993   Where injecting drug users receive HIV counseling and testing. *Public Health Reports* 108:294-298.

Part 1
Dimensions of the Problem

1

The Epidemiology of HIV and AIDS

The picture we can draw of the HIV/AIDS epidemic is limited by the data available. To date, the AIDS case reporting system of the Centers for Disease Control and Prevention (CDC) is the only complete national population-based data available to monitor the epidemic. Although data are useful in evaluating disease prevalence and incidence, reported AIDS cases are only the clinical tip of the iceberg of effects produced by HIV infection. HIV seroprevalence surveys are informative for their description of the magnitude of the epidemic, but they represent people whose date of infection is unknown; these surveys are thus limited in their ability to characterize the current direction of the epidemic. HIV incidence data are far more informative for monitoring the current course of the epidemic. Nevertheless, because HIV infection is not reportable in all states, and because most studies of HIV have not included representative samples, these data are of limited value for generalizing to other specific populations or to the entire U.S. population. HIV surveillance data also provide information that is of limited value in forecasting the future of the epidemic. To address this limitation, some have argued (e.g., Centers for Disease Control and Prevention, 1994a; Turner et al., 1989) that a broader monitoring system of the epidemic should include precursors to AIDS and HIV infection. Better-developed behavioral epidemiologic data on known risk behaviors (i.e., sexual behavior and drug use) could provide data on sites of potential transmission and future spread.

Despite these limitations, current epidemiologic data provide valuable insights into the HIV/AIDS epidemic in the United States. This chapter reviews these data with particular emphasis on the role of injection drug users. However, before reviewing these data, the panel thought it critical to provide the reader with a brief review of current knowledge of the underlying biological mechanisms involved in the transmission of the virus. The details of these behaviors and processes are important to developing an appreciation for the complexity of the issues at hand.

BIOLOGICAL MECHANISMS OF TRANSMISSION

Although the consensus among the research community is that the development of an effective vaccine for the human immunodeficiency virus (HIV) is still years away, significant strides have been made in biomedical research. As Rogers (1992:522) stated, "We now know quite precisely how the virus is transmitted and how it is not and what it does to human cells and the immune mechanism, and we know enough about its structure and life-cycle to have identified multiple potential points to get at it."

HIV transmission is limited to sharing of contaminated injection drug paraphernalia, sexual contact, transmission from infected mother to child, exposure to infected blood or blood products, and transplantation of infected organs or tissues. As of December 31, 1993, injection drug use and sexual contact accounted for approximately 92 percent of all adult and adolescent AIDS cases reported to CDC. We review here postulated mechanisms for transmission through activities associated with injection drug use, sexual, and perinatal transmission and detail the associated human behaviors.

Injection Drug Use Transmission

Injection drug use involves practices that facilitate the transmission of HIV infection. The primary category of such practices is *direct needle sharing*, which involves the reuse of needles and syringes that have been contaminated through prior use by an infected individual. Penetration of the needle through the skin is sufficient for contamination and subsequent transmission of HIV infection, as has been demonstrated in cases of needlestick injuries among health care workers (McCray, 1986). In instances of occupational exposure of health care workers, in which the amount of blood exposure frequently is small (Napoli and McGowan, 1987), the risk of transmission is about 3/1,000 exposures (Ippolito et al., 1994).

Direct Needle Sharing

The higher rates of HIV infection in injection drug users than in health care workers are due to much more frequent injections (an average of one to two injections per day, according to some published surveys) and the practice of *registering*. Registering means that once a needle is inserted, the drug user will draw back the plunger of the syringe to examine for the presence of blood to ensure that the needle has been properly placed into a vein. Registering, then, involves contamination of both the needle itself and the hub, barrel, and plunger of the syringe. Although the syringe is typically rinsed before reuse, residual blood may adhere or remain, which may be released into the next person who uses the syringe by subsequent agitation (by drawing up and administrating the drug solution). Studies of the survivability of HIV in dried or aqueous states (Resnick et al., 1986) suggest that transmission may occur even if there is a delay of a day or more before the needle and syringe are reused by a different person.

A related practice of *direct needle sharing* has been termed *booting* (Inciardi, 1990; Ouellet et al., 1991), which involves additional steps in the basic injection pattern described above. Booting is the practice performed after registering and administering the drug solution. In this process, with the needle still in the vein, the injector draws back on the plunger of the syringe to fill the barrel with blood and then reinjects the blood, sometimes repeating this practice several times. More commonly reported with cocaine than with heroin injection, this practice allegedly enhances the euphoria associated with the drug's effects. Others, however, describe the motivation for engaging in this practice as economic, that is, to wash out all traces of the drug when administering it. The volume of blood that remains in the barrel of the syringe following booting is greater than that for the practice of registering and, at least theoretically, may be associated with a higher risk of transmission to anyone who subsequently uses a booted syringe. Empirical data on the risk of transmission for the practice of booting are sparse because few injection drug users can report reliably on whether previously used syringes were booted. Nevertheless, in one study, booting was associated with increased HIV seropositivity among injection drug users (Lamothe et al., 1993).

The setting in which drug injection takes place can also be related to direct sharing. A *shooting gallery* is a clandestine location where injection drug users go to rent needles and syringes. As used syringes are returned to a common container to be rented again, this process amounts to sequential anonymous sharing of needles and syringes (Friedland and Klein, 1987; Ouellet et al., 1991). Results of a study in which researchers tested used syringes collected from shooting galleries in Miami shed some light on the potential risk associated with injection drug use in the context of a shooting gallery. They showed that 20 percent of those syringes that had visible blood residue were positive for HIV, compared with 5.1 percent of those that had no visible blood residue (Chitwood et al., 1990). In a follow-up study carried out 2 years later (McCoy et al., 1994), researchers reported that 52 percent of the syringes showing visible traces of blood tested positive for HIV.

Indirect Needle Sharing

A separate category of drug injection practices can be termed *indirect needle sharing* because they do not directly involve passing a contaminated needle and syringe between individuals. Instead, indirect sharing involves common use of other drug preparation or injection equipment that can become contaminated. Examples include cookers, cotton, rinse water, and the drug-sharing practices called *frontloading* and *backloading*.

The *cooker* is a small container, typically a spoon or a metal soda bottle cap, in which a drug in the form of powder is mixed with water and heated into a solution. The heat is applied only to the point of allowing the drug to become soluble; additional heating (which might have a sterilizing effect) is not applied, as this would require time to cool that a drug user in partial withdrawal is often unwilling to tolerate. Although two drug injectors might each possess their own needle and syringe (and therefore deny that they are needle sharing), a potential for cross-contamination of needles and syringes is possible if each dips and draws solution from the same cooker in the same, or possibly later, injection episodes.

Cotton—sometimes cotton balls and other times cigarette filters or other similar materials—is placed into a cooker. Injectors draw up drug solution into their needles and syringes through the cotton, which is used to filter out particulate matter from the cooker. Cotton, which is submerged into the drug solution, typically is not discarded after each use. Instead, it is saved in containers to be soaked later to release residual drugs during periods when their availability is scarce. If contaminated needles are submerged in cotton, there is at least a theoretical possibility of contamination with viable virus that might lead to transmission.

Rinse water refers to containers of water from which one injector will draw up and squirt out tap water between the use of needles and syringes by different individuals. As needles and syringes are dipped into this rinse water, the water becomes contaminated. Contamination increases with greater use, especially over protracted periods between water changes, and also if rinse water that has been drawn into a syringe is squirted back into the same container that is to be reused for additional rinses. Moreover, rinse water is commonly used not only for rinsing, but also for the mixing of the drug solution to be injected. With regard to sharing rinse water, it is the injection of this contaminated water that poses the greatest threat for HIV transmission, especially in the case of cocaine injection, because cocaine is water soluble and does not always require heating in a cooker to be dissolved (depending on the dilutants and adulterants used).

Frontloading involves the parceling out of individual portions from a mixer/distributor's syringe to the other participants' syringes by removing the needles from the receiving syringes. *Backloading* involves transferring the drug from one syringe to another by removing the plunger from the receiving syringes. The drug solution can also be divided by having the mixer/distributor squirt all but his or her own portion back into the cooker for each participant to draw up his or her own agreed-on individual portion. These behaviors have been described in some detail in the professional literature (Inciardi and Page, 1991; Koester et al., 1990; Koester, 1994; Turner et al., 1989; Grund et al., 1990, 1991; Jose et al., 1993; McCoy et al., 1994; Samuels et al., 1991; Zule, 1992; Page et al., 1990; Auerbach et al., 1994).

Risk Behaviors and Interventions

Little attention has been given to these risk behaviors in most HIV/ AIDS prevention interventions aimed at injection drug users. In an in-depth ethnographic study, Koester and Hoffer (1994) reported that only 7 percent of the injectors they interviewed in their study were aware that these behaviors represented any type of risk of becoming infected. These findings are disturbing, given that over 70 percent of their study participants were participating or had participated in an HIV/AIDS intervention program.

The distinction between direct and indirect needle sharing is not merely academic but reflects a dichotomy that must be considered when evaluating needle exchange and bleach distribution programs. These intervention programs are aimed at direct needle-sharing practices by providing new sterile needles or disinfectant for them. However, neither sterile needles nor their disinfection can be expected to prevent transmission due to sharing of cookers, cotton, rinse water, or frontloading/backloading. Any assessment of the reductions in HIV seroconversion rates for specific programs needs to consider these points. It would seem prudent for prevention programs to educate people about the potential dangers of indirect sharing methods and supply sterile equipment whenever possible.

Finally, it must be noted that infectious agents other than HIV can be transmitted by contaminated injection equipment. Other blood-borne pathogens that have been associated with injection drug use include malaria, syphilis, hepatitis B and C viruses, and human T-lymphotropic virus type II, as well as other bacterial pathogens that cause sepsis and endocarditis (Cherubin, 1967; Sapira, 1968; Louria et al., 1967; Levine and Sobel, 1991; Stein, 1990; Haverkos and Lange, 1990; Cherubin and Sapira, 1993; Stimmel et al., 1975; Novick et al., 1988; Kreek, 1983; Esteban et al., 1989; Donahue et al., 1991; Des Jarlais et al., 1992; Selwyn and Alcabes, 1994). The recognition of multiple pathogens that can be transmitted parenterally by injection drug users is important, because development and implementation of prevention programs directed at HIV infection can be viewed more broadly as prevention programs for blood-borne pathogens in general.

Sexual Transmission

Sexual intercourse was implicated as a primary mode of transmission of the virus even before the etiologic agent (HIV) had been identified (Jaffe et al., 1983a, 1983b; Centers for Disease Control, 1981, 1982). However, the sexual transmission of the virus is not highly efficient, and the risk of acquiring the infection as a result of a single sexual exposure is relatively low (Friedland and Klein, 1987; Institute of Medicine, 1988; Holmberg et al., 1989). That does not mean that documented evidence of people becoming infected after one or only a few sexual contacts does not exist (Padian et al., 1988). Sexual transmission depends on the type and frequency of sexual encounters, as well as the prevalence of other risk factors (e.g., condom use). Receptive anal intercourse is particularly dangerous regardless of the sexual orientation of the individuals (Kingsley et al., 1987; Winkelstein et al., 1987), and frequent sexual exposures (vaginal or anal) to an infected partner also increase the likelihood of transmission (Padian et al., 1990; Lazzarin et al., 1991).

With respect to heterosexual transmission, as with other sexually transmitted diseases, women are at higher risk than men (Aral, 1993). Nonetheless, as is also the case with other sexually transmitted diseases, transmission occurs in both directions (male-to-female and female-to-male). The differential efficiency of transmission between the sexes has led to some debate about whether current estimates of female-to-male transmission rates are accurate (Redfield et al., 1985; Haverkos and Edelman, 1985, 1988; Polk, 1985; Handsfield, 1988; Padian et al., 1991; Haverkos and Battjes, 1992; Haverkos and Needle, 1994; Haverkos, 1994).

Transmission rates may also vary depending on the risk group of the originally infected partner. The risk of transmission has been shown to be lower for female partners of hemophiliacs and bisexual men and for partners of transfusion-infected persons than it is for female or male partners of injection drug users (Padian, 1987; Padian et al., 1987; Curran et al., 1988; De Gruttola and Mayer, 1988; Johnson, 1988).

Delineation of the precise biological mechanisms involved in the heterosexual transmission of HIV has been complicated by the difficulty of identifying a potential series of sexual encounters in which exposure to HIV is known to have occurred each time. We know that cell-free virus is infectious for blood product recipients and that cell-associated virus can infect cell lines in vitro. We simply do not know the relative contributions of cell-free and cell-associated HIV transmission in various at-risk circumstances, including drug injection and sexual contact. Furthermore, viral factors that may influence the efficiency of transmission are so far poorly understood, i.e., certain strains of HIV may be more easily transmitted than other strains. It is not yet known whether specific viral genotypic or phenotypic attributes influence the efficiency of viral transmission.

Transmission is known to be facilitated by a compromise of the integrity of mucosal surfaces and the presence of other sexually transmitted diseases, such as syphilis and chancroid, particularly in the recipient (Johnson and Laga, 1988). By increasing circulating lymphocytes and macrophages that may harbor HIV at the site of local infection, the presence of sexually transmitted diseases may potentially increase infectiousness as well. As a result, the prevalence of sexually transmitted diseases in a population of individuals at risk for HIV infection can significantly alter the efficiency of virus spread.

If a virus-transmitting donor has advanced HIV disease, the recipient may also be more likely to become infected. Furthermore, infection by an advanced-stage donor is associated with a higher incidence of acute viral syndrome in the recipient (Laga et al., 1989). These phenomena may be due to increased viral load in the transmitter or to increased virulence of the transmitted strains of HIV (which may be present after a long period of infection), or both. Infectiousness may also increase over time because plasma-associated and cell-associated viral load increases with disease progression, and studies show that the presence of HIV RNA is more likely to occur in the semen of men with lower $CD4^+$ cell counts.

Perinatal Transmission

Female injection drug users or partners of male injection drug users represent the largest number of HIV-infected women of childbearing age, constituting a sizable threat for perinatal transmission of HIV. The transmission of HIV from an infected mother to her offspring may occur in utero, during the birth process (intrapartum), or at some time following birth (postpartum) by breast-feeding. The relative frequency of the different timings of infection has not been clearly defined and may vary among different populations and locales. Approximately 25 to 30 percent of neonates born to HIV-seropositive mothers become infected (Boylan and Stein, 1991; Vermund et al., 1992; Mofenson, 1992).

For infants born to HIV-seropositive mothers, the transplacental transfer of maternal anti-HIV antibodies complicates the accurate estimate of the number of infants infected in utero versus those infected during or after birth.[1] Furthermore, because many HIV-infected pregnant women are unaware of their infection, the opportunity for the early diagnosis and treatment of their infected infants frequently may be missed. Similarly, interventions to prevent postpartum transmission, such as avoidance of breast-feeding, are not available to women who do not know that they are infected with HIV. Such interventions may also not be recommended in regions of the world where risks of HIV transmission are overshadowed by risks for other adverse health outcomes (e.g., diarrheal disease) among infants who are not breast-fed.

In perinatal transmission, a variety of factors, usually associated with latter-stage disease, including the presence of maternal p24 antigenemia and low maternal $CD4^+$ lymphocyte counts at the time of conception, correlate with the likelihood of infection of a neonate. Additional risk factors in perinatal transmission include high maternal $CD8^+$ T-lymphocyte counts, placental membrane inflammation, and maternal fever. It is likely that many HIV infections in infants are acquired at birth through contact with contaminated blood or secretions. Among twins born to HIV-infected mothers, a higher risk of HIV infection is seen in the firstborn, even for twins delivered by cesarean section, suggesting that factors related to the delivery process affect the risk of infection.

The fact that both the virus donor and the recipient are known in the case of perinatal HIV infection provides potential opportunities for interventions to decrease the risk of viral transmission. Recent studies have shown that antiviral treatment of an HIV-infected mother with zidovudine (AZT) can significantly decrease the likelihood of HIV infection in her offspring (Connor et al., 1994). The availability of an effective intervention to decrease perinatal HIV transmission has increased interest in screening pregnant women for the presence of HIV infection so that perinatal HIV infection may be limited.

Conclusion

In summary, much is known about the various modes of HIV transmission. However, it is not possible to provide accurate estimates of their relative efficiency. It is difficult to identify accurate denominators for the numbers of individuals and encounters in which exposure has occurred; moreover, transmission of the virus depends on factors other than the mode of exposure. The dose of virus transferred (inoculum size), the frequency of exposure, differences in host susceptibility, variations in infectiousness of an infected person over time, and the differences in virulence among HIV isolates, as well as the presence of factors such as particular sexual practices and the presence of sexually transmitted diseases, may all influence the likelihood of transmission.

EPIDEMIOLOGIC DATA

In this section we first review general epidemiologic trends in HIV and AIDS and then review data particular to injection drug users.

HIV and AIDS Surveillance

As of June 1994, AIDS had claimed over 243,000 lives in the United States, and 401,749 cases of AIDS had been reported to CDC. On January 1, 1993, CDC revised its AIDS surveillance case definition for adolescents and adults to include three additional clinical conditions and one laboratory marker of immunosuppression.[2] This expansion made for a broader case definition, resulting in a large increase in AIDS cases reported across all subpopulation groups. In 1993, 105,990 new adolescent and adult AIDS cases were reported, representing a 127 percent increase over the 46,791 cases reported in 1992.

There were 5,228 pediatric AIDS cases reported to CDC as of December 31, 1993. In 39 percent of cases, the mother was an injection drug user, and in an additional 17 percent of cases she had sex with an injection drug user. Thus, over half of all pediatric AIDS cases are associated with the HIV epidemic among injection drug users. This is likely to be a lower bound estimate because the risk factors for the mother were unknown for an additional 21 percent of pediatric cases.

In 1992, AIDS had become the eighth leading cause of death in the United States. Among women ages 25 to 44, AIDS was the fourth leading cause of death; for men in this age group, AIDS was the leading cause of death, surpassing unintentional injuries, heart disease, cancer, suicide, and homicide (Centers for Disease Control and Prevention, 1994b). Moreover, in New Jersey and New York, AIDS has been reported to be the leading killer among African American women between the ages of 20 and 40 (Kaplan, 1993). In addition to race, the risk to women also appears to be heavily skewed by social class (Epstein et al., 1993; Hu et al., 1993; Kaplan, 1993; Phillips et al., 1993; Fife and Mode, 1992). As discussed below, the largest recent increases in case reporting were observed for adolescents, women, racial/ethnic minorities, and individuals infected through injection drug use and heterosexual contact.

The dynamic nature of the epidemic is illustrated by the temporal changes in dissemination within the United States. In 1984, two cities—New York and San Francisco—reported half of all AIDS cases in this country; as of December 1993, those two cities accounted for 18 percent of new cases. These two cities have also differed in the distribution of AIDS cases by mode of exposure: in San Francisco the majority of cases are related to men who have sex with men; in New York the majority of cases are related to injection drug use. Figure 1.1 illustrates the variation in AIDS incidence rates across states. Moreover, a closer look at selected metropolitan area AIDS cases reported in 1993 reveals some substantial variations within and across regions (Table 1.1).

In contrast to surveillance data on AIDS, precise estimates of HIV infection rates in the total U.S. population remain problematic. National estimates rely on mathematical models that backcalculate HIV incidence from AIDS surveillance data as well as a composite of HIV seroprevalence data from numerous sources: states' reporting and screening of newborns, blood donors, armed forces recruits, Job Corps participants, persons attending alternative testing sites and sexually transmitted disease clinics, admissions to drug abuse treatment centers and prisons, and various other sentinel populations.[3] Over the years, the Public Health Service (PHS) has estimated that there are between 600,000 and 1.2 million HIV-infected people in the United States and that approximately 40,000 new infections occur each year among adults and adolescents (U.S. Public Health Service, 1986; Centers for Disease Control, 1987, 1990a; MacQuillan et al., 1993). A discussion of the large observed variations in PHS estimates over the years is presented in Vermund (1991).

Mode of Acquisition of Infection

Important trends in the mode of acquisition of the HIV infection can be discerned. In this country and throughout the world, the majority of HIV infections are sexually transmitted (Roper et al., 1993). In most of the world, over 75 percent of HIV infections are due to heterosexual behavior, approximately 15 percent to homosexual behavior, and a relatively small proportion to injection drug use. However, in the United States, men who have sex with men account for the largest number of reported AIDS cases (54 percent of all reported cases, that is, 193,652 cases as of December 31, 1993). Yet a review of the percentage of annual AIDS cases (Figure 1.2), classified according to CDC's exposure categories, reveals that the proportion of cases of *men who have sex with men* has decreased steadily over the years (from 74 percent in 1981 to 47 percent in 1993), while the proportion of cases of exposure from *injection drug use* has steadily increased over the last 13 years (from 12 percent in 1981 to 28 percent in 1993).

In the United States, gay and bisexual men are still the largest risk group for HIV infection and disease. Drug users constitute the next-largest risk group, although there is a large overlap between these groups. Recent CDC estimates of HIV prevalence and incidence (Holmberg, 1993, 1994) indicate that the HIV/AIDS epidemic in the United States is being driven by three subepidemics: (1) injection drug users and their sexual partners and offspring (especially in the northeastern United States; Miami, Florida; and

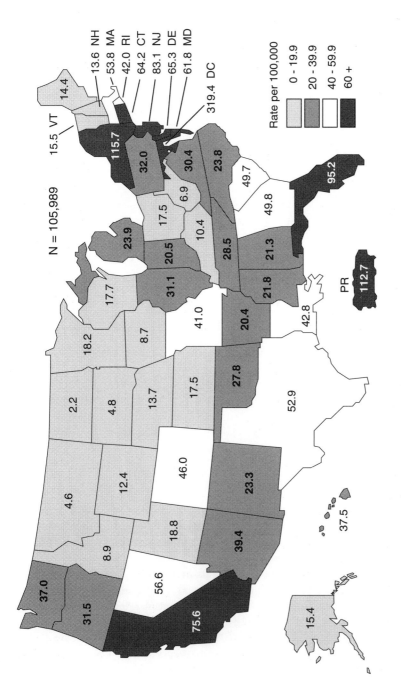

FIGURE 1.1   Annual incidence rates of AIDS for adults and adolescents per 100,000 population, for cases reported in 1993 in the United States.   SOURCE: Valdiserri, 1994.

TABLE 1.1 Newly Reported AIDS Cases by Select Metropolitan Areas, 1993

Metropolitan Area of Residence	Number	Percent of Total Cases	Local Annual Rate per 100,000 Population
Central United States			
Chicago, Illinois	2,497	2.3	32.7
Cincinnati, Ohio	273	0.3	17.3
Cleveland, Ohio	454	0.4	20.4
Dayton, Ohio	153	0.1	15.9
Denver, Colorado	1,111	1.0	62.8
Detroit, Michigan	1,272	1.2	29.5
Indianapolis, Indiana	499	0.5	34.5
Kansas City, Missouri	771	0.7	47.2
Milwaukee, Wisconsin	369	0.3	25.3
Minneapolis-Saint Paul, Minnesota	576	0.5	21.7
Saint Louis, Missouri	886	0.8	35.0
Salt Lake City, Utah	237	0.2	20.5
SUBTOTAL		8.3	
Northeastern United States			
Baltimore, Maryland	1,780	1.7	72.7
Boston, Massachusetts	2,426	2.3	42.6
Hartford, Connecticut	632	0.6	56.4
Jersey City, New Jersey	735	0.7	132.0
Nassau-Suffolk, New York	992	0.9	37.3
New Haven, Connecticut	974	0.9	59.8
New York, New York	14,716	13.8	171.8
Newark, New Jersey	2,109	2.0	109.3
Philadelphia, Pennsylvania	2,656	2.5	53.6
Pittsburgh, Pennsylvania	293	0.3	12.2
Providence, Rhode Island	325	0.3	35.6
Washington, District of Columbia	2,788	2.6	63.0
SUBTOTAL		28.6	

San Juan, Puerto Rico); (2) young and minority men who have sex with men; and (3) heterosexual women who use crack. Of these three subepidemics, two are directly linked with drug use, which underscores its catalytic role in the transmission of HIV infection.

Another noteworthy trend depicted in Figure 1.2 is the substantial increase in the proportion of new AIDS cases attributed to heterosexual transmission (from 1 percent in 1984 to 9 percent in 1993). The proportion of reported heterosexually acquired AIDS cases in women increased from 28 to 37 percent between 1987 and 1991, compared with an increase of 1.1 to 2.7 percent among men during the same years (Neal et al., 1993). Between 1991 and 1992, the annual reported AIDS cases among women in-

TABLE 1.1 Continued

Metropolitan Area of Residence	Number	Percent of Total Cases	Local Annual Rate Per 100,000 Population
Southern United States			
Atlanta, Georgia	1,912	1.8	59.1
Dallas, Texas	1,880	1.8	65.9
Fort Lauderdale, Florida	1,274	1.2	96.7
Fort Worth, Texas	440	0.4	30.4
Jacksonville, Florida	909	0.8	93.7
Miami, Florida	3,514	3.3	172.9
New Orleans, Louisiana	750	0.7	57.4
Orlando, Florida	924	0.9	69.1
Phoenix, Arizona	875	0.8	36.6
San Juan, Puerto Rico	1,960	1.8	103.4
Tampa-Saint Petersburg, Florida	1,437	1.3	67.9
West Palm Beach, Florida	858	0.8	93.9
SUBTOTAL		15.6	
Western United States			
Honolulu, Hawaii	276	0.3	31.7
Houston, Texas	2,569	2.4	70.7
Los Angeles, California	6,040	5.6	66.6
Oakland, California	1,285	1.2	59.4
Orange County, California	759	0.7	30.3
Portland, Oregon	280	0.6	41.3
Riverside-San Bernardino, California	1,201	1.1	41.2
Sacramento, California	491	0.5	34.0
San Diego, California	1,695	1.6	64.4
San Francisco, California	4,670	4.4	287.5
San Jose, California	555	0.5	36.2
Seattle, Washington	1,116	1.0	51.7
SUBTOTAL		19.9	
Total AIDS Cases in 1993—106,949			

SOURCE: *HIV/AIDS Surveillance Report* (Centers for Disease Control and Prevention, 1994b:5-7).

creased another 9.1 percent, compared with an observed increase of 2.5 percent among men during the same period (U.S. Public Health Service, 1994). During the latest time period for which annual data are available (1992 to 1993), the number of reported AIDS cases among women increased 167 percent (from 6,295 in 1992 to 16,824 in 1993), compared with a 120 percent increase among men (from 40,496 in 1992 to 89,165 in 1993).[4]

Whereas heterosexual contact accounted for 4 percent of reported AIDS cases among men in 1993, the figure was 37 percent among women. The majority of new AIDS cases among women occurred among African Ameri-

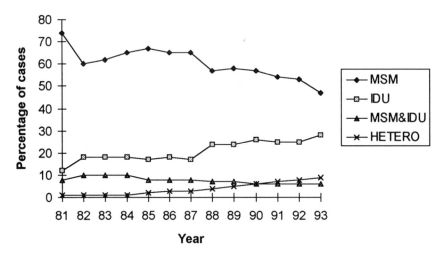

FIGURE 1.2. Annual percentage of new AIDS cases per mode of exposure, 1981 to 1993. NOTE: *MSM* = men who have sex with men; *MSM & IDU* = men who have sex with men and inject drugs; *IDU* = injection drug use; *HETERO* = heterosexual contact. SOURCE: Unpublished data from the Centers for Disease Control and Prevention, National Center for Infectious Diseases, 1994.

cans (54 percent). Figure 1.3 illustrates that this ethnic/racial disparity also was observed in new pediatric cases (55 percent were African American). A closer examination of cases by exposure category reveals that 71 percent of the newly reported cases among African American women were related to injection drug use; 52 percent of African American women diagnosed with AIDS in 1993 injected drugs, and an additional 19 percent of those cases were attributed to "sex with injecting drug user" (i.e., heterosexual contact). That same year, for other racial/ethnic categories of women diagnosed with AIDS linked with injection drug use, the corresponding proportions were 61 percent of white women (44 percent injected drugs and 17 percent reported sexual contact with an injection drug user) and 76 percent of Hispanic women (48 percent injected drugs and 28 percent reported sexual contact with an injection drug user). Among both male and female injection drug users, this ethnic disparity is greatest in the northeastern United States.

In sum, these epidemiologic data indicate that injection drug users are currently a major component of the HIV epidemic in the United States and a key bridge to the heterosexual populations. They underscore the critical importance of directing prevention efforts to injection drug users and their sexual partners.

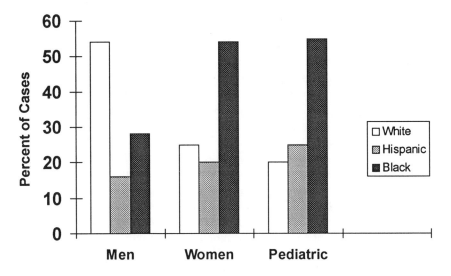

FIGURE 1.3 Proportion of adult men, women, and pediatric AIDS cases by race. SOURCE: Data from *HIV/AIDS Surveillance Report* (Centers for Disease Control and Prevention, 1994b).

HIV AND AIDS AMONG INJECTION DRUG USERS

Surveillance

Prevalence and incidence rates of HIV among injection drug users vary considerably by geographic location, so the experiences of different communities also vary. In a 1988 review of 92 studies of intravenous drug users in treatment, Hahn and colleagues (1989) reported HIV seroprevalence rates that range from 0 to 65 percent. Marked geographic differences were noted: HIV rates were highest in the Northeast (ranging from 10 to 65 percent), and lower in the West, the Midwest, and the South—5 percent or lower.

More recent information concerning the prevalence of HIV infection among injection drug users has been consistent with the findings reported by Hahn et al. (1989). In updates (Prevots et al., 1995) of CDC's HIV seroprevalence surveys of injection drug users entering drug treatment centers (most sites were methadone maintenance programs) from 1988 through 1993, seroprevalence rates of 27 percent in the Northeast, 12 percent in the South, 7 percent in the Midwest, and 3 percent in the West were reported for all years combined. Although seroprevalence rates were similar among women and men, observed rates among women were consistently higher than among men in all geographic areas. The South was the only region in which seroprevalence rates among women were found to be statistically higher than among men (i.e., 18 percent and 10 percent, respectively). Moreover, in all regions, seroprevalence rates among African Americans were higher than among whites; African Americans had a two- to sixfold increased seroprevalence compared with whites (rates ranged from 8 percent among African Americans compared with 3 percent among whites in the Midwest to 38 percent compared with 21 percent, respectively, in the Northeast). Hispanics in the Northeast were found to have prevalence rates similar to those of African Americans in the same region, but they were found to have higher rates than African Americans in the Midwest. These same surveillance data indicate that HIV seroprevalence has stabilized in most U.S. metropolitan areas. Although a moderate decline in HIV seroprevalence among the young (<30) white injection drug users was observed in high-seroprevalence areas (>10 percent), trends in annual seroprevalence were found to be stable among age and racial/ethnic subgroups. Des Jarlais et al. (1994) have also reported such declines in a cross-sectional survey among young injection drug users entering a detoxification unit in a high-seroprevalence area.

Similar patterns of seroprevalence by geographic areas have been reported by researchers at the National Institute on Drug Abuse (Battjes et al., 1991) from data collected as part of a series on nonblind point-prevalence surveys among injection drug users admitted to methadone treatment in seven areas (New York City; Trenton and Asbury Park, New Jersey; Baltimore, Maryland; Chicago, Illinois; San Antonio, Texas; and Los Angeles, California) over a 2-year period (from late 1987 through early 1989). These researchers reported significant variations in seroprevalence across geographical locations. The highest rates were observed in the Northeast: New York City and Asbury Park had rates ranging from 28.6 to 58.6 percent. Los Angeles (West) had low prevalence rates ranging from 0.9 to 3.4 percent over the course of this 2-year study. With the exception of Chicago, the multiple data points across time revealed stable seroprevalence rates within geographic location. In a more recent look (i.e., 1987 through 1991) at the seroprevalence rates in five of those original cities (i.e., New York City, Asbury Park, Trenton, Baltimore, and Chicago), Battjes et al. (1994) reported similar seroprevalence rates by location.

This reported stabilization of seroprevalence rates within geographical areas is comparable to the results of mathematical modeling studies that indicate that HIV incidence among injection drug users has shown a slight to moderate decline since the mid-1980s (Brookmeyer, 1991). Moreover, Drucker and Vermund (1989) have provided a mathematical model that allows the estimation of prevalence rates for population subgroups and overcomes some of the limitations that are associated with large-scale national cross-sectional surveys. National seroprevalence surveys are expensive, and they can mask significant variations and changes in small local population subgroups. However, the Drucker and Vermund model allows the use of local serosurvey data among various injection drug user subgroups to estimate seroprevalence among key population subgroups in a given geographic area.

Despite the wide variation by geographic location, evidence suggests that, even in areas in which prevalence is low among injection drug users, the risk of HIV infection should not be viewed with complacency. In Milan, Edinburgh, New York City, and Bangkok, once HIV became established in a community of injection drug users (i.e., a prevalence of less than 10 percent), prevalence subsequently rose dramatically within the next 2 to 4 years (Angarano et al., 1985; Robertson et al., 1986; Des Jarlais and Friedman, 1988a; Des Jarlais et al., 1994; Kitayaporn et al., 1994). Although this pattern has not been observed universally (some cities, such as Los Angeles, stabilize prevalence at lower levels), these examples suggest the need for HIV prevention programs not only when prevalence is moderate or high, but also when prevalence is low (especially when injection drug users frequently engage in high-risk behaviors). It is interesting to note, in a study of four cities with sustained low seroprevalence of HIV in injection drug users, all cities had extensive HIV prevention efforts (Des Jarlais, 1994).

Hahn and colleagues' review of injection drug users in treatment (Hahn et al., 1989) reported that the HIV seroincidence data available from some sites revealed rates of 0 to 14 percent per year, again, with the highest incidence reported in the Northeast, especially in New York City. Similar trends were observed among surveys conducted nationwide (again, in a variety of treatment settings) by CDC (Allen et al., 1992). Here, annual seroincidence rates ranged from 0 to 43 percent, the highest rates (ranging from 15 to 44 percent) again reported in the Northeast.

One study provided prevalence and incidence rates for HIV infection among intravenous drug users in and out of treatment in Philadelphia (Metzger et al., 1993). In 1989, prevalence was 10 percent among intravenous drug users in methadone treatment and 16 percent among those out of treatment. Eighteen months later, follow-up rates revealed incidence rates of 3.5 percent for those intravenous drug users in treatment, and 22 percent for those out of treatment. These data, although subject to possible selection bias, suggest that treatment for drug abuse is probably an important intervention for HIV prevention.

Efficiency of transmission among injection drug users varies according to many behavioral risk characteristics, which vary among individuals. They include: frequency of injection, sharing injection equipment, the number of needle-sharing partners, and risky sexual practices (discussed below). However, in most studies that have examined risk factors and seroconversion or prevalent infection, the sharing of drug injection equipment, including needle sharing and the use of shooting galleries, was the most significant predictor of HIV (Marmor et al., 1987; Vlahov et al., 1990; Solomon et al., 1993; Schoenbaum et al., 1989; Nicolosi et al., 1992). The type of drug administered intravenously is also associated with HIV infection. After controlling for other known risk factors, intravenous drug users who inject cocaine are more likely to be infected than intravenous drug users who inject heroin (Anthony et al., 1991; Chaisson et al., 1989; Novick et al., 1989). This may be partly because cocaine injectors are known to inject more frequently than other injectors in any given drug session.

Certain demographic factors are also associated with infection. As mentioned above, there are dramatic geographic differences in the distribution of AIDS in general, and HIV infection among intravenous drug users in particular (Des Jarlais et al., 1991; Lange et al., 1988). In general, rates are also higher among minority intravenous drug users (Friedman et al., 1987; Schoenbaum et al., 1989), women (Nelson et al., 1991, in press), and younger users (Nicolosi et al., 1992; Solomon et al., 1993; Nelson et al., 1993). These factors highlight the importance of directing prevention activities to these groups. In addition to minority women, such at-risk individuals include young, recent initiates into drug use, many of whom may be excluded from programs in which evidence of chronic use is a criterion for participation.

Sexual Transmission Among Injection Drug Users

As mentioned above, gay and bisexual intravenous drug users are not rare, and bisexual intravenous drug users may act as a conduit for transmission from both the homosexual and the intravenous drug user communities to heterosexuals, particularly women. In a survey of intravenous drug users recruited in San Francisco from street outreach and drug treatment programs (Lewis and Watters, 1991), 12 percent (49/396) of intravenous drug-using men were bisexual, based on reports of female partners prior to entry into the study. However, fewer than half of these men identified themselves as being bisexual, highlighting the difficulties that female partners have in assessing their male sexual partner's risk history. This may be particularly important because, in at least one study (Mandell et al., 1994), bisexual men (along with homosexual men) were more likely to report needle sharing than their heterosexual counterparts. Bisexual men may also have been important by acting as a conduit for HIV infection between homosexual men and the injection drug user community, at least in some areas. For example, in Chicago (Lampinen, 1992), the first reported AIDS case from injection drug use occurred in a bisexual man, and large numbers of cases involving users who were also gay and bisexual men continued for several years.

As discussed above, sexual transmission from intravenous drug users to their sexual partners may pose a greater risk for women than for men. The likelihood that an injection drug user has an injection drug-using partner is generally quite high, particularly among women (Mandell et al., 1994; Ross et al., 1992; Dwyer et al., 1994). As estimated, 75 to 90 percent of female injection drug users have a male injection drug-using partner compared with 20 to 50 percent of male users who have female drug-using partners (Cohen et al., 1989; Mondanaro, 1990; Donoghoe, 1992). In one survey in New York City (Fordyce et al., 1991), 2 percent of all currently sexually active women in 1990 reported that they knew they had a sexual partner who injected drugs. In another survey of risk factors for HIV infection among female injection drug users in methadone treatment (Schoenbaum et al., 1989), the number of male sexual partners who used drugs was strongly associated with HIV infection and was the only risk factor associated with acquisition of HIV for those women who had not used drugs since 1982.

Female sexual partners of male injection drug users may use sex as a way to obtain drugs (Donoghoe, 1992). They may also share needles with partners, thus exposing themselves to two sources of risk. Such women may be at even greater risk for sexual transmission of HIV than female partners of male injection drug users who do not themselves inject drugs— who may, in fact, be less likely to use condoms with male injection drug-using partners than with their partners who do not inject (Klee et al., 1990; Cohen, 1991; Worth, 1989).

Trading sex for drugs or money increases infection rates between injection drug users and the heterosexual community. Approximately 25 percent of female injection drug users engage in prostitution (Cohen et al., 1989; Donoghoe, 1992; Saxon et al., 1991). According to one survey in Baltimore (Astemborski et al., 1994), women who traded sex for drugs with more than 50 men over the 10 years prior to entry into the study were more likely to be infected with HIV than other female injection drug users. This finding remained significant after controlling for a range of risk factors for HIV.

In addition, women who use crack (whether or not they use injection drugs) may also trade sex for drugs and may also serve to bridge the gap between injection drug use and the heterosexual risk of HIV transmission (Des Jarlais and Friedman, 1988b; Edlin et al., 1994). Through acquisition of large numbers of partners, many of whom are also injection drug users, women who engage in this practice also expose themselves to HIV. This problem may be confounded by the profound disinhibition associated with cocaine use, resulting in little concern for safe sex or safe needle use (Donoghoe, 1992; Hartel et al., 1992). This may be due in part to the direct effects of crack as a sexual stimulant (Grinspoon and Bakalar, 1985; Weiss and Mirin, 1987). However, the relative magnitude of the pharmacologic causal effect of crack (or cocaine) on increased sexual activity is still not well understood. Although there may be increased sexual activity associated with early stages of use, as use of the drug increases, sexual dysfunction follows. Even then, there may be heightened sexual activity—sex for crack exchanges— but at this more advanced stage of drug abuse, the increase in sexual activity appears to be driven by the compulsion to use the drug and tends to be devoid of pleasurable sensation. Hence, if infected by their injection drug-using partners, these noninjection drug-using sexual partners also constitute a conduit into the heterosexual community. Crack may also amplify the spread of HIV because of its strong association with syphilis. Trading sex for crack has resulted in a large increase in syphilis (Centers for Disease Control and Prevention, 1992; Greenberg et al., 1992), which may in turn facilitate HIV transmission by increasing either infectiousness or susceptibility.

Some of the increased rates of transmission from injection drug users to their sexual partners, compared with transmission rates from infected people from other risk groups to their sexual partners, may also be attributed to high-risk sexual practices. In one survey of injection drug users who were not in treatment but who were recruited and interviewed on the street in San Francisco (Lewis and Watters, 1991), 67 percent of the sample reported never using condoms, 15 percent had more than 10 partners, and approximately 35 percent engaged in prostitution or practiced anal sex (or both). In a similar nationwide survey, 70 percent of injection drug users reported never using condoms, and more than 25 percent practiced anal sex (Centers for Disease Control and Prevention, 1990b). In a survey of injection drug users in treatment taken in the Northeast, Texas, and California, only 14 percent reported using condoms (Battjes and Pickens, 1988). In another similar study in New York City, only 5 percent reported condom use at all (Primm et al., 1988); among those who did use condoms, fewer than half used them for all sexual encounters. In the San Francisco survey described above (Lewis and Watters, 1991), more than a third of both bisexual and heterosexual male injection drug users reported that they never used condoms.

In a variety of studies that attempted risk reduction programs among injection drug users, success was greater in influencing participants to change risky injection behavior than sexual behavior (Des Jarlais and Friedman, 1988b). Again, for women this may be particularly difficult because the change to safe sex practices requires the cooperation of the male partner, which may not always be a feasible proposition (Worth, 1988). An additional concern related to power dynamics in sexual partnerships is the disclosure of HIV status. In particular, women may fear disclosing their HIV infection to male partners, thus increasing the likelihood of unsafe sexual practices (North and Rothenberg, 1993).

Part of the increase in transmission rates from injection drug users may be attributed to misclassification of modes of transmission. What is called sexual transmission may actually be transmission associated with injection drug use in the partner. Many noninjection drug-using partners of injection drug users report past injection drug use and recent use of noninjection drugs such as cocaine or crack (Centers for Disease Control and Prevention, 1991), and many of these partners also report having traded sex for drugs or money. Furthermore, as mentioned above, because female injection drug users are more likely to have a male injection drug-using partner, misclassification of female-to-male transmission is probably more severe than that for male-to-female transmission. Of course, what is labeled as transmission attributed to injection drug use may in fact be due to heterosexual contact; it is nearly impossible to separate these effects. The confluence of high-risk sexual practices with injection drug-using behavior may make it more difficult to intervene because of sources of uncertainty in the mechanisms of transmission. Nevertheless, simply acknowledging high transmission rates in areas characterized by injection drug use may be sufficient to justify proper allocation of health care resources and targeting of prevention messages.

Finally, it is possible that increased rates of transmission may also result from the fact that injection drug users may be more infectious than individuals from other risk groups or, conversely, their partners may be more susceptible. In one heterosexual partner study (Padian et al., 1994), rates of male-to-female transmission were higher from injection drug users to their partners compared with transmission from men in other risk groups, after controlling for all known risk factors in a multivariate model. An improved understanding of the postulated biological mechanisms for heterosexual transmission might shed light on this issue.

Perinatal Transmission from Injection Drug Users

Several studies have demonstrated an association between HIV infection in newborns and drug use in their mothers. Such studies have examined risk factors either using the individual as the unit of analysis (Hand et al., 1992) or in ecologic studies that correlate HIV incidence in neonates with drug use, as determined by either hospital discharge data (Morse et al., 1991) or drug-use rates by zip code (Novick et al., 1989).

Female injection drug users (regardless of their serostatus) may be more likely to become pregnant than their counterparts who do not inject drugs. Researchers (Caskey and Wathey, 1982) found that, in New York City, birth rates for addicted women were higher than those for nonaddicted women.

Female injection drug users may also be poorer users of contraception, as demonstrated in one study (Ralph and Spigner, 1986), in which female injection drug users were less likely to use condoms than a comparable group of women matched on age, ethnicity, and marital status.

In one study that was able to extricate the effects of injection drug use from HIV infection in association with pregnancy among a group of female injection drug users (all of whom were recruited at a methadone treatment clinic), 24 percent of the 70 who were seropositive and 22 percent of the 115 who were seronegative became pregnant during the course of follow-up (Selwyn et al., 1989). Similar numbers of infected and uninfected women chose to terminate their pregnancy. When comparing those who did elect to terminate with those who did not (among HIV-positive women), the reasons for termination were not unlike those reported for uninfected women, including lack of a planned pregnancy, negative feelings toward the pregnancy, and having a difficult time deciding whether to continue the pregnancy (Selwyn et al., 1989).

SUMMARY

In summary, an injection drug user infected with HIV can cause a cascade of new infections in many other individuals through needle sharing, sexual transmission, and perinatal transmission. In fact, HIV infection among injection drug users is driving the epidemic among women and among children (Des Jarlais et al., 1989; Des Jarlais and Friedman, 1988a; Fordyce et al., 1991; Turner et al., 1989). Obviously, then, any reduction in infection among injection drug users would also result in a reduction of infection among their sexual partners and future offspring. Each of these newly infected individuals can in turn cause a cascade of additional infections, again, through needle sharing, sexual transmission, and perinatal transmission. Each female of childbearing age who becomes infected is at risk of infecting a newborn. Thus, prevention of infections among injection drug users affects the growth rates of the epidemic not only among themselves, but also among adults and children in the community of noninjection drug users.

As this chapter notes, the sharing of contaminated needles is responsible for a substantial proportion of HIV infection among injection drug users. Provision of sterile needles and adequate disinfection of used needles would seem to have some merit as strategies to reduce the risk of HIV transmission in this population. However, other drug injection practices involving indirect sharing and sexual practices that are capable of transmitting HIV infection cannot be affected by the provision of sterile needles, syringes, and disinfectants.

As a result, evaluation of needle exchange and bleach distribution programs that use HIV seroconversion as an outcome probably cannot be expected to find absolute or complete reductions in HIV seroincidence. Programs that are more comprehensive in orientation and that include components on the prevention of sexual transmission would seem to have greater impact in terms of HIV prevention. However, it must be kept in mind that injection drug users are at risk for a wide variety of blood-borne pathogens, including the hepatitis viruses. Strategies to prevent transmission of the HIV infection by injecting drugs in this population might have broader public health impact in terms of prevention of other blood-borne pathogens as well. In evaluating HIV prevention programs, it is important to consider whenever possible their impact on other infectious diseases.

Finally, in order to assess the needs of a community, better methods of monitoring epidemic spread and the potential for such spread must be developed. Consequently, the panel supports the creation of more active epidemiologic surveillance of HIV prevalence and incidence so that the current progress of the epidemic can be accurately monitored. We also strongly encourage development of surveillance for behavioral data on known risk behaviors (i.e., sexual behavior and drug use), as well as surrogate markers for HIV risk, such as incident sexually transmitted diseases. This is needed so that intervention programs can be appropriately selected and evaluated.

The panel's review of the available epidemiologic data lead to the following specific conclusions and recommendations.

Conclusions

• The spread of HIV among injection drug users, their sexual partners, and offspring accounts for a major proportion of new HIV infections in the United States, and the resultant propagation of the AIDS epidemic.

• Throughout the United States, the epidemiology of HIV and AIDS differs, depending on geography, inherent differences in the population at risk, and the distribution of risk behaviors associated with transmission.

• Injection drug use with contaminated injecting equipment contributes significantly to the spread of HIV infection and thereby to the AIDS epidemic.

Recommendations

The panel recommends that:

• The Assistant Secretary for Health should charge appropriate agencies to develop improved ways of monitoring and reporting the prevalence of HIV in population subgroups of injection drug users (e.g., youth, women) in the United States.

• Given the serious public health threat associated with HIV infection among injection drug users, their sexual partners and offspring, the Assistant Secretary for Health should ensure that AIDS prevention efforts targeted to injection drug users are expanded specifically to include behavioral interventions in order to limit the further spread of HIV infection.

• AIDS behavioral prevention efforts need to target direct and indirect needle sharing and the sexual practices of injection drug users and their sex partners.

NOTES

1. The presence of maternal anti-HIV antibodies precludes an accurate diagnosis of HIV infection in infants by serologic methods. Other methods for diagnosis of neonatal infection, including HIV culture, immune-complex dissociated p24 (a viral core protein) assays, and polymerase chain reaction analyses permit the early diagnosis of HIV infection, but these techniques are expensive and not universally available.

2. The additional clinical conditions are pulmonary tuberculosis, recurrent pneumonia, and invasive cervical cancer, whereas the new laboratory marker of severe immunosuppression consists of a $CD4^+$ T-lymphocyte count <200 per milliliter.

3. A detailed presentation of CDC's family of seroprevalence surveys is presented in a special issue of *Public Health Reports* (1990).

4. These disproportionately large increases in AIDS cases in 1993 were due to CDC's revised definition of AIDS.

REFERENCES

Allen, D.M., I.M. Onorato, and T.A. Green
  1992   HIV infection in intravenous drug users entering drug treatment, United States,
          1988 to 1989. *American Journal of Public Health* 82(4):541-545.
Angarano, G., G. Pastore, L. Monno, T. Santantonio, N. Luchena, and O. Schiraldi
  1985   Rapid spread of HTLV-III infection among drug addicts in Italy. *Lancet* 2(8467):1302.
Anthony, J.C., D. Vlahov, K.E. Nelson, S. Cohn, J. Astemborski, and L. Solomon
  1991   New evidence on intravenous cocaine use and the risk of infection with human
          immunodeficiency virus type 1. *American Journal of Epidemiology* 134(10):1175-
          1189.
Aral, S.O.
  1993   Heterosexual transmission of HIV: The role of other sexually transmitted infec-
          tions and behavior in its epidemiology, prevention and control. *Annual Review of
          Public Health* 14:451-467.
Astemborski, J., D. Vlahov, D. Warren, L. Solomon, and K.E. Nelson
  1994   The trading of sex for drugs or money and HIV seropositivity among female
          intravenous drug users. *American Journal of Public Health* 84(3):382-387.

Auerbach, J.D., C. Wypijewska, and H.K.H. Brodie, eds.
1994   *AIDS and Behavior: An Integrated Approach.* Washington, DC: National Academy Press.
Battjes, R.J., and R. Pickens
1988   AIDS Transmission Risk Behaviors Among Intravenous Drug Abusers (IVDAs). Presented at the Fourth International AIDS Conference, Stockholm, June 12-16.
Battjes, R.J., R.W. Pickens, and Z. Amsel
1991   HIV infection and AIDS risk behaviors among intravenous drug users entering methadone treatment in selected U.S. cities. *Journal of Acquired Immune Deficiency Syndromes* 4:1148-1154.
Battjes, R.J., R.W. Pickens, H.W. Haverkos, and Z. Sloboda
1994   HIV risk factors among injecting drug users in five U.S. cities. *AIDS* 8:681-687.
Boylan, L., and Z.A. Stein
1991   The epidemiology of HIV infection in children and their mothers—Vertical transmission. *Epidemiology Reviews* 13:143-177.
Brookmeyer, R.
1991   Reconstruction and future trends of the AIDS epidemic in the United States. *Science* 253:37-42.
Caskey, W.R., and R.B. Wathey
1982   *Female Addiction: A Longitudinal Study.* Lexington, MA: Lexington Books.
Centers for Disease Control
1981   Kaposi's sarcoma and *Pneumocystis* pneumonia among homosexual men—New York City and California. *Morbidity and Mortality Weekly Report* 30:305-308.
1982   Persistent, generalized lymphadenopathy among homosexual males. *Morbidity and Mortality Weekly Report* 31:249-252.
1987   Human immunodeficiency virus infection in the United States: A review of current knowledge. *Morbidity and Mortality Weekly Report* 36(suppl. S-6):1-48.
1990a   HIV prevalence estimates and AIDS case projections for the United States: Report based upon a workshop. *Morbidity and Mortality Weekly Report* 39(RR-16):1-31.
1990b   Behaviors for HIV transmission among intravenous-drug users not in drug treatment—United States, 1987-1989. *Morbidity and Mortality Weekly Report* 39(16):273-276.
1991   Drug use and sexual behaviors among sex partners of injecting-drug users—United States, 1988-1990. *Morbidity and Mortality Weekly Report* 40(49):855-860.
1992   Update: Acquired immunodeficiency syndrome—United States, 1992. *Morbidity and Mortality Weekly Report* 42:547-551, 557.
1994a   *CDC HIV/AIDS Prevention* 5(2).
1994b   *HIV/AIDS Surveillance Report* 5(4).
Chaisson, R.E., P. Bacchetti, D. Osmond, B. Brodie, M.A. Sande, and A.R. Moss
1989   Cocaine use and HIV infection in intravenous drug users in San Francisco. *Journal of the American Medical Association* 261(4):561-565.
Cherubin, C.
1967   The medical sequelae of narcotic addiction. *Archives of Internal Medicine* 67:23-33.
Cherubin, C.E., and J.D. Sapira
1993   The medical complications of drug addiction and the medical assessment of the IV drug users: Twenty-five years later. *Archives of Internal Medicine* 119:1017-1028.

Chitwood, D.D., C.B. McCoy, J.A. Inciardi, D.C. McBride, M. Comerford, E. Trapido, H.V.
McCoy, J.B. Page, J. Griffin, M.A. Fletcher, et al.
    1990   HIV seropositivity of needles from shooting galleries in South Florida. *American
            Journal of Public Health* 80:150-152.
Cohen, J.B.
    1991   Why women partners of drug users will continue to be at high risk for HIV
            infection. *Journal of Addiction Diseases* 10:99-110.
Cohen, J., L. Hauer, and C. Wofsy
    1989   Women and intravenous drugs: Parenteral and heterosexual transmission of HIV.
            Journal of Drug Issues 19:39-56.
Connor, E.M., R.S. Sperling, R. Gelber, P. Kiselev, G. Scott, J.J. O'Sullivan, R. Van Dyke, M.
Bey, W. Shearer, R.L. Jacobson, E. Jimenez, E. O'Neill, B. Bazin, J.-F. Delfraissy, M. Culnane,
R. Coombs, M. Elkins, J. Moye, P. Stratton, and J. Balsley
    1994   Reduction of maternal-infant transmission of human immunodeficiency virus type
            1 with zidovudine treatment. *New England Journal of Medicine* 331(18):1173-
            1180.
Curran, J.W., H.W. Jaffe, A.M. Hardy, W.M. Morgan, R. M. Selik, and T.J. Dondero
    1988   Epidemiology of HIV infection and AIDS in the United States. *Science* 239:610-
            616.
De Gruttola, V., and K.H. Mayer
    1988   Assessing and modeling heterosexual spread of the human immunodeficiency vi-
            rus in the United States. *Review of Infectious Diseases* 10:138-150.
Des Jarlais, D.C.
    1994   Epidemiology of HIV Among Intravenous Drug Users. Presentation at the meet-
            ing of the Panel on Needle Exchange and Bleach Distribution Programs, January
            7.
Des Jarlais, D.C., and S.R. Friedman
    1988a   HIV infection among persons who inject illicit drugs: Problems and prospects.
            Journal of Acquired Immune Deficiency Syndromes 1:267-273.
    1988b   HIV and intravenous drug use. *AIDS* 2(1):S65-S69.
Des Jarlais, D.C., S.R. Friedman, D.M. Novick, J.L. Sotheran, P. Thomas, S.R. Yancovitz, D.
Mildvan, J. Weber, M.J. Kreek, and R. Maslansky
    1989   HIV-1 infection among intravenous drug users in Manhattan, New York City,
            from 1977 through 1987. *Journal of the American Medical Association* 261(7):1008-
            1012.
Des Jarlais, D.C., S.R. Friedman, K. Choopanya, S. Vanichseni, and T.P. Ward
    1992   International epidemiology of HIV and AIDS among injecting drug users. *AIDS*
            6:1053-1068.
Des Jarlais, D.C., S.R. Friedman, J.L. Sotheran, J. Wenston, M. Marmor, S.R. Yancovitz, B.
Frank, S. Beatrice, and D. Mildvan
    1994   Continuity and change within an HIV epidemic. Injecting drug users in New York
            City, 1984 through 1992. *Journal of the American Medical Association* 271(2):121-
            127.
Donahue, J.G., K.E. Nelson, A. Muñoz, D. Vlahov, L.L. Rennie, E.L. Taylor, A.J. Saah, S.
Cohn, N.J. Odaka, and H. Farzadegan
    1991   Antibody to hepatitis C virus among cardiac surgery patients, homosexual men,
            and intravenous drug users in Baltimore, Maryland. *American Journal of Epide-
            miology* 134(10):1206-1211.
Donoghoe, M.C.
    1992   Sex, HIV and the injecting drug user. *British Journal of Addiction* 87:405-416.

Drucker, E., and S.H. Vermund
1989   Estimating population prevalence of human immunodeficiency virus infection in urban areas with high rates of intravenous drug use: A model of the Bronx in 1988. *American Journal of Epidemiology* 130(1):133-142.

Dwyer, R., D. Richardson, M.W. Ross, A. Wodak, M.E. Miller, and J. Gold
1994   A comparison of HIV risk between women and men who inject drugs. *AIDS Education and Prevention* 6(5):379-389.

Edlin, B.R., K.L. Irwin, S. Faruque, et al.
1994   Intersecting epidemics: Crack cocaine use and HIV infection among inner-city young adults. Multicenter Crack Cocaine and HIV Infection Study Team. *New England Journal of Medicine* 331(21):1422-1427.

Epstein, M.R., G.A. Conway, C.R. Hayman, et al.
1993   Youth, Poverty and HIV: Trends in HIV Prevalence in a National Job Training Program, 1988-1992. Paper presented at the 121st meeting of the American Public Health Association, San Francisco, CA.

Esteban, J.I., R. Esteban, Viladomiu, J.C. Talavera-Lupez, A. Gonzalez, J.M. Hernandez, M. Roget, V. Vargas, J. Genesca, M. Buti, et al.
1989   Hepatitis C antibodies among risk groups in Spain. *Lancet* 2(8658):294-297.

Fife, D., and C. Mode
1992   AIDS prevalence by income group in Philadelphia. *Journal of Acquired Immune Deficiency Syndromes* 6:1111-2225.

Fordyce, E.J., S. Blum, A. Balanon, and R.L. Stoneburner
1991   A method for estimating HIV transmission rates among female sex partners of male intravenous drug users. *American Journal of Epidemiology* 133(6):590-598.

Friedland, G.H., and R.S. Klein
1987   Transmission of the human immunodeficiency virus. *New England Journal of Medicine* 317(18):1125-1135.

Friedman, S.R., J.L. Sotheran, A. Abdul-Quader, B.J. Primm, D.C. Des Jarlais, P. Kleinman, C. Mauge, D.S. Goldsmith, W. el-Sadr, and R. Maslansky
1987   The AIDS epidemic among blacks and Hispanics. *Millbank Quarterly* 65(Suppl 2):455-499.

Greenberg, J., D. Schnell, and R. Colon
1992   Behavior of crack cocaine users and their impact on early syphilis intervention. *Sexually Transmitted Diseases* 19:346-350.

Grinspoon, L., and J. Bakalar
1985   *Cocaine: A Drug and Its Social Evolution.* New York, NY: Basic Books.

Grund, J.P., C.D. Kaplan, N.F. Adiraans, P. Blanken, and J. Huisman
1990   The limitations of the concept of needle sharing: The practice of frontloading. *AIDS* 4(8):819-821.

Grund, J.P. C.D. Kaplan, and N.F.P. Adriaans
1991   Needle sharing in the Netherlands: An ethnographic analysis. *American Journal of Public Health* 81(12):1602-1607.

Hahn, R.A., I.M. Onorato, S. Jones, and J. Dougherty
1989   Prevalence of HIV infection among intravenous drug users in the United States. *Journal of the American Medical Association* 261(18):2677-2684.

Hand, I.L, A. Wiznia, R.T. Checola, M.H. Kim, L.M. Noble, T.J. Daley, and J.J. Yoon
1992   Human immunodeficiency virus seropositivity in critically ill neonates in the South Bronx. *Pediatric Infectious Disease Journal* 11(1):39-42.

Handsfield, H.H.
1988   Heterosexual transmission of human immunodeficiency virus. *Journal of the American Medical Association* 260(13):1943-1944.

Hartel, D., E. Schoenbaum, P. Selwyn, I. Fleming, A. Gapuchin, and G. Friedland
1992   Gender Differences in Drug Use and AIDS Mortality Among Intravenous Drug Users. Eighth International Conference on AIDS, Amsterdam.
Haverkos, H.
1994   Reporting AIDS in New York City. *Journal of the American Medical Association* 271(4):273-274.
Haverkos, H, and R. Battjes
1992   Female-to-male transmission of HIV. *Journal of the American Medical Association* 268:1855.
Haverkos, H.W., and R. Edelman
1985   Female-to-male transmission of AIDS. *Journal of the American Medical Association* 254(8):1035-1036.
1988   The epidemiology of acquired immunodeficiency syndrome among heterosexuals. *Journal of the American Medical Association* 260(13):1922-1929.
Haverkos, H.W., and W.R. Lange
1990   Serious infections other than human immunodeficiency virus among intravenous drug users. *Journal of Infectious Diseases* 161:894-902.
Haverkos, H., and R. Needle
1994   Reporting AIDS in New York City. *Journal of the American Medical Association* 271(4):273-274.
Holmberg, S.D.
1993   Emerging epidemiological patterns in the USA. Presented at the Sixth Annual Meeting of the National Cooperative Vaccine Development Group for AIDS, Alexandria, Va., October 30-November 4.
1994   Panel on Injection Drug Users and the HIV Epidemic: Understanding the Regional Differences in Prevalence, Incidence, and Risk Factors for Transmission. Public Health and Diversity: Opportunities for Equity, American Public Health Association's 122nd Annual Meeting and Exhibition, Washington, D.C., November 2.
Holmberg, S.D., C.R. Horsburgh, Jr., J.W. Ward, and H.W. Jaffe
1989   Biologic factors in the sexual transmission of human immunodeficiency virus. *Journal of Infectious Diseases* 1601(1):116-125.
Hu, D.J., R. Frey, S. Costa, et al.
1993   AIDS Rates and Sociodemographic Variables in the Newark, New Jersey, Metropolitan Area. Paper presented at the Ninth International Conference on AIDS, Berlin, Germany.
Inciardi, J.
1990   AIDS—A strange disease of uncertain origins. *American Behavioral Scientist* 33:397-407.
Inciardi, J., and J. Page
1991   Drug sharing among intravenous drug users. *AIDS* 5(6):772-773.
Institute of Medicine
1988   *Confronting AIDS: Update 1988.* Washington, DC: National Academy Press.
Ippolito, G., G. DeCarli, V. Puro, N. Petrosillo, C. Arici, B. Bertucci, L. Bianciardi, L. Bonazzi, A. Cestrone, M. Daglio, et al.
1994   Device-specific risk of needlestick injury in health care workers. *Journal of the American Medical Association* 272(8):607-610.
Jaffe, H.W., D.J. Bregman, and R.M. Selik
1983a   Acquired immune deficiency syndrome in the United States: The first 1,000 cases. *Journal of Infectious Disease* 48:339-345.
Jaffe, H.W., K. Choi, P.A. Thomas, H.W. Haverkos, D.M. Auerbach, M.E. Guinan, M.F.

Rogers, T.J. Spira, W.W. Darrow, M.A. Kramer, S.M. Friedman, J.M. Monroe, A.E. Friedman-Kien, L.J. Laubenstein, M. Marmor, B. Safai, S.K. Dritz, S.J. Crispi, S.L. Fannin, J.P. Orkwis, A. Kelter, W.R. Rushing, S.B. Thacker, and J.W. Curran
  1983b   National case-control study of Kaposi's sarcoma and *Pneumocystis carinii* pneumonia in homosexual men: Part I. Epidemiologic results. *Annals of Internal Medicine* 99:145-151.
Jaffe, H.W., W.W. Darrow, D.F. Echenberg, P.M. O'Malley, J.P. Getchell, V.S. Kalyanaraman, R.H. Byers, D.P. Drennan, E.H. Braff, J.W. Curran, and D.P. Francis
  1985   The acquired immunodeficiency syndrome in a cohort of homosexual men. A six-year follow-up study. *Annals of Internal Medicine* 103:210-214.
Johnson, A.M.
  1988   Heterosexual transmission of human immunodeficiency virus. *British Medical Journal* 296:1017-1020.
Johnson, A.M., and M. Laga
  1988   Heterosexual transmission of HIV. *AIDS* Suppl 1:S49-S56.
Jose, B., S.R. Friedman, A. Neaigus, R. Curtis, J.P. Grund, M.F. Goldstein, T.P. Ward, and D.C. Des Jarlais
  1993   Syringe-mediated drug-sharing (backloading): A new risk factor for HIV among injecting drug users. *AIDS* 7(12):1653-1660.
Kaplan, M.S.
  1993   Women and AIDS: Toward a Feminist Conception of Social Prevention. Paper presented at the 121st annual meeting of the American Public Health Association, San Francisco, CA.
Kingsley, L.A., R. Detels, R. Kaslow, B.F. Polk, C.R. Rinaldo, Jr., J. Chmiel, K. Detre, S.F. Kelsey, N. Odaka, D. Ostrow, et al.
  1987   Risk factors for seroconversion to human immunodeficiency virus among male homosexuals: Results from the Multicenter AIDS Cohort Study. *Lancet* 1(8529):345-349.
Kitayaporn, D., C. Uneklabh, B.G. Weninger, et al.
  1994   Incidence determined retrospectively among drug users in Bangkok, Thailand. *AIDS 1994*:1443-1450.
Klee, H., J. Faughier, C. Hayes, T. Boulton, and J. Morris
  1990   Factors associated with risk behavior among injecting drug users. *AIDS* 2:133-145.
Koester, S.K.
  1994   Copping, running and paraphernalia laws: Contextual variables and needle risk behavior among injection drug users in Denver. *Human Organization* 53(3).
Koester, S.K., and L. Hoffer
  1994   Indirect sharing: Additional HIV risks associated with drug injection. *AIDS and Public Policy Journal* Summer:100-105.
Koester, S.K., R. Booth, and W. Wiebel
  1990   The risk of transmission from sharing water, drug mixing containers, and cotton filters among intravenous drug users. *International Journal on Drug Policy* 1(6):28-30.
Kreek, M.J.
  1983   Health consequences associated with the use of methadone. Pp. 456-482 in *Research on the Treatment of Narcotic Addiction*, J.R. Cooper, F. Altman, B.S. Brown, and D. Czechowicz, eds. Rockville, MD: National Institute on Drug Abuse.
Laga, M., H. Taelman, P. Van der Stuyft, et al.
  1989   Advanced immunodeficiency as a risk factor for heterosexual transmission of HIV. *AIDS* 3:361-366.

Lamothe, F., J. Bruneau, R. Coates, J.G. Rankin, J. Soto, R. Arshinoff, M. Brabant, J. Vincelette, and M. Fauvel
1993   Seroprevalence of and risk factors for HIV-1 infection in injection drug users in Montréal and Toronto: A collaborative study. *Canadian Medical Association Journal* 149(7):945-951.
Lampinen, T.M.
1992   Prevalence of Human Immunodeficiency Virus Type I Among Chicago Injecting Drug Users. Thesis submitted in partial fulfillment of the requirements of the Master of Science in Public Health Sciences in the Graduate College of the University of Illinois at Chicago School of Public Health, Chicago.
Lange, W.R., F.R. Snyder, D. Lozovsky, V. Kaistha, M.A. Kaczaniuk, and J.H. Jaffe
1988   Geographic distribution of human immunodeficiency virus markers in parenteral drug abusers. *American Journal of Public Health* 7(4):443-446.
Lazzarin, A., A. Saracco, M. Musicco, and A. Nicolosi
1991   Man-to-woman transmission of the human immunodeficiency virus. Risk factors related to sexual behavior, man's infectiousness, and woman's susceptibility. Italian Study Group on HIV Heterosexual Transmission (published erratum appears in *Archives of Internal Medicine* April 1992, 152[4]:876). *Archives of Internal Medicine* 151(12):2411-2416.
Levine, D.P., and J.D. Sobel, eds.
1991   *Infections in Intravenous Drug Abusers*. New York, NY: Oxford University Press.
Lewis, D.K., and J.K. Watters
1991   Sexual risk behavior among heterosexual intravenous drug users: Ethnic and gender variations. *AIDS* 5:77-83.
Louria, D.B., T. Hensle, and J. Rose
1967   The major medical complications of narcotic addition. *Annals of Internal Medicine* 67:1-32.
MacQuillan, G.M., M. Khare, T.M. Ezzati, et al.
1993   The seroepidemiology of human immunodeficiency virus in the United States household population: NHANES III, 1988-1991 [abstract 21]. P. 59 in *Program and Abstracts: The First National Conference on Human Retroviruses and Related Infections*. Washington, DC: National Foundation for Infectious Diseases, American Society for Microbiology.
Mandell, W., D. Vlahov, C. Latkin, M. Oziemkowska, and S. Cohn
1994   Correlates of needle sharing among injection drug users. *American Journal of Public Health* 84(6): 920-923.
Marmor, M., D.C. Des Jarlais, H. Cohen, S.R. Friedman, S.T. Beatrice, N. Dubin, W. El-Sadr, D. Mildvan, S. Yancovitz, U. Mathur, and R. Holzman
1987   Risk factors for infection with human immunodeficiency virus among drug abusers in New York City. *AIDS* 1:39-44.
McCoy, C.B., P. Shapshak, S.M. Shah, H.V. McCoy, J.E. Rivers, J.B. Page, D.D. Chitwood, N.L. Weatherby, J.A. Inciardi, D.C. McBride, D.C. Mash, and J.K. Watters
1994   HIV-1 Prevention: Interdisciplinary studies and reviews on efficacy of bleach and compliance to bleach prevention protocols. Pp. 255-283 in *Proceedings, Workshop on Needle Exchange and Bleach Distribution Programs*. Washington, DC: National Academy Press.
McCray, E.
1986   Occupational risk of the acquired immunodeficiency syndrome among health care workers. *New England Journal of Medicine* 314(17):1127-1132.

Metzger, D.S., G.E. Woody, A.T. McLellan, C.P. O'Brien, P. Druley, H. Navaline, D. DePhilippis, P. Stolley, and E. Abrutyn
1993   Human immunodeficiency virus seroconversion among intravenous drug users in- and out-of-treatment: An 18-month prospective follow-up. *Journal of Acquired Immune Deficiency Syndromes* 6:1049-1056.

Mofenson, L.M.
1992   Preventing mother to infant HIV transmission: What we know so far. *The AIDS Reader* March/April:42-51.

Mondanaro, J.
1990   *Treatment of Women with Chemical Dependency Problems.* Lexington, MA: Lexington Press.

Morse, D.L., L. Lessner, M.G. Medvesky, D.M. Glebatis, and L.F. Novick
1991   Geographic distribution of newborn HIV seroprevalence in relation to four sociodemographic variables. *American Journal of Public Health* 81(Suppl):25-29.

Napoli, V.M., and J.E. McGowan, Jr.
1987   How much blood is in a needlestick? [letter] *Journal of Infectious Diseases* 155(4):828.

Neal, J.J., C.A. Ciesielski, and P.L. Fleming
1993   Heterosexually Acquired AIDS in the United States: The Next Epidemic Wave. Paper presented at the 121st annual meeting of the American Public Health Associations, San Francisco, CA.

Nelson, K., D. Vlahov, and S. Cohn
1991   Sexually transmitted diseases in a population of intravenous drug users: Association with seropositivity to the human immunodeficiency virus (HIV). *Journal of Infectious Diseases* 164:457-463.

Nelson, K.E., D. Vlahov, L. Solomon, S. Cohn, and A. Muñoz
in press Temporal trends of incident HIV infection in a cohort of injection drug users in Baltimore, Maryland. *Archives of Internal Medicine.*

Nicolosi, A., M.L. Correa Leite, M. Musicco, S. Molinari, and A. Lazzarin
1992   Parenteral and sexual transmission of human immunodeficiency virus in intravenous drug users: A study of seroconversion. *American Journal of Epidemiology* 135(3):225-233.

North, R.L., and K.H. Rothenberg
1993   Partner notification and the threat of domestic violence against women with HIV infection. *New England Journal of Medicine* 329:1194-1196.

Novick, D.M., P. Farci, T.S. Croxsan, M.B. Taylor, C.W. Schneebaum, M.E. Lai, N. Bach, R.T. Senie, A.M. Gelb, and M.J. Kreek
1988   Hepatitis D virus and human immunodeficiency virus antibodies in parenteral drug abusers who are hepatitis B surface antigen positive. *Journal of Infectious Diseases* 158(4):795-803.

Novick, D.M., H.L Trigg, D.C. Des Jarlais, S.R. Friedman, D. Vlahov, and M.J. Kreek
1989   Cocaine injection and ethnicity in parenteral drug users during the early years of the human immunodeficiency virus (HIV) epidemic in New York City. *Journal of Medical Virology* 29:181-185.

Ouellet, L., A. Jimenez, W. Johnson, et al.
1991   Shooting galleries and HIV disease: Variations in places for injecting illicit drugs. *Crime and Delinquency* 37:64-85.

Padian, N.S.
1987   Heterosexual transmission of acquired immunodeficiency syndrome: International perspectives and national projections. *Review of Infectious Diseases* 9:947-960.

Padian, N., L. Marquis, D.P. Francis, R.E. Anderson, G.W. Rutherford, P.M. O'Malley, and
W. Winkelstein, Jr.
    1987   Male-to-female transmission of human immunodeficiency virus. *Journal of the
            American Medical Association* 258(6):788-790.
Padian, N., J. Wiley, and S. Glass
    1988   Anomalies of Infectivity in the Heterosexual Transmission of HIV. Paper pre-
            sented at the Fourth International Conference on AIDS, Stockholm.
Padian, N., P.J. Hitchcock, R.E. Fullilove, 3d, V. Kohlstadt, and R. Burnham
    1990   Report of the NIAID Study Group on Integrated Behavioral Research for Preven-
            tion and Control of Sexually Transmitted Diseases. Part I: Issues in defining
            behavioral risk factors and their distribution. *Sexually Transmitted Diseases* 17(4):200-
            204.
Padian, N.S., S.C. Shiboski, and N.P. Jewell
    1991   Female-to-male transmission of human immunodeficiency virus. *Journal of the
            American Medical Association* 266(12):1664-1667.
Padian, N., S. Shiboski, E. Vittinghoff, and N. Hessol
    1994   Heterosexual transmission of HIV in Northern California: 1984-1993. Presented
            at the Society for Epidemiologic Research, Miami.
Page, J.B., D. Chitwood, P. Smith, N. Kane, and D. McBride
    1990   Intravenous drug use and HIV infection in Miami. *Medical Anthropology Quar-
            terly* 4(4):56-71.
Phillips, R.K., N. Salem, and S.R. Novey
    1993   Targeting HIV/AIDS Services to Meet Growing Needs of Underserved Popula-
            tions in Los Angeles County. Paper presented at the 121st annual meeting of the
            American Public Health Association, San Francisco, CA.
Polk, B.F.
    1985   Female-to-male transmission of AIDS. *Journal of the American Medical Associa-
            tion* 254(22):3177-3178.
Prevots, D.R., D.M. Allen, J.S. Lehman, T.A. Green, L.R. Petersen, and M. Gwinn
    1995   Trends in HIV Seroprevalence Among Injection Drug Users Entering Drug Treat-
            ment Centers, United States, 1988-1993. Paper presented at the Second National
            Conference on Human Retroviruses and Related Infections, Abstract 312. In press,
            American Journal of Epidemiology.
Primm, B.J., L.S. Brown, B.S. Gibson, and A. Chu
    1988   The Range of Sexual Behaviors of Intravenous Drug Abusers. Presented at the
            Fourth International AIDS Conference, Stockholm, June 12-16.
Ralph, N., and C. Spigner
    1986   Contraceptive practices among female heroin addicts. *American Journal of Public
            Health* 76:1016-1017.
Redfield, R.R., P.D. Markham, S.Z. Salahuddin, M.G. Sarngadharan, A.J. Bodner, T.M. Folks,
W.R. Ballou, D.C. Wright, and R.C. Gallo
    1985   Frequent transmission of HTLV-III among spouses of patients with AIDS-related
            complex and AIDS. *Journal of the American Medical Association* 253(11):1571-
            1573.
Resnick, L., K. Veren, S.Z. Salahuddin, et al.
    1986   Stability and inactivation of HTLV-III/LAV under clinical and laboratory environ-
            ments. *Journal of the American Medical Association* 255:53-68.
Robertson, J.R., A.B.V. Bucknall, P.D. Welsby, J.J. Roberts, J.M. Inglis, J.F. Peutherer, and
R.P. Brettle
    1986   Epidemic of AIDS-related virus (HTLV-III/LAV) infection among intravenous
            drug users. *British Medical Journal* 292(6519):527-529.

Rogers, D.E.
1992   Report card on our national response to the AIDS epidemic: Some A's, too many D's. *American Journal of Public Health* 82(4):522-524.
Roper, W. L., H. B. Peterson, and J. W. Curran
1993   Commentary: Condoms and HIV/STD prevention—Clarifying the message. *American Journal of Public Health* 83(4):501-503.
Ross, M.W., A. Wodak, and J. Gold
1992   Sexual behaviour in injecting drug users. *Journal of Psychology and Human Sexuality* 5:89-104.
Samuels, J.F., D. Vlahov, J.C. Anthony, L. Solomon, and D.D. Celentano
1991   The practice of "frontloading" among intravenous drug users: Association with HIV-antibody. *AIDS* 5(3):343.
Sapira, J.D.
1968   The narcotic addict as a medical patient. *American Journal of Medicine* 45:555-588.
Saxon, A., D.A. Calsyn, S. Whittaker, and G. Freeman
1991   Sexual behavior of intravenous drug users in treatment. *Journal of Acquired Immune Deficiency Syndromes* 4:938-944
Schoenbaum, E.E., D. Hartel, P.A. Selwyn, R.S. Klein, K. Davenny, M. Rogers, C. Feiner, and G. Friedland
1989   Risk factors for human immunodeficiency virus infection in intravenous drug users. *New England Journal of Medicine* 321(13):874-879.
Selwyn, P.A., and P.A. Alcabes
1994   The Potential Impact of Needle Exchange Programs on Health Outcomes Other Than HIV and Drug Use. Paper commissioned by the Panel on Needle Exchange and Bleach Distribution Programs.
Selwyn, P.A., R.J. Carter, E.E. Schoenbaum, V.J. Robertson, R.S. Klein, and M.F. Rogers
1989   Knowledge of HIV antibody status and decisions to continue or terminate pregnancy among intravenous drug users. *Journal of the American Medical Association* 261(24):3567-3571.
Solomon, L., J. Astemborski, D. Warren, A. Muñoz, S. Cohn, D. Vlahov, and K. Nelson
1993   Difference in risk factors for human immunodeficiency virus type-1 seroconversion among male and female intravenous drug users. *American Journal of Epidemiology* 137(8):892-898.
Stein, M.D.
1990   Medical complications of intravenous drug use. *Journal of General Internal Medicine* 5:249-257.
Stimmel, B., S. Vernace, and F. Schaffner
1975   Hepatitis B surface antigen and antibody in asymptomatic drug users. *Journal of the American Medical Association* 243:1135-1138.
Turner, C., H. Miller, and L. Moses, eds.
1989   *AIDS: Sexual Behavior and Intravenous Drug Use.* National Research Council. Washington, DC: National Academy Press.
U.S. Public Health Service
1986   Coolfont report: A PHS plan for prevention and control of AIDS and the AIDS virus. *Public Health Reports* 101:341-348.
1994   Fight against HIV/AIDS moves to new fronts. *Prevention Report*, Office of Disease Prevention and Health Promotion. Washington, DC: U.S. Department of Health and Human Services.
Valdiserri, R.
1994   Presentation at HIV Prevention: Looking Back, Looking Ahead: Targeted and

Universal Approaches to Reducing the Risk of HIV Transmission, New York Academy of Medicine, September 20.

Vermund, S.H.
1991   Changing estimates of HIV-1 seroprevalence in the United States. *Journal of NIH Research* 3:77-81.

Vermund, S.H., M.A. Galbraith, S.C. Ebner, A.R. Sheon, and R.A. Kaslow
1992   Human immunodeficiency virus/acquired immunodeficiency syndrome in pregnant women. *Annals of Epidemiology* 2(6):773-803.

Vlahov, D., A. Muñoz, J.C. Anthony, S. Cohn, D.D. Celentano, and K.E. Nelson
1990   Association of drug injection patterns with antibody to human immunodeficiency virus type 1 among intravenous drug users in Baltimore, Maryland. *New England Journal of Medicine* 123(5):847-856.

Weiss, R., and S. Mirin
1987   *Cocaine.* Washington, DC: American Psychiatric Press.

Winkelstein, W., Jr., M. Samuel, N.S. Padian, J.A. Wiley, W. Lang, R.E. Anderson, and J.A. Levy
1987   The San Francisco Men's Health Study, III: Reduction in human immunodeficiency virus transmission among homosexual/bisexual men, 1982-86. *American Journal of Public Health* 77(6):685-689.

Worth, D.
1988   Self-Help Interventions with Women at High Risk of HIV Infection. Montefiore Medical Center, New York City.
1989   Sexual decision-making and AIDS: Why condom promotion among vulnerable women is likely to fail. *Studies in Family Planning* 20(6):297-307.

Zule, W.A.
1992   Risk and reciprocity: HIV and the injection drug user. *Journal of Psychoactive Drugs* 24(3):243-249.

2

The Epidemiology of Injection Drug Use

Estimating the numbers of injection drug users in the United States is an important part of planning the nation's response to the public health threat posed by the AIDS epidemic. At federal, state, and local levels, policy planners need reasonably accurate estimates regarding the size, characteristics, and geographical distribution of the drug-injecting population within their jurisdictions in order to establish a sound rationale for allocating limited resources. Although there have been some advances, it remains true that precise estimation of the numbers of injection drug users remains extraordinarily difficult. Given the illegal and covert nature of the behavior, the situation could hardly be otherwise.

A critical issue in counting injection drug users is definitional: injection drug users vary greatly in the type and combinations of drugs they use, the frequency of injection, the settings in which injections occur, the amount of sharing of injection equipment that takes place, and so forth. The National Research Council dealt with this issue in a previous report, *AIDS, Sexual Behavior, and Intravenous Drug Use* (Turner et al., 1989).

One particularly important example concerns the injection of cocaine. Because of the shorter duration of euphoria associated with this drug, users who inject cocaine tend to go on binges or "runs," in which they inject repeatedly in a relatively short time; that is, cocaine is sometimes taken in discrete episodes of high-intensity use (Gawin and Kleber, 1985). A binge episode may be followed by an extended period of no injection at all. This pattern is quite different from the typical pattern for a heroin injector, who may inject a few times throughout the day to forestall physical withdrawal. The cocaine user on a run may be more likely to share needles, due to the need for repeated administration of the drug within a short time in order to satisfy the intense craving to consume more of the drug. This illustrates the point that merely counting the number of injection drug users, defined in some fashion, may not be sufficient to adequately address the prevention needs of certain subgroups of injection drug users.

The National Research Council report found "the current estimates of the prevalence of IV drug use to be seriously flawed" (p. 233) and recommended that a high priority be given to research on the estimation of the number of injection drug users in the United States (Turner et al., 1989). Since that report, a special issue of the *Journal of Drug Issues* (Hser and Anglin, 1993) on prevalence estimation techniques for drug-using populations makes note of improvements in the quality and quantity of data available and convincingly documents a growing recognition of the importance of this area of inquiry. Acknowledging the imprecision of existing estimation models, Anglin et al. (1993) are more positive about the state of the field. By looking at prevalence estimation as policy research, they stress the potential of this work to inform ongoing decision making, thereby emphasizing appropriate but cautious application of estimates with less stress on absolute precision. In sum, although the continuing imprecision in estimates of the number of injection drug users remains a concern, this panel recognizes the need to make the best use of available data to inform the decisions of policy makers.

ESTIMATES OF INJECTION DRUG USERS

Despite the imprecision of available estimates in this country, most would agree that the magnitude of the population of drug injectors is a major influence on evolving patterns of HIV transmission. U.S. Public Health Service reports dating back to the 1980s all estimate the national figure for injection drug user to exceed 1 million. The Centers for Disease Control (1987a, 1987b) reported approximately 1.5 million injection drug users for 1986 and a revised figure of 1.1 million for 1987. One year later, the National Institute on Drug Abuse (NIDA) estimated that there were about 1.1 to 1.3 million injection drug users in the United States (Schuster, 1988). In its 1989 report, the National Research Council included a critique of the estimation methods used to generate these figures, suggesting that it was not unreasonable to believe that their margin of error could be as great as 100 percent (Spencer, 1989). The report cautions, "That is to say, the true number of IV drug users could be as few as half a million or as great as 2 million" (Turner et al., 1989:230).

Scott Holmberg (1993, 1994) of the Centers for Disease Control and

Prevention has recently attempted to estimate the number of "current active" injection drug users in the 96 largest metropolitan statistical areas (MSAs) in the United States—those with more than 500,000 inhabitants. Holmberg's estimated number of injection drug users in these 96 MSAs is approximately 1.5 million, which is in line with other estimates. Although the 96 MSAs have only about 160 million persons, or about 62 percent of the entire U.S. population of 260 million, it is likely that they include a much higher percentage of all injection drug users. Holmberg (1993, 1994) notes that these areas include about 85 percent of all reported AIDS cases, and it is likely that they include approximately the same proportion of injection drug users.[1] Thus, if at least 85 percent of all injection drug users are located in the 96 MSAs, that suggests a national total of injection drug users on the order of 1.7 million. Holmberg's detailed procedure for estimating the number of injection drug users in these metropolitan statistical areas consisted of compiling available information from diverse sources (i.e., published and unpublished). Specific studies of injection drug users performed by federal agencies, health departments, drug treatment services, academic institutions, and a large government contractor (i.e., Research Triangle Institute) were reviewed to arrive at estimates for individual MSAs. Holmberg's procedure included several criteria to ascertain the reasonableness of his estimates: (1) the estimated number of injection drug users should be consistent with the proportion of known injection drug users in treatment (reflecting NIDA estimates of the percentage of injection drug users in treatment); (2) the number should likewise correspond to the proportion of known injection drug users tested for HIV at confidential counseling and testing sites, where such information was available; (3) the estimated proportions of injection drug users should be consistent with the stratification of high-, medium-, and low-injection-use cities, as defined by the Drug Abuse Warning Network (DAWN) data, treatment providers, and ethnographers.

Geographic Variations

With respect to regional and geographic variation, the pattern is one of clusters of injection drug users, and the clusters are well dispersed across the country. Half of all injection drug users (in the 96 largest MSAs) are found in the top 16 MSAs. Of the top 11 MSAs, 6 are part of the Northeast corridor: Boston, New York City, Newark, Philadelphia, Baltimore, and Washington, D.C. Nearly a quarter (23.5 percent) of all injection drug users (in the 96 largest MSAs) are located in just these 6 MSAs. The other three-quarters are located in the other 10 MSAs: Los Angeles, Chicago, Houston, Detroit, Miami, Riverside, San Francisco, Atlanta, San Juan, and Fort Worth. Three of these are on the West Coast, two in the upper Midwest, two in Texas, two in the South, and the other in San Juan, Puerto Rico. Thus, it is clear that injection drug users are geographically dispersed throughout the nation, notwithstanding the density in the Northeast corridor.

Few national estimates of injection drug users as geographically specific as those provided by Holmberg have been published, making comparisons difficult; however, one estimate is that provided for New York City. In a paper commissioned by this panel, Frank and Williams (1994) review the history of narcotic use and prevalence estimation in New York. A narcotics registry was maintained in New York City from 1965 to 1974 in an attempt to approximate a census of addicts. During this period, almost 900,000 reports were recorded on nearly 300,000 individuals. More than 95 percent of the individuals reported were using heroin, which at the time was considered almost tantamount to being identified as an injector. Utilizing the registry as a foundation for the years 1970 to 1974 and then developing a synthetic estimation model to project for later years, Frank and Williams estimated the numbers of narcotic abusers in New York City to be 165,000 in 1970 and 200,000 in 1980. The authors suggest that the number of heroin injectors in New York City is now probably less than the 1980 figure of 200,000 due to AIDS mortality and the growing popularity of snorting heroin as a route of administration, but no more recent prevalence estimates have been attempted. The authors do not account for the possible shift in type of drug injected (i.e., cocaine), which might be missed by their methodology. Nonetheless, the Frank and Williams estimate is in accordance with Holmberg's New York City figure of 168,300.

National Surveys of Drug Abuse

Another source of information about the size of the injection drug use population is national surveys of substance abuse.

National Household Survey on Drug Abuse

The National Household Survey on Drug Abuse (NHSDA) of the Substance Abuse and Mental Health Services Administration (SAMHSA) provides an important source of data on drug use among the general population, although it cannot estimate the entirety of the injection drug user population in the country. In particular, it has major problems as a precise basis for estimating numbers of hard-core drug users, including injectors (National Institute on Drug Abuse, 1994a; U.S. General Accounting Office, 1993). The representative sample of households excludes injection drug users who are homeless, institutionalized, or transient, and the injection drug users who are approached may be reluctant to participate. Also, the survey relies on self-reports, and the stigma associated with drug injection may contribute to greater denial on the part of those who do participate.

Given the fact that the NHSDA is widely acknowledged to underrepresent injection drug users, it is surprising to note the magnitude of the subpopulation it has uncovered.[2] The 1991 survey revealed an estimated 3,768,000 people who have used a needle to inject a drug at some time in their lives and 1,083,000 who have done so in the past year. The 1992 estimated figures were much lower: 2,984,000 for lifetime prevalence and 659,000 for the past year. With regard to age, in 1991, 29 percent of those who reported having injected drugs in the past year were between the ages of 12 and 25 (Table 2.1). In 1992, that age group represented 44 percent of those who had reported injecting drugs in the past year.

Because the populations sampled in these 2 years were highly similar, the observed drop in lifetime prevalence and observed fluctuations by other demographic characteristics cannot be credibly attributed to the relatively minor changes in the sampling frame from one year to the next. As a consequence, this anomaly helps to underscore the imprecision with which the NHSDA is able to estimate numbers of injection drug users.

The large fluctuations in the NHSDA estimates are due in part to the nature of the targeted population. That is, the survey is designed to capture drug use among households nationwide, not specific population subgroups such as injection drug users. As a result, there are too few members of certain specific subgroups (e.g., injection drug users) to allow for the computation of reliable estimates. This is reflected in the large standard errors associated with the estimated number of injection drug users reported above.

Washington DC Metropolitan Area Drug Study

The Washington DC Metropolitan Area Drug Study (DC*MADS) was funded by the National Institute on Drug Abuse (1993, 1994b, 1994c) in an attempt to examine the nature and extent of drug abuse among all types of people residing in a single metropolitan area, with a special focus on populations that were underrepresented or unrepresented in the NHSDA (National Institute on Drug Abuse, 1994b). These special populations, including homeless people, transients, and institutionalized individuals, represent people who tend to be at risk for drug abuse.

Of particular relevance to the topic of this report, DC*MADS estimated that adding homeless and institutionalized populations to the 1991 NHSDA population of past-year injection drug use in the D.C. MSA would have increased the estimate of currently active injection drug users from 0.20 to 0.30 percent, an increase of one-third. The number of injection drug users among the population of households was estimated at 5,987; including the homeless, transient, and institutionalized populations, the number was 8,740.

TABLE 2.1 Needle Use: Ever Used and Past
Year Use by Age, Sex, and Race, 1992 and
1991 NHSDA Data[a]

	1991	1992
Age		
Ever used		
12-17	152	69
18-25	643	635
26-34	1,223	1,079
35+	1,760	1,201
Used past year		
12-17	84	42
18-25	232	250
26-34	228	169
35+	539	199
Sex		
Ever used		
Male	2,636	2,034
Female	1,233	950
Used past year		
Male	738	454
Female	345	205
Race		
Ever used		
White	2,729	2,346
Black	559	395
Hispanic	384	160
Used past year		
White	815	504
Black	154	88
Hispanic	94	59

[a]In thousands.

SOURCE: Unpublished data from National Household Survey
on Drug Abuse (1991, 1992).

(Needle use is defined as the injection of cocaine, opiates, or psychotherapeutics
for nonmedical reasons at least once in the previous 12 months.)   This
difference is too small to change prevalence estimates noticeably, but it
would result in a one-third increase in the population estimates often used
by providers for estimating the number of people in need of treatment and,
for that matter, HIV prevention services.

One noteworthy point is that most of the injection drug users were
found in the household population (about two-thirds). It is of course the
case that some unknown portion of injection drug users either denied such

use or refused to participate in either the NHSDA or the DC*MADS studies. Thus, these estimates of one-third and two-thirds have some unknown degree of associated error.[3]

Surveys of Youth

NIDA's Monitoring the Future survey provides the most accurate data available on drug use among secondary school students, but it has the same limitations as the NHSDA in its ability to estimate the hard-core subpopulation of drug users that includes injection drug users. However, like the NHSDA, the Monitoring the Future survey does pick up a small but substantial number of its sampled population who acknowledge having injected drugs. In 1992, 1.7 percent of high school seniors reported having injected a drug during their lives, and 0.8 percent did so in the past year. In 1993, 1.4 percent reported having injected during their lives, and 0.7 percent did so in the past year (O'Malley, unpublished data).

The Centers for Disease Control and Prevention conducted several nationally representative surveys of students in grades 9-12 asking about various risk behaviors, including injection of drugs (Centers for Disease Control and Prevention, 1992). The 1990 Youth Risk Behavior Survey showed 1.5 percent lifetime prevalence for grade 10, and 1.3 percent for grade 12, which are fairly close to the corresponding figures from the Monitoring the Future surveys (1.4 percent and 1.7 percent, respectively). Another noteworthy finding is that studies in both San Francisco and New York report that sharing appears to be more frequent among younger injectors (Guydish et al., 1990; Kleinman et al., 1990), who are typically not very well represented in current needle exchange programs in this country (see the section on the demographics of program participants in Chapter 3).

Conclusion

In sum, across a number of surveys of the type that would be expected to underestimate injection drug use, there is a fair amount of consistency, suggesting a prevalence rate that is clearly not zero and may be as high as 1 to 2 percent among young Americans. None of the surveys show any dramatic shifts in recent years.

Another perspective that is important to consider in light of broader population-based surveys of injection drug users is the limited number of injection drug users that are in treatment. It is estimated that between 10 and 20 percent of injection drug users are in drug treatment at any give time (Centers for Disease Control and Prevention, 1990; Office of Technology Assessment, 1990; Wiley and Samuel, 1989; Schuster, 1988).

CHARACTERISTICS OF INJECTION DRUG USERS

Given the substantial uncertainty in our ability to specify numbers of injection drug users in the United States, it is likewise problematic to estimate accurately the characteristics of this elusive population. Yet existing surveys, drug abuse indicator databases, and other research offer considerable insight in beginning to identify the composition of injection drug users within our borders.

A review of available data reveals at least two predominant themes. First, the overall population of injection drug users in the United States is quite heterogeneous in composition. It is emphatically not the case that all injection drug users are male minorities located in large urban areas, as stereotypes would imply. Second, the composition and characteristics of this population are continually evolving and have changed markedly over time. These facts suggest that the useful improvements that can be made in prevalence estimation techniques are not limited merely to reducing the margins of error for a national approximation of numbers of injectors. To offer meaningful insight, future estimation models will also need to reflect important regional differences and be generated at regular intervals so as to account for variation over time.

A National Profile

NIDA's National AIDS Demonstration Research (NADR) programs provide the most comprehensive profile of active drug injectors not in drug abuse treatment in this country (Brown and Beschner, 1993). However, their description of the characteristics of injection drug users is based on a large sample of out-of-treatment injectors, so the information may be limited by a volunteer/selection bias. As noted earlier in this chapter, it is extremely difficult, if not impossible, to get a truly representative sample of injection drug users. The most feasible approach to generating sound inferences is to obtain information from multiple sampling schemes, which includes the efficiency of sampling entrants to drug treatment programs and entrants into the criminal justice system, as well as community-based recruitment schemes, as was done for NADR. Each scheme has limitations, but in combination they allow for sound inferences (Vlahov and Polk, 1988; Alcabes et al., 1991, 1992; Watters and Biernacki, 1989). In particular, surveys of entrants into treatment for drug abuse at multiple sites (Hahn et al., 1989; Prevots et al., 1995; Battjes et al., 1994) and prison-based surveys at multiple sites (Vlahov et al., 1991a) show similar patterns of geographic diversity of risk behaviors and HIV seroprevalence, which helps to validate estimates and inferences derived from the NADR database.

In the NADR study, a review of the sociodemographic characteristics of 13,475 active injection drug users from 28 sites across the country, the diversity of this population begins to emerge. Just over half (51 percent) of the injection drug users were African American, but a cross-site comparison indicated a range from 9 to 95 percent African American. One-quarter were Hispanic (ranging from 0 to 81 percent by site), and 22 percent were white (ranging from 3 to 65 percent by site). The percentage of females was 26 percent and ranged from 12 to 37 percent by site. The percentage of high school graduates was 45 percent and ranged from 31 to 67 percent by site. The percentage unemployed was 55 percent and ranged from 29 to 75 percent. The percentage that had previously been in jail was 81 percent and ranged from 64 to 94 percent. The percentage that had previously been in substance abuse treatment was 59 percent and ranged from 29 to 75 percent). The primary drugs injected were heroin (28 percent), cocaine (21 percent), and the combination (speedball) of heroin with cocaine (35 percent); these proportions varied substantially among sites, with 6 to 57 percent injecting heroin alone, the same range injecting cocaine alone, and 6 to 75 percent injecting the combination of heroin with cocaine (all data from Brown and Beschner, 1993:529).

Further analysis of the NADR database offers additional insight into patterns of drug use and high-risk behaviors for the transmission of HIV among injection drug users. For 25,603 members of the sample, half reported injecting daily (p. 118). Daily injection among African Americans and Hispanics was similar at 45 and 46 percent, respectively, and highest among whites at 63 percent. The difference in frequency of daily injection by gender was negligible.

An examination of types of sharing behaviors that place injectors at risk of HIV infection was conducted on 17,891 injection drug users in the NADR database who had reported a history of needle sharing (pp. 124-125). The most frequently reported risk behaviors included sharing cookers for the preparation of injectable solutions and sharing the rinse water used to flush syringes following injection, 90 and 78 percent, respectively. Although both these practices are considered to be of lesser risk than the sharing of syringes, it is notable that neither practice would be directly addressed by syringe exchange, and bleach distribution would be of value only as a potential means to decontaminate shared cookers. The greater risk behavior of reusing needles was reported by 68 percent of the sample, and 41 percent had rented needles in the past.

With regard to types of needle-sharing partners among 18,918 members of the NADR sample (p. 122), 68 percent reported having shared with friends, 67 percent with "running partners," 52 percent with a spouse or partner, and 25 percent with strangers.

Although none of the NADR sites purport to have recruited a representative sample of injection drug users from the regions they covered, it is interesting to note that, by focusing on active injectors not in treatment, this program exclusively enrolled members of the hard-core drug-using population, which the major household and student surveys underrepresent. Nevertheless, the fact that the mean age of subjects in the 28-site NADR analysis ranged from ages 31 to 40 and the mean years of injection drug use ranged from 10 to 19 suggests that this database overrepresents the most long-standing and active subpopulation of hard-core injection drug users. As a consequence, it appears that NADR was more successful in recruiting well-established social networks of injection drug users than recent initiates or occasional users. Despite these limitations, the NADR study is important because it shows that a large proportion of injection drug users had no history of drug abuse treatment, despite mean duration of injection of 10 to 19 years. This suggests that there is a subgroup of injection drug users not being accessed into treatment. However, a substantial proportion of these high-risk injection drug users do have a repeated history of treatment, suggesting that treatment as an HIV prevention activity may need to be supplemented (Siegal, 1995).

Additional studies suggest that there may be a secular trend toward reductions in high-risk injection practices. Several studies have reported decreases in risk over time (Battjes et al., 1992; Selwyn et al., 1987; Celentano et al., 1991). For example, Vlahov et al. (1991c) studied an out-of-treatment sample of injection drug users in Baltimore. They focused on behaviors during the 3 months following injection incidence, examining time trends from 1982 through 1987 among successive cohorts of injection drug users classified according to the year in which they first injected. They found significant increases over time in the proportion who sometimes used sterile needles, a decrease in the proportion always using equipment that had previously been used by others, and a decrease in the number of needle-sharing partners. Another relevant finding was a dramatic shift in the first drug injected from heroin to cocaine between 1982 and 1987.

Local Drug Use Trends and Patterns

As succeeding chapters of this report will make clear, a critical aspect of drug use is that it is specific to regions and communities. Although its reports do not focus upon injection drug use alone, the proceedings of NIDA's Community Epidemiology Work Group (CEWG) further illustrate the diversity of injection drug-using patterns across the country and the extent to which these patterns change over time. The CEWG is a drug abuse surveillance network composed of researchers from 20 major U.S. metropolitan areas: Atlanta, Boston, Chicago, Dallas, Denver, Detroit, Honolulu, Los Angeles, Miami, Minneapolis, Newark, New Orleans, New York, Philadelphia, Phoenix, St. Louis, San Diego, San Francisco, Seattle, and

Washington, D.C. Its primary mission is to provide a semiannual community-level assessment of drug abuse, principally through the collection and
analysis of epidemiologic and ethnographic research data. It provides current descriptive and analytic information on the nature and patterns of drug
abuse, emerging trends, consequences of drug abuse, and characteristics of
vulnerable populations.

Every six months, the work group meets to share information on recent
trends. Sources of data include:

- reports from researchers, often ethnographic, in major metropolitan
  areas about local situations,
- DAWN data on drug-related deaths, as reported by medical examin-
  ers,
- DAWN emergency room reports of drug-related medical emergen-
  cies, treatment admissions data where available,
- data from the Drug Enforcement Administration (DEA) Domestic
  Monitor Program drug intelligence reports on seizure, price, purity,
  prescription, distribution, and arrests,
- results of urinalysis data from the Drug Use Forecast program sponsored by the National Institute of Justice, and
- data on HIV and AIDS from the Centers for Disease Control and
  Prevention.

The various sources are examined by locality and semiannual reports dis-
cussing the trends are produced.

The CEWG's greatest strength is its ability to monitor drug-use trends
and document regionally specific patterns of drug use. Helping to improve
our understanding of injection drug use, its reports include the history of
the shift from heroin alone as a primary drug of injection in the late 1970s
to the integration of cocaine during the 1980s, both as an independent drug
of injection and as used in combination with heroin. Also reported was the
emergence and eventual decline some 10 years ago of a midwestern epidemic of pentazocine and tripelennamine (Ts and blues) injection. Whereas
the injection of stimulant drugs other than cocaine has remained a relatively
isolated phenomenon across much of the country, a series of CEWG publications reveals that amphetamine injection has been a major problem in San
Diego, and the injection of stimulants in Chicago is much less common and
typified by injection of the pharmaceutical drugs phenmetrazine among whites
on the north side of the city and methylphenidate among African Americans
on the city's south side. Thus, although not directly involved in the calcu-
lation of drug-use prevalence estimates, it can be seen that the CEWG is an
invaluable resource in tracking the nature and scope of substance abuse
across major metropolitan areas.

Given our lack of ability to definitively describe the extant population of injection drug users, it should be clear that any attempts to project into the future are highly speculative. Yet drawing some sense of factors that may influence the size of the injection drug user population in the coming years seems warranted. In referring to CEWG, trend analysis would seem to hold some promise as a basis of forecasting; however, many of the secondary indicator databases relating to substance abuse do not currently report on route of drug administration. As a consequence, CEWG does not currently monitor trends in injection drug use as an independent focus of analysis. Recent proceedings nevertheless include discussion of at least two trends, previously noted by Frank and Williams (1994), that may significantly influence future injection drug user prevalence. The first is AIDS-related mortality, which has already begun to deplete the numbers in this population. The second, and potentially countervailing trend, is a resurgence in the prevalence of heroin use, which has been associated with an increasing number of initiates who are using the drug intranasally.

The proceedings of the CEWG meeting in December 1993 show the trend of increasing intranasal heroin use to be most pronounced in Newark, Chicago, and New York City (National Institute on Drug Abuse, 1994a). Newark reported 66 percent of heroin admissions to be snorters (French and Mammo, 1994). In Chicago, intranasal consumption accounted for 60 percent of treatment admissions for heroin dependence (Wiebel et al., 1994), and in New York City, 51 percent of heroin admissions reported a primary intranasal route of drug administration (Frank and Galea, 1994). DEA's Domestic Monitor Program (Drug Enforcement Administration, 1994), which analyzes the price and purity of heroin in major metropolitan areas, has documented substantial increases in the purity of heroin sold on the streets over the past half decade. Some have noted a direct association between the availability of higher-quality heroin and its intranasal consumption (Ouellet et al., 1993; Des Jarlais et al., 1994; Friedman et al., 1994; Frank and Williams, 1994); however, it is not yet clear whether this regionally emergent epidemic will spread across the entire country. It is also uncertain as to the proportion of current intranasal heroin users who are or will become physically dependent, or the numbers likely to ultimately progress to injecting the drug. Ouellet et al. (1993) in Chicago noted that current younger snorters of heroin do not see themselves as being at any risk for progressing to injection, unlike older injectors, who consider intranasal heroin use as merely a transitional phase leading up to injection. As cautioned by Friedman et al. (1994) in a commissioned paper for this panel on the etiology of drug injection, "Heroin snorters represent a real but unknown risk for progressing to injection drug use."

SUMMARY

As some have suggested (Anglin et al., 1993), accurate estimates of injection drug use may be less important to policy makers than a constellation of data that helps to assess need and allocate limited resources. If this is the case, then more systematic efforts need to be directed toward monitoring patterns and trends in injection drug use, including improvements in recording the route of administration in secondary drug abuse indicator reporting systems. NIDA's Community Epidemiology Work Group provides one mechanism that may prove useful, particularly if expanded to incorporate more specific data on route of administration in its monitoring purview. This would provide policy planners with periodic updates as to whether the pool of injector drug users is likely to increase or decrease and whether there are any substantial shifts in the composition of the pool, including the emergence of injection as a route of drug administration among any previously unafflicted subpopulations.

Recommendation

The panel recommends that:

• The Assistant Secretary for Health should charge appropriate agencies (i.e., the National Institutes of Health and the Centers for Disease Control and Prevention), in consultation with academic departments of epidemiology, to develop more effective surveillance of drug use, particularly for local areas. The data collected should move beyond gross prevalence estimation of drug use and toward detailed information about users. This should include data on behavioral dynamics (e.g., pattern of drug use, sharing of drugs and drug paraphernalia, social context of drug use) by drugs of choice, routes of administration for each, and the flow of injection drug users into and out of drug treatment programs.

NOTES

1. The logic is that there are relatively fewer injection drug users in less populated rural areas. Note also that population centers that may sometimes be thought of as rather small are included within MSAs of more than 500,000 inhabitants. For example, the city of Ann Arbor, Michigan, with a population of about 110,000 is included because it is located within a metropolitan area that includes over 500,000 persons; similarly, Tacoma, Washington, Bridgeport, Connecticut, and Nashua, New Hampshire, are all represented within these 96 MSAs.

2. These data were made available to the panel by Joseph Gfroerer, who performed special analyses of the NHSDA.

3. Note that the DC*MADS survey did not cover the same geographical area as covered by Holmberg's review, which precludes a direct comparison between the two estimated numbers of injection drug users.

REFERENCES

Alcabes, P., G. Friedland, D. Vlahov, and A. Muñoz
1991   Estimation of Seroconversion Dates for Two Seroprevalent Cohorts of Intravenous Drug Users in the United States. VII International Conference on AIDS, Florence, Italy, June 16-21.
Alcabes, P., D. Vlahov, and J.C. Anthony
1992   Characteristics of intravenous drug users by history of arrest and treatment of drug abuse. *Journal of Nervous Mental Disorders* 180:48-54.
Anglin, M.D., J.P. Caulkins, and Y. Hser
1993   Prevalence estimation: Policy needs, current status, and future potential. *Journal of Drug Issues* 23(2):345-360.
Battjes, R.J., C.G. Leukefeld, and R.W. Pickens
1992   Age at first injection and HIV risk among intravenous drug users. *American Journal of Drug and Alcohol Abuse* 18:263-273.
Battjes, R.J., R.W. Pickens, H.W. Haverkes, and Z. Sloboda
1994   HIV risk factors among injecting drug users in five U.S. cities. *AIDS* 8:681-687.
Brown, B.S., and G.M. Beschner, eds.
1993   *Handbook on Risk of AIDS: Injection Drug Users and Sexual Partners.* Westport, CT: Greenwood Press.
Celentano, D.D., D. Vlahov, S. Cohn, J.C. Anthony, L. Solomon, and K.E. Nelson
1991   Risk factors for shooting gallery use and cessation among intravenous drug users. *American Journal of Public Health* 81(10):1291-1295.
Centers for Disease Control and Prevention
1987a   Human immunodeficiency virus infection in the United States: A review of current knowledge. *Morbidity and Mortality Weekly Report* 36(Suppl. S-6):1-48.
1987b   Human Immunodeficiency Virus Infections in the United States: A Review of Current Knowledge and Plans for Expansion of HIV Surveillance Activities. Report to the Domestic Policy Council. November 30. Atlanta, GA: Centers for Disease Control.
1990   HIV prevalence estimates and AIDS case projections for the United States: Report based on a workshop. *Morbidity and Mortality Weekly Report* 39(RR-16):273-276.
1992   Chronic Disease and Health Promotion MMWR Reprints: 1990-1991 Youth Risk Behavior Surveillance System. Selected behaviors that increase risk for HIV infection among high school students - United States, 1990. *Morbidity and Mortality Weekly Report* 41:231,237-240.
Des Jarlais, D.C., S.R. Friedman, J.L. Sotheran, J. Wenston, M. Marmor, S.R. Yancovitz, B. Frank, S. Beatrice, and D. Mildvan
1994   Continuity and change within an HIV epidemic: Injecting drug users in New York City, 1984 through 1992. *Journal of the American Medical Association* 271:121-127.
Drug Enforcement Administration
1994   *Domestic Monitor Program, October-December 1993.* DEA-94058. Washington DC: U.S. Department of Justice.

Frank, B., and J. Galea
1994   Current Drug Use Trends in New York City. Pp. 159-175 in *Epidemiologic Trends in Drug Abuse, December 1993*. NIH Publication No. 94-3746(II). Rockville, MD: National Institute on Drug Abuse.

Frank, B., and N. Williams
1994   Epidemiologic Trends in Injection Drug Use in New York City. Commissioned Paper for the National Research Council.

French, J., and A. Mammo
1994   Drug Abuse in Newark and New Jersey: An Overview. Pp. 134-148 in *Epidemiologic Trends in Drug Abuse, December 1993*. NIH Publication No. 94-3746(II). Rockville, MD: National Institute on Drug Abuse.

Friedman, S.R., D.C. Doherty, D. Paone, and B. Jose
1994   Notes on Research on the Etiology of Drug Injection. Commissioned Paper for the National Research Council.

Gawin, F.H., and H.D. Kleber
1985   Cocaine use in a treatment population: Patterns and diagnostic distinctions. Pp. 182-192 in *Cocaine Use in America: Epidemiologic and Clinical Perspectives*, N.J. Kozel and E.H. Adams, eds. NIDA Research Monograph 61. Washington, DC: National Institute on Drug Abuse.

Guydish, J.R., A. Abramowitz, W. Woods, M. Black, and J.L. Sorensen
1990   Changes in needle sharing behavior among intravenous drug users: San Francisco, 1986-88. *American Journal of Public Health* 80(8):995-997.

Hahn, R.A., I.M. Onorato, S. Jones, and J. Dougherty
1989   Prevalence of HIV infection among intravenous drug users in the United States. *Journal of the American Medical Association* 261(18):2677-2684.

Holmberg, S.D.
1993   Emerging epidemiological patterns in the USA. Presented at the Sixth Annual Meeting of the National Cooperative Vaccine Development Group for AIDS, Alexandria, Virginia, October 30-November 4.

Holmberg, S.D.
1994   Panel on Injection Drug Users and the HIV Epidemic: Understanding the Regional Differences in Prevalence, Incidence, and Risk Factors for Transmission. Public Health and Diversity: Opportunities for Equity, American Public Health Association's 122nd Annual Meeting and Exhibition, Washington, DC, November 2.

Hser, Y.I., and M.D. Anglin, eds.
1993   Prevalence estimation techniques for drug-using populations. *Journal of Drug Issues* 23(2):163-360.

Kleinman, P.H., D.S. Goldsmith, S.R. Friedman, W. Hopkins, and D.C. Des Jarlais
1990   Knowledge about and behaviors affecting the spread of AIDS: A street survey of intravenous drug users and their associates in New York City. *International Journal of Addictions* 25(4):345-361.

National Institute on Drug Abuse
(1976- *Proceedings of the Community Epidemiology Work Group*. Rockville, MD.
1994)
1993   *Prevalence of Drug Use in the Washington DC Metropolitan Area Homeless and Transient Population, 1991. Technical Report #2*. Rockville, MD: National Institute on Drug Abuse.
1994a   *Epidemiologic Trends in Drug Abuse: Community Epidemiology Work Group, December 1993* (NIH Publication No. 94-3746). Rockville, MD: National Institute on Drug Abuse.

1994b   *The Washington, DC, Metropolitan Area Drug Study: Prevalence of Drug Use in the DC Metropolitan Area Household and Nonhousehold Populations: 1991* (Technical Report #8). Rockville, MD: National Institute on Drug Abuse.

1994c   *Current Treatment Client Characteristics in the Washington DC Metropolitan Area, 1991. Technical Report #5.* Rockville, MD: National Institute on Drug Abuse.

Office of Technology Assessment

1990   *The Effectiveness of Drug Abuse Treatment: Implications for Controlling AIDS/HIV Infection.* (Report Number 052-003-0120-3). Washington, DC: U.S. Government Printing Office.

O'Malley, P.M.

         Unpublished data from the Monitoring the Future Project, Institute for Social Research, University of Michigan.

Ouellet, L., A.D. Jimenez, and W.W. Wiebel

1993   Heroin Again: New Users of Heroin in Chicago. Society for the Study of Social Problems, Miami Beach, August 11-13.

Prevots, D.R., D.M. Allen, J.S. Lehman, T.A. Green, L.R. Petersen, and M. Gwinn

1995   Trends in Seroprevalence Among Injection Drug Users Entering Drug Treatment Centers, United States, 1988-1993. Paper presented at the Second National Conference on Human Retroviruses and Related Infections, American Society for Microbiology, Washington, D.C.

Schuster, C.R.

1988   Intravenous drug use and AIDS prevention. *Public Health Reports* 103(3):281-286.

Selwyn, P.A., C. Feiner, C.P. Cox, C. Lipshutz, and R.L. Cohen

1987   Knowledge about AIDS and high-risk behavior among intravenous drug users in New York City. *AIDS* 1(4):247-254.

Siegal, H.A., R.G. Carlson, R.S. Falck, and J. Wang

1995   Drug abuse treatment experience and HIV risk behaviors among active drug injectors in Ohio. *American Journal of Public Health* 85(1):105-108.

Spencer, B.D.

1989   On the accuracy of current estimates of the numbers of intravenous drug users. Pp. 429-446 in *AIDS: Sexual Behavior and Intravenous Drug Use*, C.F. Turner, H.G. Miller, and L.E. Moses, eds. Washington DC: National Academy Press.

Turner, C.F., H.G. Miller, and L.E. Moses, eds.

1989   *AIDS: Sexual Behavior and Intravenous Drug Use.* Washington, DC: National Academy Press.

U.S. General Accounting Office

1993   *Drug Use Measurement: Strengths, Limitations, and Recommendations for Improvement* (Report prepared for the Chairman, Committee on Government Operations, U.S. House of Representatives, GAO/PEMD-93-18). Washington, DC: U.S. General Accounting Office.

Vlahov, D., and B.F. Polk

1988   Intravenous drug users and human immunodeficiency virus infection in prison. *AIDS Public Policy Journal* 3:42-46.

Vlahov, D., T.F. Brewer, K.G. Castro, J.P. Narkunas, M.E. Salive, J. Ullrich, and A. Muñoz

1991a   Prevalence of antibody to HIV-1 among entrants to U.S. correctional facilities. *Journal of the American Medical Association* 265:1129-1132.

Vlahov, D., J.C. Anthony, D. Celentano, L. Solomon, and N. Chowdhury

1991b   Trends of HIV-1 risk reduction among initiates into intravenous drug use 1982-1987. *American Journal of Drug and Alcohol Abuse* 17:39-48.

Vlahov, D., A. Muñoz, D.D. Celentano, S. Cohn, J.C. Anthony, H. Chilcoat, and K.E. Nelson
   1991c   HIV seroconversion and disinfection of injection equipment among intravenous drug users, Baltimore, Maryland. *Epidemiology* 2:442-444.
Watters, J.K., and P. Biernacki
   1989   Targeted sampling: Options for the study of hidden populations. *Social Problems* 36:416-430.
Wiebel, W., A. Rahimian, A. Pach, and M. O'Brien
   1994   Nature and scope of substance abuse in Chicago. Pp. 27-45 in *Epidemiologic Trends in Drug Abuse, December 1993* (NIH Publication No. 94-3746[II]). Rockville, MD: National Institute on Drug Abuse.
Wiley, J.A., and M.C. Samuel
   1989   The prevalence of HIV infection in the United States. *AIDS* 3:71-78.

3

Needle Exchange and Bleach Distribution Programs in the United States

INTRODUCTION

In an effort to curb the rate of HIV infection among injection drug users in the United States, needle exchange programs have been instituted in 20 states. In September 1993, a total of 33 active needle exchange programs were reported by the University of California/Centers for Disease Control and Prevention (Lurie et al., 1993a) to be operating in the United States. Since that time, new programs have opened in Baltimore, Boston, Milwaukee, and Dallas, and legislation has been passed to establish needle exchange programs in Minnesota and Rhode Island. A survey conducted in October 1994 reported 76 needle exchange programs in 55 U.S. cities (North American Syringe Exchange Network, 1994).

To date, no systematic survey of bleach distribution programs in the United States has been reported. However, information about bleach distribution is described in a report by the National Institute on Drug Abuse (NIDA), which covers 41 projects in 50 cities nationwide (National Institute on Drug Abuse, 1994).

The purpose of this chapter is to describe the needle exchange and bleach distribution programs that are currently active in the United States, their operational characteristics, and the on-site services offered. In addition, whenever available, the demographic characteristics of program participants are described.

Although information about individual programs is accessible, comparative studies across programs are sparse. It also is clear from the data on individual programs that some recruit small and others large numbers of participants. If prevention programs are to be effective, it seems reasonable to suggest that they need to be able to recruit large numbers of individuals at risk. Another purpose of this chapter is therefore to summarize case studies of selected programs to examine organizational characteristics that might affect their recruitment of participants. The chapter includes a brief discussion of the cost associated with operating a needle exchange program and cost-effectiveness estimates from the literature.

The material presented in this chapter contributes to the panel's overall assessment of the effectiveness of needle exchange and bleach distribution programs, and its findings and conclusions are integrated in the recommendations that appear in Chapter 7. As stated in the Introduction, this approach reflects the development of the panel's deliberations on the issues.

NEEDLE EXCHANGE PROGRAMS

Needle exchange programs either distribute sterile needles or exchange used needles for new ones. (The first programs were initiated by activists and advocacy groups in violation of prescription drug laws and drug paraphernalia laws.) Most also offer a variety of other services and/or referrals, including HIV screening and counseling, screening for tuberculosis and sexually transmitted diseases, substance abuse counseling, primary medical care, case management, health education, and condom and bleach distribution.

The primary sources for the information that follows are a report prepared by the School of Public Health, University of California, Berkeley, and the Institute for Health Policy Studies, University of California, San Francisco (Lurie et al., 1993a, 1993b), and reports on the Washington, D.C., and Baltimore needle exchange programs, which opened subsequent to the University of California report.

Legal Issues

The status of needle exchange programs according to existing laws primarily determines their characteristics. The most important laws affecting needle exchange programs are drug paraphernalia and prescription drug laws. A total of 45 states and the District of Columbia (Valleroy et al., in press) have paraphernalia laws that prohibit the possession of needles and syringes for the purpose of using illicit drugs (Figure 3.1). Of the states operating needle exchange programs, Alaska is the only one not restricted by such a law.

Nine states and the District of Columbia (Valleroy et al., in press) have

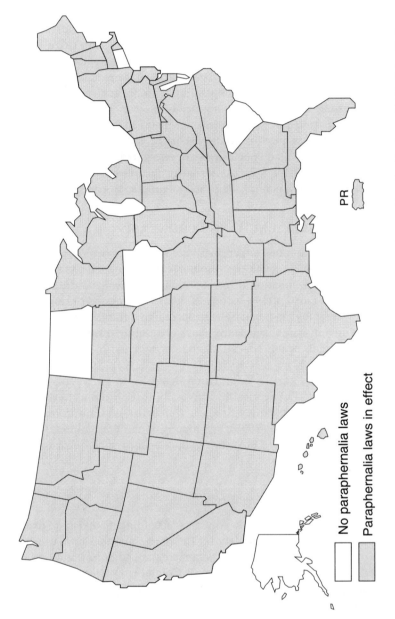

FIGURE 3.1 States that prohibit nonmedical needle and syringe possession and/or distribution. SOURCE: Update on Upcoming Research Activities Pertaining to Needle Exchange and Bleach Distribution (Jones, 1994).

laws requiring a prescription to purchase needles and syringes (Figure 3.2). Four of these states—California, Illinois, Massachusetts, and New York—have needle exchange programs. In this report, a needle exchange program is defined as legally authorized when it has been specifically authorized by statute, regulation, or case law in the state.

Other laws affecting the operation of needle exchange programs involve drug-free zones and prostitution-free zones. These are city ordinances that prohibit persons convicted of a drug-related crime or prostitution from entering certain areas during certain times of the day. They tend to be areas with high drug trafficking, which are precisely the areas that needle exchange programs target in order to reach the most people. The ordinances impede injection drug users from obtaining sterile injection equipment from needle exchange programs operating in these areas and limit the operating capabilities of the programs (see Chapter 5 for an in-depth discussion of legal issues).

The administrative structures and funding sources of the programs are closely related to whether they are legally authorized. The programs that are not legally authorized tend to be operated by activists and funded by private donations and, occasionally, by foundation grants; however, this is not universal. Although legally authorized needle exchange programs are more likely than those not legally authorized to receive local or state government funding, not all of them do. Activists continue to administer many of the currently operating programs. The remainder are administered by either government agencies or community-based organizations, some with and some without local or state government involvement.

Program Operations

Sites

As described by Lurie et al. (1993a), needle exchange sites can be broadly classified into two categories: *fixed* and *mobile*. Fixed sites operate at a consistent and predictable location at the same time each week. Mobile sites include deliveries and persons roving either on foot or in a vehicle. Roving sites usually cover a specific geographic area and often follow a consistent route, but they do not stay at any one location for very long. Fixed sites have the advantage of being relatively predictable, whereas mobile sites can cover a greater geographic area and can more readily accommodate changes in local conditions.

In their systematic survey, Lurie et al. (1993a) identified seven types of exchange sites: four types of fixed sites (stationary van, storefront, street, and health facility) and three types of mobile sites (walk route, deliveries, and roving van).

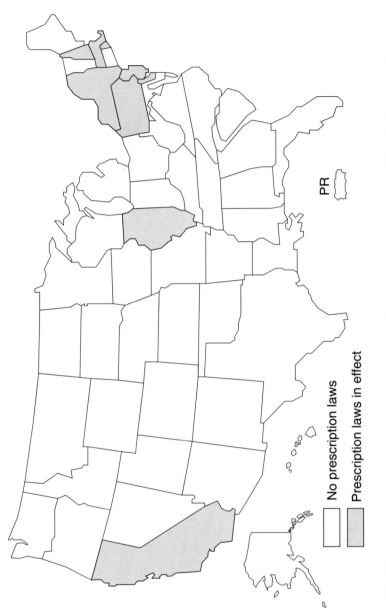

FIGURE 3.2 States that require a prescription for needle and syringe purchase. SOURCE: Update on Upcoming Research Activities Pertaining to Needle Exchange and Bleach Distribution (Jones, 1994).

A *stationary van* site consists of a van parked at a predictable location at a predictable time. One van may visit multiple fixed sites in a single outing. A van exchange is a way for needle exchange programs to provide the benefits of both a fixed and a mobile site. It can provide shelter for staff, some privacy for clients, and consistent service while covering a large geographic area.

A *storefront* program provides shelter for participants and staff. It can also provide privacy for injection drug users, especially if the storefront houses other programs and services not directly related to injection drug use. Storefront sites can also house telephones, facsimile machines, computers, desks, and chairs, which can make it easier for needle exchange program staff to provide services to injection drug users and facilitate referrals to other services. Storefront needle exchange programs may involve significant rental costs.

A *street* site is located on a sidewalk with either a card table to hold the items to be distributed or persons holding bags containing the items. Participants can blend in with the foot traffic as they approach the table to pick up condoms, peruse the available literature, or ask a question about AIDS. Injection drug users are not the only persons to approach the needle exchange program table and thus their privacy can be protected.

Housing a needle exchange program in a *health facility* can also provide shelter and privacy. Such sites also facilitate referral of injection drug users to other services, especially if these services are also provided within the health facility. However, health facilities can present geographic and psychological barriers to injection drug users. The needle exchange program may be located in a public health building in an area of low injection drug use activity. Many injection drug users may not feel comfortable entering institutional buildings, particularly ones in close proximity to other government buildings (e.g., police headquarters).

Needle exchange program services provided on *walk routes* generally target areas known to have high concentrations of injection drug users. A roving site of this sort generally follows a relatively consistent route, although it can change in response to immediate neighborhood conditions (e.g., increased police presence) or to incorporate additional populations of injection drug users.

Deliveries bring needle exchange program services directly to injection drug users. In many ways, deliveries are the most private type of site, in that they meet the injection drug user at a location of his or her choice. However, deliveries require access to transportation, are labor intensive, and may present many logistical challenges.

Roving vans allow a needle exchange program to cover a greater geographic area. A roving site keeps staff members relatively inconspicuous to neighbors, local businesspeople, and police officers.

In summary, needle exchange programs are operated from a variety of locations, some mobile, some fixed, and some with both fixed and mobile sites. Sites range from health department pharmacies to mobile vans to tables set up on city sidewalks.

Staffing

The plurality of the programs are staffed by a combination of paid employees and volunteers. As with funding, the staffing mix is related to whether exchanges are legally authorized and the administering body of the programs. Programs administered by activists are typically staffed by volunteers. Only legally authorized programs that are administered by either local or state government agencies or community-based organizations are predominantly operated by paid staff.

Policies

According to Lurie et al. (1993a), needle exchange policies restrict the exchange of syringes, or limit eligibility to use the needle exchange programs, or both. These policies alleviate potential staff-participant conflicts by clearly delineating procedural rules that must be followed. In general, the policies seek to establish an optimal balance among the following criteria: remaining convenient to the participant, maintaining frequent contact with the participant, and alleviating community concerns over the potential of needle exchange programs to facilitate drug use or increase the numbers of needles discarded in public places.

At a *one-for-one exchange*, a new syringe is given out for each used syringe turned in. A needle exchange program that adheres to a strict one-for-one exchange rule cannot increase the total number of discarded syringes if it provides no *starter needles*. Starter needles are those distributed to participants at their first visits, even if they do not have any needles to exchange. This rule removes a potential barrier to entering a needle exchange program. The Lurie et al. (1993a) report classified needle exchange programs that give out starter needles but thereafter have a strict one-for-one exchange rule as having both rules.

An *exchange maximum* is a limit placed on the number of needles that can be exchanged per visit or per unit time. Some needle exchange programs impose an exchange maximum solely because of limited supplies. An argument sometimes offered in favor of an exchange maximum is that it brings participants back to the needle exchange program more frequently, thus increasing staff-participant contact and providing more opportunities to refer injection drug users to drug treatment and other public health services. However, an exchange maximum might lead to an increase in the reuse of dirty syringes and may be inconvenient for injection drug users who have to travel long distances to use the needle exchange program.

A *minimum age requirement* for exchanging is generally imposed in response to the concern that the needle exchange program may encourage young people to start injecting illicit drugs. A countervailing concern is that young injection drug users may have difficulties gaining access to sterile needles.

Requiring a participant to show needle "track" marks (visibly scarred veins due to repeated injection) in order to use the needle exchange program is intended to limit clientele to active users. This rule is, in part, a response to the concern that needle exchange programs may encourage noninjection drug users to start injecting drugs, but it can also be used to prevent noninjection drug users from selling syringes for a profit. However, some programs note that participants who do not have tracks may be neither new injectors nor profiteers, but may instead be surrogates exchanging syringes for friends or family members. Some programs actively encourage surrogate exchangers, believing that they act as important sources of sterile needles and, perhaps, of education for otherwise hidden injection drug user populations.

Hours of Operation

Of the surveyed programs (Lurie et al., 1993a), the number of operating hours per week, not including deliveries, typically ranged from 8 to 168, with a median of 10. Hours of operation was also found to be related to whether programs are legally authorized: legally authorized exchanges are open more hours per week.

On-Site Services Offered

The range of services offered by needle exchange programs includes

- education,
- HIV testing and counseling,
- tuberculosis screening,
- screening for sexually transmitted diseases,
- primary medical care,
- substance abuse treatment, and
- case management.

Services to educate and inform injection drug users regarding injection practices, safety steps, nonsharing behavior, and other risk reduction methods are an important part of a needle exchange program. The ability and capacity to provide such a service are somewhat dependent on site of operation (roving van versus a storefront, for example) and types and number of staff. A critical component of education involves sexual behaviors and practices and the use of condoms. The majority of the programs surveyed by Lurie et al. (1993a) reported that they distribute educational materials most often in the form of health pamphlets. The need for and value of targeted education and behavior modification efforts directed at injection drug users at risk of HIV transmission have been clearly demonstrated in programs that do not include needle exchange (Wiebel et al., 1993).

Additional services include HIV testing and counseling, tuberculosis screening, screening and treatment of sexually transmitted diseases, primary medical care and case management, drug treatment, assertiveness training focused on negotiation skills, and other health and social services. The ability to provide these additional services on site is related to space and available personnel, which are in turn related to funding and whether programs are legally authorized. At the time of the Lurie et al. (1993a) report, the only two programs to offer all of these above services were The Works (Boulder, Colorado) and the Tacoma-Pierce County Health Department (Tacoma, Washington). Both of these programs are legally authorized, are government administered and funded, have paid staff, and are open more than 10 hours per week.

For the most part, the needle exchange programs that offer primary medical care and/or substance abuse treatment have paid staff. HIV testing and counseling, however, are provided by both paid and volunteer employees.

Although a minority of programs have the capacity to provide all of the services mentioned above, the majority do refer participants to services. For instance, of all U.S. programs surveyed by Lurie et al. (1993a, 1993b), all but one program provided referrals to drug abuse treatment.

Items Distributed

In addition to sterile needles, the programs distribute other paraphernalia and supplies. These typically include cotton, sterile cookers, sterile water bottles, and alcohol wipes. With a few exceptions, all programs also distribute bleach, condoms, and health pamphlets. Because of concerns about the efficacy of bleach in inactivating HIV in injection equipment, some of the providers are reluctant to provide it (see Chapter 6).

Characteristics of Program Participants

The variation in the demographic characteristics of needle exchange program participants is one of the most notable features of the programs overall. Data from published accounts of data collection efforts at 10 U.S. programs are presented in Table 3.1. The data are notable in several respects.

Needle exchange programs attract males predominantly: the proportion of participants who are female ranges from 15 to 34 percent. However, as noted in Chapters 1 and 2, female injection drug users in general tend to show higher HIV seroincidence than their male counterparts, suggesting that the programs may not be targeting high-risk women. The sex profile of needle exchange programs is similar to that of drug abuse treatment programs and other populations used to sample injection drug users.

Needle exchange programs vary considerably in their racial/ethnic distributions. As Table 3.1 shows, the proportion of program participants who are African American ranges from 8 to 100 percent; Asian participants range from 0 to 12 percent; Hispanic participants range from 0 to 53 percent; white participants range from 0 to 70 percent; and others (primarily Native Americans) range from 0 to 28 percent. This variation across programs to some extent reflects regional differences.

The mean age at entry into needle exchange programs tends to be similar across programs, ranging from age 33 to 41.

The mean duration of injection drug use ranges from 7 to 20 years. Combined with the information available on age, these data suggest that needle exchange programs do not tend to attract recent initiates into injection drug use. A more recent report from San Francisco noted that less than 1 percent of needle exchange program participants were under age 18 (Watters et al., 1994). These data could be considered as indirect evidence that needle exchange does not encourage the initiation of injection drug use. However, considered in conjunction with the data presented in Chapter 2 on the prevalence of injection drug use by age, the overall data suggest that these programs may not be attracting the young injectors who, according to available estimates, represent a sizable portion of the injection drug user population. This is especially disconcerting in light of the findings reported in several studies that show that the risk of HIV infection is higher among younger and more recent initiates.

Before firm conclusions are drawn, it is important to note that the data presented here mostly reflect samples of program participants who agreed to be interviewed. The published descriptions of sampling procedures are incomplete, so the extent to which potential biases could have operated cannot be assessed.

When needle exchange participants were compared with nonparticipants, the participants were found to be more likely to be male and older, and less likely to be African American and to have been in drug treatment (Hagan et al., 1991; Joseph, 1989; Watters and Case, 1989).

TABLE 3.1 Demographic Characteristics of Needle Exchange Participants

City	Sample Size	Percent Female	Percent African American	Asian	Hispanic	White	Other	Mean Age (years)	Mean Years Intravenous Drug Use
Boulder, CO	118	15	10	NR	12	76	2	34	14
Chicago, IL	66	20	100	NR	NR	NR	NR	41	20
Honolulu, HI	126	20	12	12	8	41	28	35	NR
New Haven, CT	720	21	41	NR	34	25	<1	34	7
New York, NY	250	31	27	NR	53	18	2	33	NR
Portland, OR	700	14	8	1	3	79	9	34	NR
San Francisco, CA	50	34	18	8	10	58	6	NR	NR
Seattle, WA	62	18	55	NR	15	27	3	NR	NR
Tacoma, WA	265	23	25	NR	6	61	8	38	16
Washington, DC	30	20	83	NR	NR	17	0	38	18

NOTE: NR = not reported.

Original Data Sources:

The Chicago Recovery Alliance
1992   Individuals Concerned with Addiction, Recovery, and HIV Disease. *Risk Reduction Outreach with Syringe Exchange: Guidelines and Operating Procedures.* June 24.

Clark, G., D. Garcia, J. Guydish, and P. Case
1991   Street-Based Survey of Needle Exchange Clients. Abstract WC 3295 in *Final Program and Abstracts of the VII International Conference on AIDS,* Florence, Italy.

Demographics Among 700 Drug Injectors. Unpublished material.

Department of Health, State of Hawaii
1992   *Needle Exchange Evaluation Report.* January 1.

Guilfoile, A., D. Lenaway, and V. Harris
1991   Boulder County Health Department Needle Exchange Program. Unpublished material. October 15.

Hagan, H., D.C. Des Jarlais, S.R. Friedman, D. Purchase, and T.R. Reid
1992   Multiple Outcome Measures of the Impact of the Tacoma Syringe Exchange. Abstract 4283 in *Final Program and Abstracts of the VIII International Conference on AIDS,* Amsterdam, Netherlands.

Harris, N.V., M.J. Fields, D.C. Gordon, et al.
1991   HIV and Related Risk Behaviors Among Inmates and Needle Exchange and Drug Treatment Clients. Abstract WC 3362 in *Final Program and Abstracts of the VII International Conference on AIDS,* Florence, Italy.

Joseph, S.C.
1989   A bridge to treatment: The needle exchange pilot program in New York City. *AIDS Education and Prevention* 1:340-345.

O'Keefe, E., E. Kaplan, and K. Khoshnood
1991   City of New Haven. *Preliminary Report: City of New Haven Needle Exchange Program.* July 31.

Oliver, K., S.R. Friedman, H. Maynard, and D.C. Des Jarlais
1991   Behavioral Impact of the Portland Syringe Exchange Program: Some Preliminary Results. Presentation in *Third National AIDS Demonstration Research Conference.*

SOURCE: Adapted from *The Public Health Impact of Needle Exchange Programs in the United States and Abroad, Volume 1* (Lurie et al., 1993a:274).

Cost and Cost-Effectiveness

The cost of operating a needle exchange program was estimated in the University of California/Centers for Disease Control and Prevention report (Lurie et al., 1993a). Briefly, their report noted wide variation in annual cost across the 18 programs sampled, ranging from $18,628 in the Tacoma Pharmacy Exchange to $393,951 in the Lower East Side, New York City, Exchange. The median annual cost of operating a needle exchange was $168,650. The budgets reflect actual plus donated resources for personnel, consultants, equipment, supplies, transportation, travel, and space rental. The proportion of the budget specifically allocated to syringes ranged from 2 percent in Boston and New Haven to 47 percent in the Tacoma Pharmacy Exchange (median = 7 percent), with the proportion per program reflecting the volume of needles exchanged. The largest proportion of the budget was for personnel, ranging from 27 percent in Berkeley's NEED exchange to 79 to 80 percent in the Boulder, New Haven, and Portland exchange programs (median = 66 percent).

In an attempt to measure the productivity of needle exchange programs, the University of California team of investigators used the annual budget, the number of participant contacts, the number of syringes distributed, and the hours of operation for each program to calculate the cost per participant contact, the cost per syringe distributed, and the cost per hour open. The median cost per participant contact across the seven programs with available data was $17; the median cost per syringe distributed was $1.35; and the median cost per hour of program operation was $145. The median number of syringes distributed per hour was 205.

The variability across sites was attributed to differences in exchange rates of needles: higher costs per needle, contact, and hours of operation were related to activities that do not contribute directly to needle exchange. For example, Boston's ACT-UP project spent considerable time attempting to engage a scattered clientele under continual police scrutiny and had exchanged 9 syringes per hour, considerably below the median of 205.

In an attempt to measure the cost-effectiveness of programs, the University of California research team estimated absolute impact (number of HIV infections averted) and associated cost-effectiveness (program cost divided by number of HIV infections averted) on the basis of three different models. The three models included a simplified circulation model formula (Kaplan, 1993), a behavior change model (Kahn et al., 1992), and a combined circulation and behavior change model (Lurie et al., 1993a:496-499). The results summarized here are based on a hypothetical needle exchange program with specific characteristics (e.g., high volume of needle exchange, limited counseling and referrals to other services) and HIV risk determinants (e.g., high prevalence and incidence, drug and sexual risk behaviors).

Although the three models differ in many ways, the primary distinguishing factors are as follows. The simplified circulation model focuses on obtaining estimates of averted HIV infections among program participants, based on a 1-year time frame, attributable to transmission from sharing contaminated needles. The behavior change model estimates averted infections among all injection drug users in the community as well as their sexual partners and offspring over a 5-year time interval, attributable to transmissions from both sharing and sexual behavior. The combined circulation and behavior change model incorporates characteristics of both models.

As depicted in Table 3.2, all models estimated that the hypothetical needle exchange program had a substantial impact on averted HIV infections and reported significantly lower costs per HIV infection averted than the $119,000 estimated lifetime HIV medical costs associated with treating a person infected with HIV (Hellinger, 1993). One noticeable disparity is the substantially different estimates in the number of infections averted over 5 years reported by the behavior change model compared with the combined model. This disparity is due mainly to the fact, as with the circulation model, that the combined model limits its estimates to infections averted among program participants only (participants are assumed to share only with each other).

These are obviously crude estimates of the cost-effectiveness of needle exchange programs and are of limited value in assisting health policy mak-

TABLE 3.2 Comparison of Three Model Estimates of Needle Exchange Impact and Cost-Effectiveness

	Simplified Circulation Model	Behavior Change Model	Combined Model
Absolute HIV infection averted	50	46	53
Additional absolute HIV infection averted[a]	0	113	11
Cost per HIV infection averted[b]	$12,000	$3,773	$9,375

[a]Estimated drug-related (i.e., direct sharing) HIV infections averted in program participants during 1 year of program participation.

[b]Estimated drug-related and sexually related HIV infections averted among program clients, their drug and sexual partners, and their offspring over 5 years. That is, 1 year of program operation and 4 years of delayed effects (averted infections during the 1 year of program operation among program participants due to sharing are not included).

SOURCE: Adapted from *The Public Health Impact of Needle Exchange Programs in the United States and Abroad, Volume 1* (Lurie et al., 1993a:499).

ers set priorities for allocating resources across various health promotion and disease prevention programs. Nonetheless, these estimates demonstrate that multiple models lead to the conclusion that needle exchanges reduce the number of new HIV infections at a cost per infection averted far below the $119,000 lifetime cost of treating an HIV-infected person.

In order for cost-effectiveness analysis to be a useful tool in guiding the setting of priorities for the use of scarce financial resource allocations for AIDS prevention, certain critical information is needed:

- measures of program effectiveness on meaningful health outcome measures,
- estimates of costs, as well as discounting and variable cost rates, and
- a set of independent AIDS prevention programs from which to choose, each having an expected degree of effectiveness and an associated cost.

Once these elements are known, policy makers will be able to maximize program effectiveness by allocating financial resources to programs according to their respective cost-effectiveness ratio. Numerous uncertainties surround these elements, such as the parameter estimates that should be included in the models, the tenability of the underlying assumptions used to derive those estimates, the necessary level of precision, and whether collateral program effects should be included (e.g., on crime, sexually transmitted diseases, drug use). Although these issues must be carefully addressed in cost-effectiveness analyses of AIDS prevention programs, they are beyond the scope of this report. For a more detailed treatment of benefit-cost analysis of AIDS prevention programs, the interested reader is referred to a previous National Research Council report (Turner et al., 1989:471-499).

Moreover, Kaplan (1995, in press) in a recent paper provides various models for estimating the cost and benefits of HIV prevention programs and uses data from the New Haven needle exchange to illustrate how such models can assist policy makers in making resource allocation decisions. In particular, the proposed models do provide some guidance for addressing pragmatic issues, such as how a given needle exchange program, in a specific epidemiologic environment, can optimize its cost-effectiveness ratio (i.e., cost per infection averted), within a budget constraint. The author also depicts how these ratios are a function of critical program parameters (e.g., number of program participants, number of needles exchanged per participant, HIV incidence in population being served).

Organizational Characteristics

Although brief descriptions of needle exchange programs along selected dimensions are available, few studies thus far have examined the organizational characteristics of needle exchange programs themselves as potential determinants of the behavior of the injection drug users participating in the exchange. Since needle exchanges are service delivery organizations, it is reasonable to expect that the particular mode of organizing the services may in itself be a very important determinant of the HIV and AIDS risk behavior of the participants in the exchange.

In this section we review existing research on the organizational characteristics of needle exchange programs and outline possible directions for future research. Before reviewing the few available comparative studies of the organization of needle exchange programs, we briefly examine five case studies in which organizational issues were found to be critical to the effectiveness—or ineffectiveness—of needle exchange programs in reducing HIV risk behavior.

Three Simple Case Studies

Dundee-Wishart, Scotland Many of the earliest needle exchange programs implemented in the United Kingdom were operated by preexisting drug service agencies that, in some cases, were lacking both the resources and the appropriate training for this challenging new task. Perhaps the clearest example of these problems was in the experience of the needle exchange program that operated from the premises of the Wishart Drug Problems Centre in Dundee-Wishart, Scotland, in summer 1988 (Stimson et al., 1988). At that time, the Dundee-Wishart facility was not only understaffed in relation to an already full caseload, but also encumbered with an ill-suited and overly rigid set of rules for a fledgling needle exchange. In addition, it was being operated by the staff of an abstinence-oriented treatment program who clearly felt overwhelmed by the sudden influx of injection drug users seeking only to exchange used needles for new ones and who plainly did not desire abstinence treatment. Indeed, injection drug users in the area came to perceive the primary aim of the exchange as recruiting them into the treatment program. Hence, very few participated in the exchange, causing it to close within 6 weeks.

New York City The first legally authorized needle exchange program in New York City opened in 1988 as a single-site operation, although it had originally been designed and proposed as a pilot study that aimed to compare injection risk behavior and the rates of entry into treatment among injection drug users seen at four different sites (Anderson, 1991; Joseph and

Des Jarlais, 1989). Two of these planned locations were to offer needle exchange services, and two were not. Subjects were to be recruited from the waiting lists of drug treatment programs in order to better compare rates of actual entry into treatment and to place a prearranged limit on length of needle exchange participation (which was to end as soon as a treatment slot became available for the subject.)

When the scheduled opening of the needle exchange program was announced, however, the ensuing controversy led to a political compromise that no needle exchange would be located "within 1,000 feet of a school." This, however, precluded all four of the originally planned sites. Indeed, the only site that both (a) met the school distance criterion and (b) was under the control of the City Health Department was in the Health Department's own Lower Manhattan headquarters, which happened to be in an area that was not only inconvenient for injection drug users, but also conspicuously near police headquarters and the Manhattan criminal courts. Moreover, the registration procedures themselves lasted several hours and included tuberculosis screening, administration of a detailed questionnaire on risk behavior, and issuance of a photo ID card. A strict one-for-one exchange rule was in effect, whereby only one syringe at a time could be exchanged.

In a little over a year of operation, 317 injection drug users participated in the program. Many were placed into treatment programs quickly, and too few participated long enough to enable researchers to make pre- and post-program comparisons of risk behavior. Plans were being made to expand the exchange operations into areas more convenient to drug users but, at the end of 1989, a decision was made by a new mayor to close the exchange.

Washington, D.C. The Washington, D.C., program had many similarities to the first legally authorized New York City exchange program. First, the program design itself was actually the product of a delicate compromise with political opponents of needle exchange on the District of Columbia City Council. In addition, as in New York: (1) the program was obliged to operate out of a single site, a drug abuse treatment program, (2) participant eligibility was restricted to those already on a waiting list for drug abuse treatment, and (3) the cumbersome entry procedure required hours of participant and staff time (Vlahov et al., 1994). Also, as in Dundee-Wishart, some of the treatment program staff at the designated site were adamantly opposed to any distribution of needles in a treatment setting. Moreover, the Washington, D.C., needle exchange program was permitted to operate for only 60 days, during which time it was able to enroll a total of 31 injection drug users in the first month and 2 in the second month from the District's estimated 16,000 injection drug users. It was then closed, in keeping with the original agreement, while public health officials assessed the experience. The Vlahov et al. (1994) evaluation study also noted that the program was supplying both syringes and needles in a size incompatible with those used by injection drug users in the local community.

Discussion None of these three needle exchange programs would be considered user-friendly (a concept discussed below). Some of the unfriendliness in program operation stemmed from concessions to political opponents of needle exchange and some from research design requirements. Other aspects of the unfriendliness, such as tuberculosis screening, were required in a sincere belief that they were in the best interests of the participants. None of these three programs appears to have had any impact on HIV transmission in the local area, and it is not even likely that any of them had any meaningful impact on the HIV/AIDS risk behavior of the small numbers of people who participated.

Nonetheless, these three programs may provide valuable learning experiences for future exchanges. The New York City exchange in particular was the first to demonstrate that a needle exchange program could serve as a bridge to treatment (New York City Department of Health, 1989). The many similarities between the first legally authorized New York City needle exchange program (1988) and the Washington, D.C., program 4 years later (August 1992), however, raise the question of how the program planners can learn about important organizational issues from past experiences.

Two Complex Case Studies

The primary lesson to be drawn from the above three cases histories, of course, is that a needle exchange program needs to be user-friendly in order to attract participants and to have a public-health-level impact on HIV and AIDS risk behavior. This somewhat straightforward organizational lesson, however, does not illustrate any of the possible complexities involved in the organizational characteristics of a needle exchange program and its possible effectiveness. The following two case histories show some of the possible complexities.

Manchester In 1988, Klee conducted an interview study of HIV/AIDS risk behavior among injection drug users in Manchester, United Kingdom, and published results somewhat later (Klee et al., 1991). She found that some of the local injection drug users who had participated in the local needle exchange program had become known among the drug user community as sources of injection equipment. These injection drug users themselves were often socially pressured by other injection drug users to pass on injection equipment, and they actually did pass on their used injection equipment more frequently than did a comparison group of injection drug users who were not using the exchange. In the U.S. General Accounting Office (1993) review of needle exchange studies, this study was classified as showing an association between participation in a needle exchange program and increased sharing of drug injection equipment. (Indeed, this was the only study so classified.)

Klee, however, disputes this classification of her findings. She notes that the data from this study were collected at a time when local needle exchange programs were just being implemented and before they had engaged a large number of participants. Klee conducted a later study, after needle exchange programs in Manchester had reached a larger number of participants, in which she did not find that users of the exchange were more likely to pass on used injection equipment (Klee, personal communication, February 1994). Thus, the apparent relationship between participation in the program and the sharing of used injection equipment had changed from the early to the later period of the lengthy program implementation process.

Tagging Syringes in New York City Several underground needle exchanges operated in New York City between the time that the first legally authorized needle exchange program was closed in 1989 and the legal authorization of community-based organization (CBO) exchanges, which began in 1992. Three of the underground exchanges tagged the syringes they exchanged (Paone et al., 1994b); that is, marking pens or paint were used to draw a circle around the barrel of each syringe. The tagged syringes served both as a reminder to injection drug users to inject safely and as an advertisement for the needle exchanges. Rough counts of the tagged syringes that were returned also provided a means for estimating the percentages of syringes that were returned to the exchanges out of the total number of tagged syringes that had been distributed. (The exchanges also accepted syringes that drug injectors had acquired by other means.)

The legal authorization of the underground exchanges was accompanied by increased funding and regulation. The newly authorized exchange programs had to operate within regulations issued by the New York State Department of Health. The original intention of the Health Department's regulations was to require continued tagging of syringes issued through the now legally authorized exchanges, and this stipulation was included in the first versions of the regulations. The tagging, it was reasoned, would both provide information about the percentage of issued syringes that were returned to the exchanges and help law enforcement personnel to distinguish between possession of syringes obtained from legally authorized sources and those obtained from other sources of distribution.

Moreover, with the start of legalization and increased funding, there was also a wide expansion of needle exchange programs. Two of the underground exchanges, which had been serving approximately 1,000 injection drug users per year before being legally authorized, increased to serve nearly 8,000 injection drug users within the first 12 months afterward (Paone et al., 1993, 1994a, 1994b). This expansion led to considerable logistical problems in continuing to tag syringes. The volunteer staff, who did the actual tagging, complained that they were now spending all of their time tagging syringes and no longer had time to interact with the injection drug users coming to the exchanges. This personal interaction was viewed as a major benefit to the injection drug users and a primary opportunity for the volunteers to obtain a palpable sense of accomplishment.

Staff of the two largest legally authorized exchange programs in New York City had begun refusing to continue tagging when a negotiated compromise was reached between the State Health Department and the programs. An evaluation team offered to conduct a special tagging alternative study to determine the syringe return rates and thereby no longer require the programs to tag the syringes they were issuing. In this instance, then, an exchange procedure that had earlier appeared to be highly functional for small underground exchanges clearly became dysfunctional when the exchanges underwent rapid expansion.

Discussion Both the Manchester and the New York City tagging studies suggest the need to examine the organizational characteristics of needle exchange programs within the context of their entire developmental history, as well as in the larger context of drug injection and HIV and AIDS risk behavior in the surrounding community. These two case histories illustrate the possibility that a conclusion drawn from data collected at one point in time may be totally inappropriate for other points in time.

Comparisons Across Programs

It would of course be useful to compare organizational characteristics across programs. To date only two such comparative studies have been conducted (Table 3.3). Stimson and colleagues conducted an evaluation of the national system of needle exchange programs that was implemented in the United Kingdom from 1987 to 1988 (Stimson et al., 1988); it was the first to elaborate on the concept of user-friendliness in syringe exchange. Although they did not conduct formal quantitative analyses, they were able to show that user-friendliness was associated with both attracting and retaining injection drug users in needle exchange programs. (It should be noted that the participation of injection drug users in the U.K. needle exchanges was within a context of legal authorization that permitted both over-the-counter sales of needles and syringes and personal possession of equipment to inject illicit drugs.) As indicated in the first three case histo-

TABLE 3.3 Organizational Characteristics of Needle Exchange Programs

Comparative Study	Characteristics	Components
Stimson et al. (1988)	User-friendliness	—Nonjudgmental staff attitude
		—Convenient location
		—Convenient hours of operation
		—Willingness to exchange large numbers of syringes at one time
Lurie et al. (1993a)	Legal status	—Legal
		—Illegal—tolerated
		—Illegal—underground
	Administrative body	—Activist run
		—Community-based organization run
		—Community-based organization with government support
		—Government run
	Funding source	—Private donations
		—Foundation grants
		—Community-based organization
		—City, county, and/or state government
	Sites	—Fixed sites
		—Stationary van
		—Streetfront
		—Street
		—Health facility
		—Mobile sites
		—Walk route
		—Deliveries
		—Roving van
	Staff	—Paid
		—Volunteers
		—Both paid and volunteers
	On-site services	—Educational material
		—HIV testing and counseling
		—Primary medical care
		—Tuberculosis screening
		—Sexually transmitted diseases screening
		—Drug treatment
		—Referrals to above services
		—Referrals to social services
	On-site items provided	—Needles/syringes
		—Bleach
		—Alcohol wipes
		—Cotton
		—Cookers
		—Water
		—Condoms
		—Lubricant

ries presented above, the concept of user-friendliness appears to be fundamental to at least the initial effectiveness of needle exchange programs.

The University of California, San Francisco, collected organizational data on 33 U.S. and 4 Canadian needle exchange programs (Lurie et al., 1993a). As the table shows, this study arrayed the programs according to a number of different organizational characteristics (e.g., status of legal authorization, funding sources, staffing) and was able to show some meaningful associations among them. *Unfortunately, this study was not able to associate any of the organizational characteristics with any measures of effectiveness in behavior change or HIV transmission.*

Although valuable in depicting the diversity in the type of needle exchange programs, there are certain limitations of this study that should be noted. First, the cost data used in the descriptions and analyses did not separate the costs of exchanging needles from the costs of other services. For this reason, these cost data should be used with extreme caution. Second, given the rapidly changing circumstances of needle exchange programs in the United States, the information provided by this study, as with any cross-sectional survey, represents a snapshot of a complex picture in a state of flux. As of October 1994, there were at least 76 needle exchange programs in the United States—a 130 percent increase over the number of exchanges itemized in the 1993 University of California, San Francisco, report (North American Syringe Exchange Network, 1994). In addition, many of the needle exchange programs included in the study have since undergone substantial changes. Data for the New York City exchanges, for example, do not take account of the legal authorization and expansion noted in the tagging case study presented above.

BLEACH DISTRIBUTION PROGRAMS

Unlike the situation for needle exchange programs, to date there has been no comprehensive survey of the total number of programs in the United States to distribute bleach or other disinfectants for the purpose of cleaning needles and syringes between uses. An extensive review of the literature has resulted in multiple studies that questioned injecting drug users about needle-cleaning practices, but these reports typically do not include descriptions of the characteristics of the bleach distribution programs per se (Longshore et al., 1993; Neaigus et al., 1990).

The most systematic information about bleach distribution programs in the United States comes from the National AIDS Demonstration Research (NADR) program, which was initiated in 1987 by NIDA.

The purpose of NADR was to assess the efficacy of different strategies of AIDS prevention with out-of-treatment injection drug users and their sexual partners. All these strategies—except those initiated in New Jersey—were to make use of the newly developed bleach distribution technology. All were to rely on the skills of ex-addict staff trained to conduct case finding and engagement and to provide AIDS prevention materials and counseling. NADR came to involve a total of 41 projects in nearly 50 cities nationwide. Over the life of the program, data were collected on more than 43,000 injection drug users and nearly 10,000 sexual partners, although many more tens of thousands of participants received outreach and intervention services (AIDS prevention services) but were not referred for study (Brown and Beschner, 1993).

Characteristics of Program Participants

The demographic characteristics of NADR program participants vary considerably across participating program sites. Data from 13,475 participants in the 28 sites that contributed demographic data for the final data analysis indicate that the average age of participants is 35. On average, participants had been injecting drugs for 14 years (ranging from 10 to 19 years across sites). NADR recruited predominantly men: 74 percent of the sample at intake were men. The proportion of women by site ranges from 12 to 37 percent.

NADR participants also vary considerably by site in their racial/ethnic distributions. The proportion of African American participants ranges from 9 to 95 percent; Hispanic participants range from 0 to 81 percent; and white participants range from 3 to 65 percent. As is the case with needle exchange programs, this variation across sites to some extent reflects regional differences. Overall the sample was 51 percent African American, 25 percent Latino, and 22 percent white.

Other noteworthy observations are that 81 percent of NADR participants had spent time in jail or prison, 41 percent had never been in a drug treatment program, and participants reported an average of 12 different sex partners in the past 6 months. However, it is again important to note that the demographic data presented here mostly reflect the demographics of participants who provided data for the final NADR analysis and, as a consequence, there may be a bias in the representation of the original NADR sites. Moreover, descriptions of sampling procedures (outreach workers recruited out-of-treatment injection drug users) make it unlikely that the studied sample is statistically representative of the out-of-treatment injection drug user population in this country. Nonetheless, this effort is the most extensive description of the demographic characteristics of out-of-treatment drug users to date. The similarity in demographic patterns, between NADR participants and the needle exchange participants reported earlier in this chapter, is notable.

Outreach Strategies

The outreach strategies used in bleach distribution programs are characterized by their emphasis either on (a) the development of individual behavioral skills to limit risk taking or (b) the modification of community norms to support changed behavior. Those concerned with the former are focused on counseling and behavioral skills training, and those concerned with the latter are focused on peer intervention and social contagion.

For programs that emphasize counseling and behavioral skills training, outreach mainly involves referring injection drug users to a community site at which they typically receive structured counseling and skills-building sessions (Rhodes, 1993). For programs that emphasize the peer intervention and social contagion approach, outreach workers, chosen for their knowledge of and status in the injection drug-using community, play a key role in the work of HIV and AIDS prevention by inserting themselves into the social network of injection drug users (Wiebel et al., 1993).

Outreach at the sites in the NADR project varied in terms of techniques used, from written instructions about the use of bleach to disinfect injection equipment, to demonstration of the technique in person, reverse demonstration (by the drug user to measure comprehension and competence), and videotapes. Information summarized from eight NADR sites is presented in Table 3.4. Two cities—San Francisco and Denver—reported ancillary techniques to promote the use of bleach to disinfect needles. In San Francisco, an individual was costumed as an 8-foot-tall superhero named "Bleachman," with a plastic bottle for a head and a Clorox logo on his torso. Bleachman appeared on city streets to distribute small bottles of bleach (Broadhead, 1991). In Denver, outdoor murals were painted in the city to encourage risk reduction and the bleaching of needles and syringes.

There are limitations on the NADR data, which are discussed in Chapter 6. Although the NADR program provides information to describe and evaluate bleach distribution programs in the United States, it does not describe all existing bleach distribution programs. Also, the NADR programs used outreach workers to establish trust and rapport with injection drug users outside treatment for drug abuse; bleach distribution is thus intertwined with the intervention of community health outreach workers. Other bleach distribution occurs in the setting of needle exchange programs. The panel found no instance in the literature of self-service bleach bottles with printed instructions as the sole intervention.

One further limitation: reports from San Francisco describe the instructions provided by the NADR projects for the use of bleach to disinfect needles. Undiluted bleach was packaged in 1-ounce vials, to be flushed through a used syringe twice before injecting and following each bleach flushing with a flushing of water. The extent to which instructions varied

TABLE 3.4 Percentage of Clients Receiving Intervention Components

Intervention Components	Total (n = 3,886)	Site 1	2	3	4	5	6	7	8
Give bleach	82	33	100	100	100	100	35	100	100
Demonstrate bleach use	61	33	100	100	51	44	34	37	100
Practice condom use	61	33	100	100	49	44	34	37	100
Give condom	91	100	100	100	100	100	34	100	100
Demonstrate condom use	61	33	100	100	51	44	34	37	100
Practice condom use	61	33	100	100	49	44	34	37	100
Video/slide presentation	67	44	100	100	73	100	34	37	54
One-on-one session	72	100	—	100	100	—	100	100	46
Group session (not specific)	10	43	—	—	—	—	34	—	—
Group session: problem solving	26	30	—	41	—	46	45	—	54
Group session: risk avoidance	29	33	—	41	—	100	23	—	54
Group session: negotiation	27	—	100	36	—	46	—	—	54
Role-playing: problem solving	24	—	38	35	24	—	45	—	54
Role-playing: risk avoidance	22	—	43	—	48	46	—	—	54
Role-playing: negotiation	23	—	35	35	24	46	—	—	54
Didactic session: risk avoidance	73	—	100	37	100	100	100	100	54
Booklet/brochure	50	—	100	100	100	—	—	100	100
Referral (HIV or non-HIV)	49	—	100	100	100	—	—	37	54

SOURCE: Outreach/Risk Reduction Strategies for Changing HIV-Related Risk Behaviors Among Injection Drug Users: The National AIDS Demonstration Research (NADR) Project (National Institute on Drug Abuse, 1994:58).

from this at other sites before 1993 has not been summarized systematically.

CONCLUSIONS

1. By 1994, 76 needle exchange programs had been established in the United States, an increase from 33 at the time of the University of California report in 1993. More are planned.

2. Needle exchange programs vary considerably in terms of whether they are legally authorized, their sources of funding, site characteristics, on-site services offered, and other items distributed.

3. Needle exchange programs vary in terms of the racial/ethnic distributions of the participants served. The majority served are men. The distribution of participants by age and duration of drug use shows that a wide cross section of drug injectors are attracted to needle exchange.

4. The cost of needle exchange programs varies widely, depending on their organizational aspects. The median annual cost for operation of a needle exchange program has been estimated at $168,650.

5. Needle exchange programs vary in their ability to attract clients. Factors that promote recruitment of participants include:

• An "ideal" needle exchange and bleach distribution site. This should be (1) in an area frequented by injection drug users, (2) unlikely to be noticed by passersby, (3) unlikely to engender opposition from local residents or businesses, (4) able to provide privacy for injection drug users and protection from the weather, (5) in a predictable location, (6) accessible to diverse communities of injection drug users, and (7) able to be relocated easily, if necessary. Some of these characteristics may be mutually incompatible.

• Programs that provide for an exchange of injection equipment, not a unilateral distribution. This greatly increases the likelihood that the programs will reduce the number of discarded syringes found in parks and alleys and other public sites. It also helps to ensure that existing injection drug users, not new users, are the ones using the program. Conducting the programs as an exchange also increases the possibilities for evaluating program effectiveness through tracking exchanged syringes and conducting surveys of exchange participants to ensure safe practices (Lurie et al., 1993a).

• User-friendly policies and procedures and staff that are nonjudgmental and flexible.

6. Bleach distribution and needle exchange programs are not and should not be viewed as discrete entities. They typically include a variety of prevention services (including outreach and education) that are intertwined.

REFERENCES

Anderson, W.
1991   The New York needle trial: The politics of public health in the age of AIDS. *American Journal of Public Health* 81(11):1506-1517.

Broadhead, R.S.
1991   Social constructions of bleach in combating AIDS among injection drug users. *Journal of Drug Issues* 21:713-737.

Brown, B.S., and G.M. Beschner, eds.
1993   *Handbook on Risk of AIDS: Injection Drug Users and Sexual Partners.* Westport, CT: Greenwood Press.

Hagan, H., D. Des Jarlais, D. Purchase, T. Reid, and S.R. Friedman
1991   The Tacoma syringe exchange. *Journal of Addictive Diseases* 10:81-88.

Hellinger, F.J.
1993   The lifetime cost of treating a person with HIV. *Journal of the American Medical Association* 270(4):474-478.

Jones, T.S.
1994   Update on Upcoming Research Activities Pertaining to Needle Exchange and Bleach Distribution. Presentation at the September meeting of the Panel on Needle Exchange and Bleach Distribution Programs, Woods Hole, MA.

Joseph, S.C.
1989   A bridge to treatment: The needle exchange pilot program in New York City. *AIDS Education and Prevention* 1:340-345.

Joseph, S.C., and D.C. Des Jarlais
1989   Needle and syringe exchange as a method of AIDS epidemic control. *AIDS Updates* 2(5):1-8.

Kahn, J.G., A.E. Washington, J.A. Sowstack, M. Berlin, and K. Phillips
1992   *Updated Estimates of the Impact and Cost of HIV Prevention in Injection Drug Users.* San Francisco, CA: Institute for Health Policy Studies, University of California.

Kaplan, E.H.
1993   Back-of-the-Envelope Estimates of Needle Exchange Effectiveness. Unpublished material.
in press   Economic analysis of needle exchange. *AIDS.* 9:1113-1119, 1995.

Klee, H., J. Faugier, C. Hayes, and J. Morris
1991   The sharing of injecting equipment among drug users attending prescribing clinics and those using needle-exchanges. *British Journal of Addiction* 86:217-223.

Longshore, D., M.D. Anglin, K. Annon, and S. Hsiehs
1993   Trends in self-reported HIV risk behavior: Injection drug users in Los Angeles. *Journal of Acquired Immune Deficiency Syndromes* 6:82-90.

Lurie, P., A.L. Reingold, B. Bowser, D. Chen, J. Foley, J. Guydish, J.G. Kahn, S. Land, and J. Sorensen
1993a   *The Public Health Impact of Needle Exchange Programs in the United States and Abroad, Volume 1.* San Francisco, CA: University of California.

Lurie, P., A.L. Reingold, B. Bowser, D. Chen, J. Foley, J. Guydish, J.G. Kahn, S. Land, and J. Sorensen
1993b   *The Public Health Impact of Needle Exchange Programs in the United States and Abroad: Volume 2.* San Francisco, CA: University of California, San Francisco.

National Institute on Drug Abuse
1994   *Outreach/Risk Reduction Strategies for Changing HIV-Related Risk Behaviors Among Injection Drug Users: The National AIDS Demonstration Research (NADR) Project.* NIH Publication No. 94-3726. Bethesda, MD: National Institutes of Health.
Neaigus, A., M. Sufian, S.R. Friedman, D.S. Goldsmith, B. Stephenson, P. Mota, J. Pascal, and D.C. Des Jarlais
1990   Effects of outreach intervention on AIDS risk reduction among injection drug users. *AIDS Education and Prevention* 2:253-271.
New York City Department of Health
1989   *The Pilot Needle Exchange Study in New York City: A Bridge to Treatment. A Report on the First Ten Months of Operation.* New York: New York City Department of Health.
North American Syringe Exchange Network
1994   Surveys, surveys, surveys. *Newsworks* 3(December 16):1.
Paone, D., D.C. Des Jarlais, S. Caloir, and P.B. Friedmann
1993   AIDS risk reduction behaviors among participants of syringe-exchange programs in New York City. Presented at the Ninth International Conference on AIDS, Berlin, June 6-11 [abstract PO-C24-3188].
Paone, D., D.C. Des Jarlais, S. Caloir, P.B. Freidmann, I. Ness, and S.R. Friedman
1994a   New York City syringe exchange: An Overview. Pp. 47-63 in *Proceedings, Workshop on Needle Exchange and Bleach Distribution Programs.* Washington, DC: National Academy Press.
Paone, D., S. Caloir, J. Clark, E. Gonzalez, B. Jose, and D.C. Des Jarlais
1994b   Tagging Alternative Study (TAS): A Substudy of the New York City Syringe Exchange Evaluation. Presented at the North American Needle Exchange Network Conference, Santa Cruz, CA, March 3-5.
Rhodes, F.
1993   *The Behavioral Counseling Model for Injection Drug Users.* Rockville, MD: National Institute on Drug Abuse.
Stimson, G.V., L.J. Aldritt, K.A. Dolan, M.S. Donoghoe, and R.A. Lart
1988   *Injecting Equipment Exchange Schemes. Final Report.* London: Monitoring Research Group, Goldsmith's College.
Turner, C.F., H.G. Miller, and L.E. Moses, eds.
1989   *AIDS: Sexual Behavior and Intravenous Drug Use.* Washington, DC: National Academy Press.
U.S. General Accounting Office
1993   *Needle Exchange Programs: Research Suggests Promise as an AIDS Prevention Strategy.* Washington, DC: U.S. Government Printing Office.
Valleroy, L.A., B. Weinstein, T.S. Jones, S.L. Groseclose, R.T. Rolfs, and W.J. Kassler
in press Impact of increased legal access to needles and syringes on community pharmacies' needle and syringe sales—Connecticut, 1992-1993. *Journal of Acquired Immune Deficiency Syndromes.*
Vlahov, D., C. Ryan, L. Solomon, S. Cohn, M.R. Holt, and M.N. Akhter
1994   A pilot syringe exchange program in Washington, D.C. *American Journal of Public Health* 84(2):303-304.
Watters, J.K.
1994   Trends in risk behavior and HIV seroprevalence in heterosexual injection drug users in San Francisco, 1986-1992. *Journal of Acquired Immune Deficiency Syndromes* 7:1276-1281.

Watters, J.K., and P. Case
    1989   Preliminary Study of an Illicit Needle Exchange Program in San Francisco. Pre-
               sentation in American Public Health Association Annual Meeting, Chicago.
Watters, J.K., M. Downing, P. Casse, J. Lorvick, T.Y. Cheng, and B. Fergusson
    1990   AIDS prevention for injection drug users in the community: Street-based educa-
               tion and risk behavior. *American Journal of Community Psychology* 18:587-596.
Wiebel, W., A. Jiminez, W. Johnson, L. Ouellet, T. Lampinen, J. Murray, B. Jovanovic, and
M.U. O'Brien
    1993   Positive Effect on HIV Seroconversion on Street-Outreach Intervention with IDU
               in Chicago: 1988-1992. Paper presented at the Ninth International Conference on
               AIDS, June 6-11.

4

Community Views

In the evaluation of needle exchange and bleach distribution programs, one dimension involves scientific evidence on whether the behavior of injection drug users changes and rates of new infection are reduced. However, these issues cannot be viewed in isolation, because injection drug users inhabit communities that are affected by and have already developed responses to the behavior and consequences of drug abuse. Whether HIV prevention programs, such as needle exchanges, are established and what forms they take are shaped by multiple forces in the community. The sheer variety among the operational characteristics of needle exchange programs described in the previous chapter is to some extent a function of local

Note: Some of the information used in this chapter is from a paper prepared for the panel by Stephen Thomas and Sandra Crouse Quinn, *Community Response to the Implementation of Needle Exchange and Bleach Distribution Programs* (1994). Their paper discusses the primary historical, social, and political factors that have shaped community responses to the implementation of needle exchange and bleach distribution programs. It also presents results from cross-sectional surveys of selected African American populations to demonstrate how deficits in AIDS knowledge and attitudinal barriers have shaped the perceptions of African Americans toward needle exchange programs as an HIV prevention strategy advocated by public health authorities. In addition, some of the discussion is based on information from another paper prepared for the panel by David Metzger and Dominick DePhilippis, *Treatment Community Views on Needle Exchange and Bleach Distribution Programs* (1994). Their paper explores the basis for the dilemma faced by the large and diverse drug treatment community regarding the public debate and political controversy surrounding the brief and turbulent history of needle exchange programs in this country.

responses to such programs. The *community* is not some monolith; rather, it is a dynamic interaction of groups whose views and actions vary with location and time.

The panel undertook a wide range of activities to gather pertinent information about the views of various groups on the issues relating to the implementation of needle exchange and bleach distribution programs. We reviewed the literature systematically to gather the range and extent of opinions for two groups in which the expression of viewpoints has been extensive: the African American community and the treatment community. In fact, a special workshop was held, to which representatives of the community groups covered in this chapter were invited. The panel members conducted site visits to Chicago and San Francisco to discuss issues with community outreach workers. We also solicited information from pertinent professional organizations to identify formal positions on needle exchange and bleach distribution programs. Finally, a number of public opinion surveys were identified and reviewed.

In this report, we embrace a broad definition of *community*, which includes ethnic groups, business and religious organizations, government bodies, and professional groups. Understandably, the information presented in this chapter focuses primarily on those who have been most vocal in expressing their concerns about needle and bleach distribution programs. Other views have not been overlooked intentionally.

The chapter begins with a brief consideration of the moral and ethical arguments that come into play in these issues. We then discuss *public opinion polls*, which are informative to broadly gauge community attitudes toward needle exchange and bleach distribution programs over time. The chapter goes on to discuss the perspectives of a number of community groups and their responses to needle exchange and bleach distribution programs:

- *minority communities*, which are disproportionately affected by drug abuse,
- *law enforcement officials*, who are sworn to enforce laws,
- *pharmacists*, who hold supplies of sterile needles, and
- *drug abuse treatment providers*, who work with limited funding to impact the difficult processes of addiction.

The material presented in this chapter contributes to the panel's overall assessment of the effectiveness of needle exchange and bleach distribution programs, and its findings and conclusions are integrated in the recommendations that appear in Chapter 7. As stated in the Introduction, this approach reflects the development of the panel's deliberations on the issues.

MORAL/ETHICAL ARGUMENTS

The moral arguments that are a common theme of community groups concerned with needle exchange and bleach distribution programs also appear in federal policy statements. A critique of the New Haven needle exchange evaluation study by the Office of National Drug Control Policy illustrates this point (1992:1): "There is no getting around the fact that distributing needles facilitates drug use and undercuts the credibility of society's message that using drugs is illegal and morally wrong."

Ideological and moral concerns are not scientific, empirically based arguments; however, this in no way dilutes their importance. Needle exchange and bleach distribution programs can be established only within the context of communities, and their success or failure is highly dependent on the support and leadership of community members. The strength of the scientific arguments and their weight relative to the ethical case for or against these programs can be and have been debated at length by ethicists and other concerned individuals.

Although it is beyond the scope and expertise of the panel to fully examine the complex range of ethical issues that might be judged relevant to analyze the establishment of public health policies, we nonetheless present two fundamentally divergent views that may contribute to an understanding of the polarization encountered when the establishment of needle exchange and bleach distribution programs is considered.

Within the context of an ethical debate, whether needle exchange and bleach distribution programs contribute to increased drug use in society constitutes one of many harms and/or benefits that must be weighed relative to others (Pellegrino, 1990; O'Brien, 1989). Weighing the relative benefit and relative harm associated with an action before making a judgment about its ethical soundness has been called the *proportionalist approach* to ethical analysis (Fuller, 1993). Using this approach, one can argue that people are morally compelled to support a lesser harm (evil) in order to prevent a greater harm. From this perspective, the most convincing argument in favor of needle exchange programs lies in their claim as a significant strategy for reducing harm.

Two ethical traditions take the proportionalist approach. In Jewish medical ethics, the principle of *pkuach nfesh* mandates the protection of human life and holds that, when a life is at stake, all prohibitions contained in the Torah and the Talmud may be waived to save that life (Jakobovits, 1959). The other ethical tradition that supports the proportionalist position is the moral theology of Alphonsi Mariae de Ligorio (1907), which argues that it is ethical to support a less evil activity in order to prevent a more evil one. In the case of needle exchange and bleach distribution programs, according to this tradition, even if some empirically demonstrated harms were associated with program implementation, it would still not necessarily be ruled out on ethical grounds.

A fundamentally different approach to ethical analysis is the *deontologist approach*. In this approach, actions are taken because they are right within themselves, not necessarily because some good will ensue. Accordingly, if one has concluded that injection drug use is immoral, then one may not ethically cooperate in any way with this behavior. Needle exchange programs would be viewed as immoral because they provide the material means for an immoral activity and therefore share in the evil of that activity.

Given these examples of two fundamentally divergent views of what is ethically acceptable, it is not surprising that there has been and continues to be substantial public discourse about the distribution of needles, syringes, and bleach. Nonetheless, both the public health and community well-being are at stake until we find common ground on which to clarify objectives and establish appropriate ways to reduce the spread of HIV, which may include the establishment of needle exchange and bleach distribution programs. As noted by O'Brien (1989), there is value in developing common definitions and mutually agreed-on ethical standards of analysis. Until such standards are set forth, it will be difficult to engage in a constructive ethical debate.

PUBLIC OPINION POLLS

A thorough review of public opinion polls conducted between 1985 and 1991 indicates that half of the general public supports harm reduction efforts that include needle cleaning, legalizing needle sales, needle exchange, and needle distribution (Lurie et al., 1993). Approval has tended to be higher for programs that combine bleach distribution and needle exchange than for programs that focus on needle distribution (Table 4.1). More important, the available evidence indicates that this support has tended to increase over time, as the issues have been publicly debated and more programs have been implemented.

For example, the Gilmore study (Table 4.1, Panel A) showed an increase in approval between 1988 and 1991 for teaching people to use bleach. In the same interval, that study showed an increase in support for legalizing the sale of needles and syringes to drug users (Panel B), and a similar rise in approval for needle exchange (Panel C). The studies in these three panels show substantial, sometimes majority support for measures that make sterile needles more available to injection drug users. With regard to the distribution of free sterile needles to injection drug users in order to retard the spread of AIDS (Panel D), again, between 1985 and 1991 across various locations, substantial support was found, although less than a majority in each opinion study.

As another illustration, the results of a 1994 household survey showed a

12 percent increase in the proportion of Maryland residents who support needle exchange programs (Figure 4.1). These results also point to a larger increase (19 percent) in the city of Baltimore than in the state as a whole. Moreover, findings from a recent nationwide telephone survey undertaken in February 1994 showed that, among the 1,001 adults sampled, 55 percent favored implementing needle exchange programs to reduce the spread of diseases such as AIDS, 37 percent favored allowing drug users to buy sterile needles without prescriptions from pharmacies, and 40 percent favored removing criminal penalties for the simple possession of needles and syringes (Hart, 1994).

We turn now to discussion of the views of particular groups in communities across the nation.

AFRICAN AMERICAN VIEWS

Much of the voiced African American opposition to needle exchange and bleach distribution programs must be understood in the context of perceptions that historically there has been government negligence in response to the drug abuse epidemic, distrust of public health authorities, and fear—and, for some, the conviction—that the broader society considers large segments of the African American population expendable (Thomas and Quinn, 1991, 1993). Pervasive throughout the African American community are uncertainties about the motivations of what they perceive as the white establishment.

This underlying distrust is grounded in part in a history of medical neglect and significant violations of human subjects. Most specifically, the legacy of the Tuskegee Syphilis Study is a vivid reminder (Thomas and Quinn, 1991). This study, conducted by the U.S. Public Health Service from 1932 to 1972, deliberately and irresponsibly withheld treatment for syphilis from an African American community in Tuskegee, Alabama. The Tuskegee study continues to serve as the basis for much of the widespread distrust of public health and government authorities (Jones, 1981). Recently confirmed reports about other government abuses (e.g., radiation experiments, cocaine distribution) are portrayed as further evidence to support suspicions and fears about the motivation and intent of officials urging the utilization of needle exchange programs.

According to Thomas and others (Thomas and Quinn, 1993; Belgrave and Randolph, 1993), many African Americans, including many who are well educated, believe that HIV is manufactured and that drugs are being deliberately supplied to African American communities. The prevalence of AIDS itself, as well as programs purported to reduce its spread, are viewed as part of a larger genocidal conspiracy against African Americans. In a 1990 survey of the views of African American churchgoers in five cities—

TABLE 4.1 Results of U. S. Public Opinion Polls on Needle Exchange and Needle Cleaning, 1985-1991

Date of Survey	Description of Respondents	Polling Institution	Question	Results
A. NEEDLE CLEANING				
April/May 1988	Washington State n = 800	Gilmore Research for Washington State HIV/AIDS General Population Survey (Olympia, WA) (Washington State Department of Health, 1991)	Would you support a program to teach people how to clean needles with bleach?	59%—Yes 41%—No/don't know
May 1989	Utah n = 849	Survey Research Center, University of Utah (Salt Lake City, UT) (University of Utah, 1989)	Free needle cleaning kits should be available for IV drug users: agree or disagree?	43%—Agree 57%—Disagree/don't know
April/May 1991	Washington State n = 801	Gilmore Research for Washington State HIV/AIDS General Population Survey (Olympia, WA) (Washington State Department of Health, 1991)	Would you support a program to teach people how to clean needles with bleach?	65%—Yes 35%—No/don't know

B. REMOVAL OF LEGAL BARRIERS TO NEEDLE PURCHASE

Date of Survey	Description of Respondents	Polling Institution	Question	Results
April/May 1988	Washington State $n = 800$	Gilmore Research for Washington State HIV/AIDS General Population Survey (Olympia, WA) (Washington State Department of Health, 1991)	Would you support making needles and syringes legal to sell to drug users?	38%—Yes 62%—No/don't know
April/May 1991	Washington State $n = 801$	Gilmore Research for Washington State HIV/AIDS General Population Survey (Olympia, WA) (Washington State Department of Health, 1991)	Would you support making needles and syringes legal to sell to drug users?	45%—Yes 55%—No/don't know

continued on next page

TABLE 4-1 Continued

Date of Survey	Description of Respondents	Polling Institution	Question	Results
C. NEEDLE EXCHANGE				
April/May 1988	Washington State n = 800	Gilmore Research for Washington State HIV/AIDS General Population Survey (Olympia, WA) (Washington State Department of Health, 1991)	Would you support a needle exchange program where a drug user could obtain a free sterile needle in exchange for a used one?	55%—Yes 45%—No/don't know
January 1989	Pierce and South King Counties, WA n = 411	Tacoma Morning News Tribune Poll conducted by Tacoma Marketing Research (Tacoma, WA) (Eskenazi, 1989)	Do you agree with the Board of Health decision to fund a hypodermic needle exchange program designed to reduce the spread of AIDS?	67%—Agree 18%—Disagree 14%—Unsure/don't know
1989/1990	New York City, NY Members of Harlem families n = 326	Ann Brunswick Columbia University (New York City, NY) (Brunswick, 1991)	Some people have suggested that handing out clean needles, free, would be a good way to reduce AIDS among intravenous drug users. Other people say that providing free needles would encourage drug use. How do you	38%—Agree strongly 16%—Agree somewhat 35%—Disagree strongly 5%—Disagree somewhat 6%—Not sure

			personally feel about allowing drug users to exchange their used needles for clean ones?	
1989/1990	New York City, NY Injection drug users in Harlem families *n* = 38	Ann Brunswick Columbia University (New York City, NY) (Brunswick, 1991)	Some people have suggested that handing out clean needles, free, would be a good way to reduce AIDS among intravenous drug users. Other people say that providing free needles would encourage drug use. How do you personally feel about allowing drug users to exchange their used needles for clean ones?	53%—Agree strongly 19%—Agree somewhat 18%—Disagree strongly 6%—Disagree somewhat 4%—Not sure
April/May 1991	Washington State *n* = 801	Gilmore Research for Washington State HIV/AIDS General Population Survey (Olympia, WA) (Washington State Department of Health, 1991)	Would you support a needle exchange program where a drug user could obtain a free sterile needle in exchange for a used one?	68%—Yes 32%—No/don't know

continued on next page

TABLE 4-1 Continued

Date of Survey	Description of Respondents	Polling Institution	Question	Results
D. NEEDLE DISTRIBUTION				
November 1985	Maryland residents who indicated they had heard about AIDS in the news recently *n* = 1,074	Hollander, Cohen, McBride associates for the Maryland Department of Health (Baltimore, MD) (Hollander et al., 1985)	One of the ways AIDS is spread is by drug abusers who share needles. Some health authorities have suggested that clean needles be provided free to those who ask for them [to] control spreading the disease that way. Do you agree with this approach?	37%—Agree 55%—Disagree 0%—Depends 8%—Don't know 0%—Not applicable
March 1987	Connecticut *n* = 500	The Roper Center for Public Opinion Research (Storrs, CT) (1987)	Do you favor or oppose distributing free sterile needles to drug users to slow the spread of AIDS through contaminated needles?	33%—Favor 60%—Oppose 7%—Don't know
October 1988	U.S. *n* = 1,606	CBS News/New York Times Poll (New York City, NY)	Would you favor or oppose giving injection drug users sterilized needles for free if it would slow down the spread of AIDS?	40%—Favor 53%—Oppose 7%—Don't know

February 1989	New York City, NY n = 1,015	Newsday (New York City, NY) (1989)	Do you approve or disapprove of the city's programs to provide clean needles to drug users in order to prevent the spread of AIDS?	50%—Approve 40%—Disapprove 10%—Don't know
May 1989	Utah n = 849	Survey Research Center, University of Utah (Salt Lake City, UT) (University of Utah, 1989)	Free needles and syringes should be made available to intravenous drug addicts: agree or disagree?	38%—Agree 62%—Disagree/don't know
May 1989	Connecticut n = 768	Northeast Research (Orono, ME) (1989)	I'm going to read a few of the things people have suggested that might help stop the spread of AIDS in CT. For each one please tell me if you think that method should be used. You can answer yes or no, or that you have no opinion about it. Give out free needles to drug dealers.	40%—Yes 47%—No 13%—Don't know
May 1989	United States n = 1,054	Media General/Associated Press (Richmond, VA) (1989)	The AIDS virus can be transmitted when people who use drugs share needles. If giving intravenous drug abusers free needles would slow down the spread of AIDS, would you favor or oppose giving addicts sterilized needles for free?	50%—Favor 43%—Oppose 7%—Don't know

continued on next page

TABLE 4-1 Continued

Date of Survey	Description of Respondents	Polling Institution	Question	Results
October 1989	Maricopa County, AZ n = 809	Arizona Republic (Phoenix, AZ) (The Arizona Republic, 1993)	Would you favor or oppose a program that would make it possible for sterilized needles to be distributed to drug addicts as a way to slow the spread of the AIDS virus?	52%—Favor 45%—Oppose 3%—Don't know
January 1990	Massachusetts registered voters n = 405	Bannon Research (Boston, MA) (1990)	Do you strongly favor, mildly favor, mildly oppose, or strongly oppose giving clean needles to drug users so they don't spread the AIDS virus?	26%—Strongly favor 26%—Mildly favor 14%—Mildly oppose 31%—Strongly oppose 3%—Don't know/no answer
February 1990	Chicago, IL n = 449	Northwestern University Survey Laboratory (Evanston, IL) (Lavrakas, 1990)	Drug treatment centers should distribute free needles to intravenous drug users to reduce the chances of spreading AIDS: strongly agree, somewhat agree, somewhat disagree, or strongly disagree?	38%—Strongly agree 19%—Somewhat agree 10%—Somewhat disagree 29%—Strongly disagree 4%—Uncertain
Spring 1991	Black church congregation members in 5 cities	Minority Health Research Laboratory, University of	Survey participants were asked the same questions before and after a training session on AIDS issues.	*Before* 40%—Agree 41%—Disagree 19%—Unsure

		The question asked	*After*
Before: *n* = 202 After: *n* = 180	Maryland for the Southern Christian Leadership Conference (Atlanta, GA) (Thomas and Quinn, 1993b)	The question asked respondents to agree or disagree with the following statement: I would support laws to pass out free clean needles to people who shoot drugs.	47%—Agree 40%—Disagree 14%—Unsure
May 1991 Arizona *n* = 808	Arizona Republic (Phoenix, AZ) (The Arizona Republic, 1993)	Do you agree or disagree with each of the following statements about AIDS? The state should give away needles to drug addicts to prevent the spread of AIDS.	26%—Agree 73%—Disagree 1%—Don't know
June 1991 Denver, CO *n* = 303	Talmey-Drake Research Strategy, Inc., for the Denver Post/KCNC TV (Denver, CO) (1991)	Please state your opinion regarding the following statement: The city of Denver should provide clean hypodermic needles to drug addicts to help stop the spread of AIDS.	25%—Strongly agree 24%—Somewhat agree 16%—Somewhat disagree 25%—Strongly disagree 10%—Uncertain

SOURCE: *The Public Health Impact of Needle Exchange Programs in the United States and Abroad. Volume 1* (Lurie et al., 1993:330-332).

Do You Favor Setting Up Needle Exchange Programs to Reduce The Spread of AIDS?

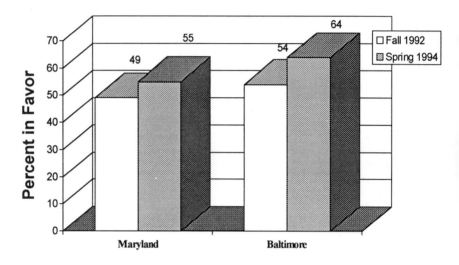

FIGURE 4.1 Needle exchange support in the state of Maryland and Baltimore city.
SOURCE: Center for Substance Abuse Research (1994).

Atlanta, Georgia; Charlotte, North Carolina; Detroit, Michigan; Kansas City, Missouri; and Tuscaloosa, Alabama—Thomas and Quinn (1993) found that only one in five persons trusts government reports on AIDS and that two-thirds consider the possibility that AIDS is a form of genocide. The study also found that 38 percent of African American college students in Washington, D.C., believe "there is some truth in reports that the AIDS virus was produced in a germ warfare laboratory"; another 26 percent said they were "unsure." Major journals focusing on issues of concern to African Americans, for example, *Essence* (Bates, 1990), have given wide attention, and therefore some degree of sanction, to these beliefs. Although these results cannot be generalized to all African Americans, they are a disturbing revelation to many who are attempting to conduct HIV and AIDS health promotion and disease prevention activities within these communities.

Proponents of genocidal theories also argue that it is not by chance that alcohol and drug abuse plague African American communities. It is pointed out that retail outlets for the sale of alcohol are controlled by government policy. The Reverend Graylan Ellis-Hagler of Plymouth Congregational Church in Washington, D.C., sounds a common theme heard in this community (Ellis-Hagler, 1993, as cited in Thomas and Quinn, 1994):

Drugs are not in our community by coincidence, but by [design]. Just like you can find a liquor store on every corner [in the inner city], you can find a dope house on every street and it's not there by coincidence, it is there by [design].

Similarly, news from sources such as *60 Minutes* (cited in Thomas and Quinn, 1994) and *The New York Times* (Weiner, 1993) is presented as evidence that illegal drugs are not in the community by coincidence. *The New York Times* reported that the Central Intelligence Agency's antidrug program in Venezuela used public monies to ship a ton of cocaine to the United States and allowed it to be sold on the streets. No criminal charges were brought in the case, and the government officials responsible declared the matter a "most regrettable incident." Many African Americans and Latinos declared it to be "genocide" (Weiner, 1993).

Church leaders and elected officials have been the primary sources of expressed opposition by the African American community to needle exchange and bleach distribution programs. The church is a central and important influence in the African American community, and its moral teachings generally forbid the kind of sexual and drug-use behaviors that are associated with the transmission of HIV and AIDS. Much of the initial opposition of the African American clergy to the idea of needle exchange and bleach distribution programs focused on the immorality of the underlying risk behaviors. Certain high-profile and prominent clergy in the African American community have joined forces with politicians, business executives, and health care providers who have determined that these interventions represent a grave risk to the community.

Influenced by the historical legacy described above, these opponents have described the idea of making sterile needles available to drug users as misguided and dangerous. Politicians and public health officials are accused of irresponsibility in their failure to concentrate exclusively on increasing funding and programs for comprehensive drug treatment. Needle exchange programs and bleach distribution are viewed, at best, as makeshift responses and, at worst, as the deliberate continuation and support of drug dependence within the African American community.

Reverend Graylan Ellis-Hagler has said, for example (Kirp and Bayer, 1993:39):

First they (the white establishment) push drugs into the community. They cripple the community politically and economically with drugs. They send the males to jail. THEN someone hands out needles to maintain the dependency.

These sentiments have been echoed by several African American leaders, including member of Congress Charles Rangel (D-New York) and activist minister Dr. Calvin O. Butts. It is significant that Ellis-Hagler's position was influenced by the leadership of recovering addicts in his congregation. Originally, he had been supportive of needle exchange programs. He has indicated that his switch to an opposing stance was in response to his recognition that issues of empowerment and local control were more important than "pushing forth some social policy that came out of some liberal think tank somewhere in America" (Ellis-Hagler, 1993).

The image of African American injection drug users reaching out for drug treatment only to receive clean needles from public health authorities provides additional support for the genocide theory (Thomas and Quinn, 1993). These sentiments have been eloquently expressed by Dalton (1989):

> For us (African Americans) drug abuse is a curse far worse than you can imagine. Addicts prey on our neighborhoods, sell drugs to our children, steal our possessions, and rob us of hope. We despise them because they hurt us and because they ARE us. They are a constant reminder of how close we all are to the edge. And "they" are "us" literally as well as figuratively; they are our sons and daughters, our sisters and brothers. Can we possibly cast out the demons without casting out our own kin? (p. 217)

> Why can't WE choose which of the many problems facing us to tackle first? Suppose we think that crack is more of a menace than AIDS. Are you willing to help us take on that one? Why do you want US to take all the risks? You say that making drug use safer (by giving away bleach or distributing clean needles) won't make it more attractive to our children or our neighbors' children? But what if you are wrong? What if as a result, we have even more addicts to contend with? Will you be around to help us then, especially if the link between addiction and AIDS has not been severed? . . . Instead of asking us to accept on faith that we won't be abandoned and possibly worse off once you move on to a new issue, why not demonstrate your commitment by empowering us to carry on the struggle whether you are there or not? (p. 219)

Although individual religious leaders express strongly held views, African American church organizations have to date not taken formal positions either in support of or in opposition to needle exchange programs (Malone, 1994). And several of the more vocal religious and political leaders in such places as New York, Boston, New Haven, and Chicago have been convinced to allow certain needle exchange programs to operate in their cities.

The views of religious leaders in the African American community have been complemented by the views of politicians. For example, in March 1993, Congressman Charles Rangel, in response to a report from the U.S. General Accounting Office (1993), commented (Select Committee on Narcotics Abuse and Control, U.S. House of Representatives News Release, March 26, 1993):

> I cannot condone my government telling communities ravaged by the twin epidemics of drugs and AIDS that clean needles are the best we can do for

you. Many of those hardest hit are minority communities like the ones I represent. I believe government has an obligation to do more than just help people use illegal drugs more safely . . . . To my way of thinking, the continuing debate over needle exchange programs only diverts us from the real issue . . . that is expanding our capacity to get drug users into effective comprehensive treatment.

When the African American religious and political leaders who have expressed opposition to needle exchange and bleach distribution programs have been convinced that these programs can be valuable in reducing HIV infection and the spread of AIDS and that the commitment to support drug treatment programs will be continued, they have been more willing to give their support. Essentially, their objections are less grounded in moral arguments than in political and practical ones.

The African American church has a long history of addressing the health and human service needs of its members. Awareness of the mounting toll of deaths within a particular community and the need for drastic action to counter the trend, therefore, has sometimes overridden community objections that were at least partly founded in moral and religious views. Some African American church leaders, like Dr. Calvin O. Butts in New York City, have stated that they would not oppose distributing clean needles (Shipp and Navarro, 1991). Butts stated (as cited in Elovich and Sorge, 1991:168):

I'm one who spoke out very harshly against the distribution of condoms and the distribution of needles saying that it's cooperation with evil but sometimes I think that God can mean what people think is evil for good. And if it's going to save lives and it's going to allow for an arresting of this disease in our community . . . then I think that these measures are not bad measures and a lot of us are going to have to think real hard about how we oppose things that could stop this disease. In drastic times, you have to take drastic actions.

African American mayors of several large cities—such as New York, Baltimore, New Haven, and Washington, D.C.—have supported needle exchange programs. It should be noted that a good number of African American clergy are also politicians. The church plays and will continue to play a pivotal role in policy debates and legislative action concerning these issues. According to Billingsley and Caldwell (1991), 84 percent of African American adults consider themselves to be religious, and almost 70 percent are members of a church. Lincoln and Mamiya (1990) estimated African American church membership at 24 million. Since 65,000 to 75,000 African American churches of various denominations exist in the United States, it is certainly possible that a wider diversity of opinion exists than has been apparent to date. Findings from the Black Election Study demonstrated that churches were a vehicle for political mobilization and that "exposure to political information in a church setting is highly correlated with church based campaign activism" (Brown, 1991:255).

LATINO/HISPANIC VIEWS

The Latino/Hispanic population in this country is extraordinarily diverse and comprises a number of groups that differ significantly from one another (e.g., Cubans, Mexicans, Puerto Ricans). The panel's limited assessment of potential concerns within the Latino/Hispanic populations did not reveal any organized opposition to needle exchange programs from these communities. On the contrary, some individual community leaders, political figures, and health care providers have been instrumental in their advocacy of needle exchange programs.

First, second, and third generations of Dominicans, Puerto Ricans, Cubans, Mexicans, and new immigrants from Central America constitute a far more complex cultural web than the term *Latino community* implies. There is no single voice, nor is there a single cultural response. Nonetheless, it is worth noting that almost all of the legal needle exchange programs in New York City are located in Latino/Hispanic neighborhoods, largely due to the advocacy of Yolanda Serrano, a Puerto Rican community worker who served as executive director of the Association for Drug Abuse Prevention and Treatment.

In a recent press release, Latino elected officials, Latino clergy, and the Latino Commission on AIDS called on the Governor of New York and the Mayor of New York City to provide funding for the expansion of needle exchange programs (Latino Commission on AIDS, 1994). Several Latino leaders have confirmed their support for the message of that press release; they include (but are not limited to) members of Congress Jose Serrano and Nydia Velasquez; Assembly members Vito Lopez, Hector Diaz, and Roberto Ramírez; and City Council members Adam Clayton Powell, Guillermo Linares, Lucy Cruz, José Rivera, and Israel Ruiz. Dennis DeLeón, executive director of the Latino Commission on AIDS, stated (Latino Commission on AIDS, 1994:1):

> Considering that HIV infection associated with IV drug use is the common route of transmission of the virus among Latinos and Latinas in New York City, it would be criminal to delay expansion of needle exchange programs. Our lives are at stake.

Latino community members have also urged that, if AIDS prevention programs are to be effective, issues of family and children's safety are critical and require that the programs address sexual and perinatal transmission issues as well as transmission through injection drug users (Rodriguez,

1994). Given the importance of the Roman Catholic Church in Latino/ Hispanic communities, the recent Latino clergy endorsement for expanding needle exchange programs in New York City may contribute to strengthening community support. However, overgeneralization across Latino/Hispanic communities regarding the above finding should be avoided, because much of the information presented reflects primarily the New York City experience, which was highly influenced by Yolanda Serrano, a respected and charismatic community leader.

LAW ENFORCEMENT VIEWS

As is the case with any controversial issue, there is substantial diversity in opinions within a given community, and law enforcement is no exception. Police departments have often been a major source of opposition to needle exchange programs, and many view needle exchange programs as inconsistent with the war declared on drugs. In some cities, such as San Francisco, where police and elected officials have shown support for the establishment of needle exchange programs and agreed to make the enforcement of drug paraphernalia laws against program clients and staff a low priority (e.g., New Haven and Portland), needle exchange participants have reported being harassed or arrested by police officers (Lurie et al., 1993:151; Stryker, 1989). Enforcement of prescription laws may result in police harassment of drug users in some cities, which in turn contributes to needle sharing among injection drug users (see Chapter 5 for further discussion of legal issues).

The police rank and file understandably have practical concerns about the potential presence of more needles. The fear of sustaining a needlestick injury while searching an injection drug user (or his or her residence) is based on the potential danger for a police officer, and the wearing of rubber gloves provides no protection from this risk.

As part of its effort to gather relevant information, the panel invited representatives of diverse communities with a stake in the outcome to participate in a workshop to discuss their views. Among those who briefed the panel were representatives of the Fraternal Order of Police and the California Bureau of Narcotic Enforcement. Their participation provided insight on the views of two distinct law enforcement entities: the street police officer (local police) and the career drug enforcement or undercover state narcotics officer. The remarks of these individuals reflect mutual agreement on many matters pertaining to needle exchange and bleach distribution programs. The expressed main areas of agreement and concerns can be summarized as follows:

• In recent years, law enforcement officers have come to adopt a much broader view of drug addiction; they do not view drug abuse as exclusively a criminal justice issue. Addiction is seen as a health care problem with many negative medical and social consequences. The risk of HIV infection is one of many consequences of injection drug use, and needle exchange programs should be viewed as one strategy that may help reduce that risk. However, these programs should not deflect attention from addressing the underlying causes of addiction. As such, treatment and prevention strategies must be the critical components of any drug abuse policy.

• Within the law enforcement community, the prevailing reaction to needle exchange is negative. The primary reasons for such a reaction are that: (1) police officers understandably have difficulty endorsing something that is illegal, (2) it sends a mixed message and may worsen society's drug problem, and (3) needlesticks to police officers may increase due to an increase in the number of needles in circulation.

• Given that drug addiction is a health issue, the requirement of a prescription to purchase needles and syringes in pharmacies does provide for at least some degree of control. Medical supervision does provide some assurance that the users are properly instructed about how to use these devices.

The following comment by one of the participants illustrates the complexity of the needle exchange issues as perceived by career law enforcement officers:

> When I look at needle exchange, I split it into two sides. One side is a poor public drug abuse policy and the other is a public health care policy that has some merit. So it becomes a war of priorities in terms of which problem is worse, the drug problem or the AIDS problem? I don't feel that needle exchange is good for both of these problems. Being a police officer I cannot support anything illegal, but I also realize that people are dying of AIDS and that is about as serious as you can get. I cannot come out and say that I am absolutely opposed, but I can say I am very concerned about it. Also, there is so much diversity in this country that federally permissive programs will not work unless it is able to be tailored to specific regions. . . . If someone could convince me that legalizing needle exchange programs will not make the drug problem worse, then I could probably move more toward the support side.

Another important issue raised at the workshop was whether prescription and paraphernalia laws are a practical tool for police officers and prosecutors to use to convict drug offenders. These laws are tangential to the problem at hand, which is to prohibit the sale, possession, and use of controlled substances. However, they do provide police officers and prosecutors with another tool for charging drug dealers and users with a criminal offense when there is no direct evidence of a sale, possession, or use of the controlled substance itself. Still, as indicated by one workshop participant, most prosecutor's offices would not view these cases as high priority given the limited resources of the criminal justice system.

Reflecting on the dilemmas presented by legislation in the area of needle exchange and bleach distribution programs, another workshop participant commented:

> If officials pass legislation to legalize needle exchange programs, police personnel will need to be educated before it will be effective.

HEALTH PROFESSIONAL VIEWS

Two groups of health professionals have direct impact on the behavior of injection drug users and, consequently, on the potential effects of needle exchange and bleach distribution programs: pharmacists and providers of drug abuse treatment services. Their perspectives on these programs differ according to their respective interactions with the injection drug user population. Pharmacists play a critical role in the access of injection drug users to injection equipment, whereas drug treatment service providers can have an impact on the drug addiction and associated drug-use risk behaviors of individuals.

In this section, we briefly summarize the views of both of these health professional groups. As was the case with other community groups whose views were sought, no consensus opinion emerged within or across groups on the potential value of these intervention programs or on the respective role each of these groups should play in the implementation of such programs.

Pharmacists

As we discussed in Chapter 1, several studies have shown a meaningful association between sharing injection equipment and increased rates of HIV transmission (Magura et al., 1989; Calsyn et al., 1991; DePhilippis and Metzger, 1993; Selwyn et al., 1987; Feldman and Biernacki, 1988; Donoghoe et al., 1992; Metzger et al., 1991; Murphy, 1987). Monitoring of pharmacy sales in Connecticut by the Centers for Disease Control and Prevention (CDC) has shown that partial revocation of prescription and paraphernalia laws has had a substantial impact on making sterile needles more readily available and has contributed to observable reductions in sharing behavior (Groseclose et al., in press). One important finding of the CDC Connecticut evaluation project highlighted the critical role of pharmacists in facilitating needle availability. The cooperation of these health professionals is crucial to eliminating important barriers to the availability of needles. However, their disposition to cooperate is at issue.

Various surveys of pharmacists and pharmacy owner-managers have been undertaken to assess their attitudes toward over-the-counter sales and pharmacy-based needle exchange programs. However, as noted by the University of California study (Lurie et al., 1993), a limited number of surveys has been conducted in the United States; to date, only one has been published. The New Orleans survey results reveal that a small portion of pharmacists (14.5 percent) indicated that they sold needles to anyone requesting them. The majority of respondents sold needles only to clients who had a valid medical prescription, even though Louisiana has no prescription law (Lawrence et al., 1991).

Other countries (the United Kingdom, France, Belgium, Australia, and Canada) have conducted surveys of pharmacists and pharmacy owner-managers (see Lurie et al., 1993). The results show similar concerns across countries with regard to selling needles over the counter and participating in a pharmacy-based needle exchange program. The main concerns include potential negative effects on business revenues and the quality of overall services provided to other customers. For example, Glanz et al. (1989) reported that pharmacies believed that the presence of injection drug users would adversely affect business (68 percent) and would lead to an increase in theft (63 percent). Similar concerns were raised in surveys in other countries (e.g., in Australia, Tsai et al., 1988). An additional issue raised by the survey respondents relates to the disposal of needles returned to pharmacies. Survey results also indicate that disposal of used needles represents a disincentive for pharmacies to participate in pharmacy-based needle exchange programs.

These concerns were also voiced by two professional pharmaceutical industry representatives at the panel's workshop on community views. They represented the National Association of Chain Drug Stores (pharmacy retailers) and the American Pharmaceutical Association (professional pharmacists).

The representative of pharmacy retailers indicated that, although the retailers support the establishment of needle exchange and bleach distribution programs, their association does not feel that pharmacies are the most appropriate sites. Areas of concern include:

• quality of health care services (i.e., providing advice, education, counseling about medications) to customers other than injection drug users may be adversely affected;
• liability;
• collection and disposal of dirty needles; and
• economic implications.

In clarifying that position, it was stated that, if pharmacies were turned into collection sites for dirty needles by encouraging injection drug users to exchange their needles in drugstores, adverse consequences could result because of reduced quality of services provided to other customers. That is, other customers would not receive the needed medical and prescription-related information they have come to expect. Moreover, the retailer representative pointed out that liability concerns arise from having to adhere to rules and regulations set forth by the Drug Enforcement Agency (DEA), the Environmental Protection Agency (EPA), the Food and Drug Administration (FDA), and the Occupational Safety and Health Administration (OSHA), as well as state and local health departments.

For example, OSHA adopted the blood-borne pathogen standard in December 1991. This consists of a comprehensive set of requirements with which an employer must comply to protect employees from exposure to blood-borne pathogens in the workplace. The standards include, among other things, a workplace evaluation for hazard potential, a written plan for treatment and follow-up, and other record-keeping requirements.

If pharmacies were to serve as exchange sites, employees would be placed at potential risk of occupational exposure to blood-borne pathogens. OSHA standards would require that all staff be properly trained on how to handle the contaminated needles. With regard to the economic implications of having pharmacy-based needle exchange programs, it was noted that the costs associated with complying with federal and state regulations would be substantial. This would not include the potential adverse effect of these programs on profit margins caused by increased thefts.

The representative from the American Pharmaceutical Association, whose membership numbers 40,000 professionals, stated that the association has an official policy statement that supports needle exchange programs as part of a comprehensive approach to HIV infection. This approach also includes outreach, counseling, treatment, and community involvement in decisions about how the program should be implemented. Moreover, it is the association's view that pharmacists are in a unique position as health care professionals in communities to play an important role in prevention efforts by expanding sales of needles, by serving as distribution sites for needle exchange (after the appropriate amendments to state and federal laws are made), or both. The association recognizes that not all pharmacists would be willing to participate in such efforts, but it believes that some would, and that a significant impact could be made even if a small proportion of pharmacies participate.

The discussion that followed the workshop presentations by health care professionals raised important issues regarding the professional discretion of individual pharmacists in the 41 states in which there are no prescription laws to determine whether to sell needles to individual customers. In states

in which it is legal to purchase needles, many pharmacists require a customer to either provide a valid medical prescription or to identify oneself
(e.g., sign a log book), thereby demonstrating that the intended use is for
legitimate medical reasons. In some states, if a pharmacist knowingly sells
needles or syringes to a customer for the purpose of injecting illicit drugs,
that pharmacist can have his or her license suspended.

Moreover, in states in which there are no legal barriers to purchasing
needles, study results have shown that this discretionary decision to sell or
not sell has led to differential access across racial groups. For example,
Compton and colleagues (1992) reported the results of a study in which two
male research assistants (one white, one African American) attempted to
purchase needles in 33 pharmacies in St. Louis. Of the surveyed pharmacies:

- 12 percent refused to sell to both purchasers,
- 12 percent refused to sell to the African American only,
- 18 percent informed study purchasers that they did not sell needles/
  syringes in small quantities, and
- 58 percent sold to both study participants.

The authors reported that the predominant reason given for refusal to sell
was store policy.

A final critical point was raised by a workshop participant regarding the
willingness of pharmacists to sell needles. We should not expect all pharmacists to be willing to sell needles to injection drug users. However, in
communities in which there is a substantial drug abuse and AIDS problem,
pharmacists may be more amenable to selling them.

Treatment Service Providers

For most practitioners in the field of substance abuse treatment, needle
exchange and bleach distribution programs present a dilemma. Support for
such programs is often perceived as a diversion of already unstable funding
away from treatment programs. Their efficacy in lowering the risk of HIV
infection and contributing to the treatment of addiction has been questioned.
Practitioners are concerned that needle exchange and bleach distribution
programs run counter to federal regulations. Many also feel that these
programs may provide a means to continue behavior that is destructive to
the individual, the family, and the community (Primm, 1990).

Drug abuse treatment programs in the United States operate in a constant state of fiscal uncertainty; it is therefore not surprising that support for
needle exchange programs is often perceived as diverting scarce financial
resources away from treatment. Furthermore, many programs are under

pressure to show evidence of their ability to effectively treat drug abuse. Although drug abuse treatment programs are for the most part funded from sources different from those that fund needle exchange and bleach distribution programs, there is concern that the latter will become attractive alternatives to drug abuse treatment because of their relatively low costs. These views have been publicly expressed by members of the treatment community. For example, Primm[1] (1990) states:

> There are some theoretical benefits, of course, in providing sterile needles. It's inexpensive, relative to drug treatment. This is why so many people are embracing it and why public health officials are talking of potential control of HIV transmission as being more important than drug treatment. . . . Needles, syringes, and drugs have been destructive forces.

For some drug treatment professionals and indigenous outreach workers who are attempting to help clients in their struggle to remain drug free, the increased access to needles dispensed by needle exchange programs represents a threat that attention will be diverted from their efforts. The major initial objection of the treatment community to the programs appears to derive from its primary orientation of strict abstinence. Needle exchange programs pose an apparent contradiction to this principal goal of treatment (Wolk et al., 1990). Critics of needle exchange programs indicate that, by implicitly condoning drug use, these programs are sending conflicting messages not only to current injection drug users, but also to those who are at risk of becoming injection drug users (Singer et al., 1991).

At the time of this writing, no empirical study of the views of the drug treatment community on needle exchange and bleach distribution programs has been published. In an attempt to obtain these views, the panel contacted 25 professional and trade associations that represent service providers and asked them to provide any policy or public statements they may have on the issue of concern. Even after mailing a reminder about the original request, the panel received responses from only 13 associations (Table 4.2).

The views of those who responded can be summarized as follows. As shown in the table, of the 13 associations (52 percent) that responded, 61.5 percent support such programs; 38.5 percent have no official or formal position on the issue. A noteworthy observation is that none of the associations that responded indicated that they were against such programs. The official policies of the American Psychiatric Association, the American Public Health Association, the American Society of Addiction Medicine, the National Association of Social Workers, and the National Association of State Alcohol and Drug Abuse Directors are the most detailed (see Appendix B). It should also be noted that both the American Medical Association and the

TABLE 4.2 Views of Professional Associations: Results from a Mail Survey

Association	Responded	Formal Policy or Public Position	Position on Needle Exchange Program	Position on Bleach Distribution
Alcohol and Drug Problems Association of North America	No			
American Academy of Health Care Providers in the Addictive Disorders	No			
The American Academy of Psychiatrists in Alcoholism & Addictions	Yes	Under consideration	Supports[a]	
American Association of Public Health Physicians	No			
American College of Addiction Treatment Administrators	Yes	No		
American Medical Association	Yes	Yes	Supports[a]	Supports[a]
American Psychiatric Association	Yes	Yes	Supports[a]	
American Public Health Association	Yes	Yes	Supports[a]	Supports[a]
American Psychological Association	No			
American Society of Addiction Medicine	Yes	Yes	Supports[a]	Supports[a]
Association of Black Psychologists	No			
Association of Medical Education and Research in Substance Abuse	Yes	Under consideration		

Organization				
Black Psychiatrists of America	No			
Chemical Dependency Treatment Programs Association	Association no longer exists			
Drug and Alcohol Nursing Association	No			
National Association of Addiction Treatment Providers	Yes	No		
National Association of Alcoholism and Drug Abuse Counselors	No			
National Association of Psychiatric Health Systems	Yes	No	Supports[a]	Supports[a]
National Association of Social Workers	Yes	Yes	Supports[a]	Supports[a]
National Association of State Alcohol and Drug Abuse Directors	Yes	Yes	Supports[a]	Supports[a]
National Association of Substance Abuse Trainers and Educators	No			
National Consortium of Chemical Dependency Nurses, Inc.	Yes	No		
National Nurses Society on Addiction	No			
Social Work Administrators in Health Care	No			
Therapeutic Communities of America	No			

NOTE: Response rate: 52 percent.
[a]see Appendix A for detailed description.

American Public Health Association have recently issued a resolution that endorses needle exchange programs.

Treatment issues are complex and have engendered debates among service providers who are dedicated to helping individuals deal with their addictions and who have divergent views about the appropriateness and efficacy of various methods that could be used to accomplish their goal. The panel decided that a more detailed discussion of the views presented above was warranted to more fully explore the underlying issues of concern.

Funding

The worrisome issue of competition for funds seems to derive from the fact that services (both addiction treatment and needle exchange programs) focus on similar targeted individuals. However, the population being served is the only factor in common between needle exchange and bleach distribution programs and treatment programs. The primary focus of the former is to address the transmission of HIV as an immediate priority, whereas the latter attempt to address drug abuse, which places an individual at risk.

Treatment Efficacy

Researchers have found drug treatment to be effective (Rettig and Yarmolinsky, 1995; McLellan et al., 1992; Gerstein and Harwood, 1990; Hubbard et al., 1989). However, there is a strong tendency to think of total and permanent abstinence from drug use as the only sign of successful treatment, when in fact diminution in drug use may in itself be a valuable outcome. Drug-use disorders are a complex group of chronic conditions that vary not only according to the substance or substances abused, but also according to individual factors such as psychiatric comorbidity, heredity, gender, ethnicity, education, and occupation. Different types of patients require different types of treatment modalities (Normand et al., 1994).

Viewing these disorders as acute problems controllable by will power is a fundamental basis of the misperception that treatment is ineffective. Yet, from a medical perspective, drug abuse and dependence are chronic disorders, much like arthritis or diabetes. They develop gradually and have a course characterized by remissions and relapses, although there is often overall progression over time. Treatments reliably produce relief of symptoms and improvements in function, but not cures.

The introduction of methadone treatment in the mid-1960s represents a substantial shift in ideology by certain members of the treatment community. Abstinence was no longer the sole treatment goal; rather, it reflects an approach to treatment that attempts to minimize the negative behavioral consequences of addiction in lieu of abstinence (Gerstein and Harwood, 1990).

This approach appears to go hand in hand with the objective of most needle exchange programs: promote harm reduction while trying to encourage program participants to enter treatment. This is reflected by the evidence presented in Chapter 3 showing that some needle exchange programs are a primary source of referrals for treatment. Moreover, injection drug users with no prior treatment history have sought out treatment services as a result of their contact with needle exchange programs (Christensson and Ljungberg, 1991; Heimer et al., 1993). It would appear that needle exchange programs are serving as a bridge to treatment for a subpopulation of injection drug users for whom traditional treatment recruiting efforts have been unsuccessful.

Treatment programs for injection drug use are for the most part methadone maintenance programs. Evaluation of these programs has shown repeatedly that increased social functioning, reduced drug use, and reduced criminal involvement do follow from methadone maintenance treatment— for those who remain in treatment (Ball and Ross, 1991; Gerstein and Harwood, 1990; Hubbard et al., 1989; McLellan et al., 1993). For patients who leave methadone treatment prematurely, not many appear to maintain these gains. In a study that is considered to be one of the most careful examinations of this phenomenon, over 80 percent of patients relapsed to injection drug use within the 12 months subsequent to their leaving treatment prematurely (Ball and Ross, 1991).

Given the chronic nature of the disorder, these relapses are also to be expected of some who are in treatment. This point is reinforced by the published findings of an ongoing longitudinal study of HIV infection and risk behaviors among 152 injection drug users in treatment and 103 out of treatment: the elevated risk of out-of-treatment injection drug users was clearly evident (Metzger et al., 1993). Continued illicit drug use was reported by a substantial portion of in-treatment participants.

These data and the results of other studies have documented significant reductions in HIV drug-use risk behaviors among in-treatment injection drug users (Ball et al., 1988; Cooper, 1989; Longshore et al., 1993; Novick et al., 1990). Moreover, the reported data from the longitudinal study by Metzger et al. (1993) show that injection drug users who are not in methadone treatment were significantly more likely to become infected than comparable individuals who were enrolled in a methadone treatment program. That is, 4 percent of those who remained in treatment for the first 18 months became infected, compared with 22 percent of those who stayed out of treatment. Although selection bias cannot be excluded, it would seem that not only is methadone treatment effective in treating the disorder of drug abuse but it also reduces HIV risk behaviors (i.e., needle use) and, more importantly, HIV transmission. These data also clearly show that in-treatment injection drug users will continue to inject on occasion. Moreover, other studies have found drug treatment experience (i.e., past history of exposure to treatment) to be related to higher levels of HIV risk behaviors for certain injection drug users (Siegal et al., 1995; Ross et al., 1993; Chitwood and Morningstar, 1985).

Federal Regulations

Few treatment programs in the United States have instituted training on how to effectively decontaminate needles or provide information on how to legally obtain sterile needles. Federal regulations governing some forms of drug abuse treatment also are obstacles to drug treatment providers and their patients to make use of needle exchange and bleach distribution programs.

For example, federal regulations concerning take-home medication for patients receiving methadone therapy [21 CFR, part 291.505 (d) (6) (iv) (B) (1)] require clinicians to consider the "absence of recent abuse of drugs (narcotic and nonnarcotic), including alcohol" in determining whether to grant the privilege of reduced clinic attendance and the provision of doses of methadone (take-home medication) for the days when the patient does not attend the clinic. Consequently, for patients who have relapsed and who may consider using needle exchange and bleach distribution programs to more safely inject drugs, this federal regulation is a disincentive to admit to recent needle exchange and bleach distribution program participation. Such an admission would result in denial or revocation of reduced clinic attendance (or take-home medication) privileges.

In a similar manner, a counselor cannot advise a patient who is receiving or is eligible for take-home medication privileges to continue to abstain from any drug use, while also suggesting participation in needle exchange and bleach distribution programs if drug use does occur. Knowledge of needle exchange and bleach distribution program participation or any other activity that may be indicative of drug use would require—because of federal regulations—drug treatment clinicians to consider denying or revoking the take-home medication status of a patient.

Condoning Drug Use

As we document more fully in Chapter 7, reviews of the empirical data show no evidence to support the charge that needle availability promotes drug use among current or potential users (Schwartz, 1993; Karpen, 1990; Watters et al., 1994; U.S. General Accounting Office, 1993; Lurie and Chen, 1993). Moreover, in considering the current knowledge base on the etiology of drug use, it is not surprising that a single risk factor—availability of sterile needles—does not play a crucial role in increasing drug use or initiating noninjectors to injection drug use. This critical point was noted by the University of California researchers (Lurie and Chen, 1993) when they stated that "initiation into drug use is influenced by many social, psychological, and biological factors—and not by the simple availability of syringes" (p. 23).

Because treatment is neither quickly nor universally effective at eliminating drug use, some injection drug use may occur even if a major expansion of drug treatment programs were implemented (Joseph, 1989). Also, even if treatment were made readily available, not all injection drug users would be interested in participating. Recognizing this, the approach adopted by needle exchange and bleach distribution programs is a pragmatic one. These programs acknowledge that not all addicts demonstrate readiness for treatment, that many who enter treatment will not be completely abstinent, and that, once abstinent, relapse is endemic to chemical dependence.

SUMMARY

As with other sensitive issues, communities cannot be categorized as simply either supporting or opposing needle exchange programs. The range of views is far more complex. Members of minority communities ravaged by the effects of drug abuse and HIV infection have articulated both opposition and support for these programs. Law enforcement personnel have been divided on the concept of these programs. Health professionals have debated extensively the pros and cons of needle exchange and bleach distribution. Public opinion polls reflect division and a trend toward more favorable disposition to accept such programs as the issues are debated.

Table 4.3 summarizes the concerns of the individual community groups solicited by the panel. They range from fears of worsening drug abuse and crime to concern about promoting immoral activities. The reactions of these stakeholders are not mutually exclusive. All share the concern that handing out sterile injection equipment or bleach bottles to injection drug users does not address the underlying problems associated with drug abuse and in fact may create more negative outcomes. In sum, the main argument against needle exchange and bleach distribution programs is based on perceptions that they do more harm than good.

CONCLUSIONS

That community responses to needle exchange and bleach distribution programs have varied considerably, not only across but also within sub-

TABLE 4.3 Community Concerns

Communities	Perceptions and Concerns
Common concerns	• Drug use is illegal and immoral and should not be condoned. • Providing clean needles to drug users is misguided and dangerous. • Programs send a mixed message and may worsen society's drug problem.
Ethnic/racial African American	• Drug abuse epidemic has been consistently neglected and drug treatment programs are either not established or not funded adequately. • Drug abuse problems and crime in urban communities will be worsened by the implementation of programs. • Community leaders are not part of decision making in the establishment of programs within their own communities. • Drugs are deliberately supplied to the black community and these programs promote their continued use. • HIV is a man-made virus and AIDS may be a form of genocide. • Public health authorities cannot be trusted because of past negative experiences, e.g., Tuskegee Syphilis Study, and large segments of the black population are regarded as expendable by the white establishment.
Hispanic	• Complex cultural web in extraordinarily diverse community will require involvement of community leaders for effective implementation of programs. • Sexual practices and mores, particularly gender issues, must be addressed adequately. • Issues of family and safety are critical to the establishment of programs.
Law enforcement	• Drug use is illegal. • Needlesticks to police officers may increase due to an increase in the number of needles in circulation. • Programs should not detract attention from addressing underlying causes of addiction. • Programs must be tailored to needs of specific communities. • Drug abuse problems and crime in urban communities will be worsened by the implementation of programs. • Personnel will need to be better educated about such programs and trained to handle situations that may arise before the programs can be successful. • Question usefulness of prescription and paraphernalia laws.

TABLE 4.3 Continued

Communities	Perceptions and Concerns
Health professionals Pharmacists	• Quality of health care services provided to noninjection drug user customers may suffer. • Subsequent negative effects on revenue. • Liability for occupational exposure of workers and adherence to rules and regulations set forth by DEA, EPA, FDA, and OSHA. • Disposal of used needles/syringes. • Lack or ambiguity of prescription laws. • Personal discretion. • Involvement in the development of site-specific programs is needed. • Education and training are needed.
Treatment service providers	• These programs promote a behavior destructive to the individual, family, and community. • Funding will be diverted from treatment. • Public and professional misperceptions about lack of efficacy of treatment. • Disincentive to participate in programs because of federal regulations dealing with drug treatment and degrees of drug use. • Largely strict abstinence orientation poses apparent contradiction to programs allowing the continuation of drug use.

groups and over time, is the major conclusion of this chapter. Many of their concerns stem from the view that needle exchange and bleach distribution programs are limited to one type of activity: the exchange or distribution of drug paraphernalia to injection drug users. It is therefore possible that programs taking a comprehensive approach could respond to some of this community opposition. Such an approach would include an overall strategy to improve the delivery of health services, including drug treatment services and social services, that address other important needs. It would also include an open public approach that clarifies the concept and explains the multifaceted and multilevel components of needle exchange and bleach distribution programs.

Focusing on the impact of needle exchange and bleach distribution programs on levels of drug abuse has been central to the discussions of these programs. This underlying focus has generated a multitude of hypotheses about their possible harmful effects. It is critically important to articulate these issues, reformulated as hypotheses, in the process of considering the program effects and operationalizing them in such a way as to steer carefully between the conflicting objectives of the campaigns against the two epidemics of drug abuse and HIV.

For example, when proponents of needle distribution argue that repeal of paraphernalia laws is more important than instituting discrete needle exchange programs because pharmacies are more plentiful, have more convenient hours, and cost less to operate, community concerns need to be acknowledged. Citizen groups and police are concerned about an increase in discarded needles and accidental needlesticks. Pharmacists are concerned about the impact on their other customers if they expand business to serve injection drug users. Public opinion polls are less supportive of needle distribution than they are of needle exchange. This combination of community views suggests that needle exchange, with the systematic collection of contaminated needles, is more palatable than outright needle distribution programs.

Another observation that arises from this chapter is that community support has built gradually for needle exchange and bleach distribution programs. Repeat surveys over time in a single geographic location are consistent in showing an increase in the proportion of respondents who react favorably toward needle exchange and bleach distribution programs. The most recent surveys in Baltimore and the state of Maryland show that a majority favors needle exchange. Similarly, quotes from politicians, drug abuse treatment providers, and African American clergy reflect a change in attitude over time. The change reflects the growing discussion of needle exchange and bleach distribution programs as part of a campaign aimed at stemming the epidemic of parenteral transmission of HIV infection—rather than as an incongruous initiative amidst a broader campaign aimed at drug abuse.

As community concerns are recognized and addressed, the concept of needle exchange and bleach distribution programs is refined. Initial constraints placed by communities on needle exchange programs in New York City and Washington, D.C. (as described in Chapter 3) resulted in programs that were universally recognized as ineffective. With continued dialogue and progressive iterations of balancing community concerns, the concept of needle exchange and bleach distribution programs continues to evolve.

When needle exchange and bleach distribution services are viewed as one of many components of a comprehensive strategy against HIV, a reduction in resistance and broader coalitions for these programs can be expected to follow. At the same time, efforts to develop comprehensive programs must recognize that change or expansion of needle exchange and bleach distribution programs must be combined with significant attention to long-term societal impacts (e.g., on community-level drug use). Failure to include community members in the decision-making process about the implementation of these programs can fan the flames of fear and distrust within the community (Thomas and Quinn, 1993).

NOTE

1. Dr. Primm has reversed his original position of opposing needle exchange programs and has stated publicly that he now supports them (Primm, 1995).

REFERENCES

The Arizona Republic
1993   Poll on AIDS Concerns, January 21.
Ball, J.C., and A. Ross
1991   The Effectiveness of Methadone Maintenance Treatment. New York, NY: Springer-Verlag.
Ball, J.C., W.R. Lange, C.P. Myers, and S.R. Friedman
1988   Reducing the risk of AIDS through methadone maintenance treatment. Journal of Health and Social Behavior 29:214-226.
Bannon Research
1990   Massachusetts Telephone Survey, Politics Poll "Media #6" (unpublished material), February 19.
Bates, K.
1990   AIDS: Is it genocide? Essence 21:77-116.
Belgrave, F.Z., and S.M. Randolph, eds.
1993   Psychosocial aspects of AIDS prevention among African Americans. Special issue of The Journal of Black Psychology 19(2) May.
Billingsley, A., and C. Caldwell
1991   The church, the family, and the school in the African American community. Journal of Negro Education 60:427-440.
Brettle, R.
1990   HIV and harm reduction for injection drug users. AIDS 5:125-136.
Brown, R.
1991   Political action. In Life in Black America, J. Jackson, ed. Newbury Park, CA: Sage Publications.
Brunswick, A.
1991   Longitudinal Harlem Health Study, NIDA Research Grant R01-DA05142 (unpublished material), April.
Calsyn, D.A., A.J. Saxon, G. Freeman, and S. Whittaker
1991   Needle-use practices among intravenous drug users in an area where needle purchase is legal. AIDS 5:187-193.
Center for Substance Abuse Research
1994   Needle Exchange Programs Supported by a Majority of Marylanders. CESAR FAX 3(28): July 25 (Weekly FAX from the Center for Substance Abuse Research, University of Maryland, College Park).
Chitwood, D.D., and P.C. Morningstar
1985   Factors which differentiate cocaine users in treatment from nontreatment users. The International Journal of the Addictions 20:449-459.

Christensson, B., and B. Ljungberg
    1991   Syringe exchange for prevention of HIV infection in Sweden: Practical experi-
            ences and community reactions. *The International Journal of the Addictions* 26(12):1293-
            1302.
Compton III, W.M., L.B. Cottler, S.H. Decker, D. Mager, and R. Stringfellow
    1992   Legal needle buying in St. Louis. *American Journal of Public Health* 82(4):595-
            596.
Cooper. J.R.
    1989   Methadone treatment and acquired immunodeficiency syndrome. *Journal of the
            American Medical Association* 262:1664-1668.
Dalton, H.
    1989   AIDS in blackface. *Daedalus: Journal of the American Academy of Arts and
            Sciences* 118:205-228.
de Ligorio, A.M.
    1907   *Theologia Moralis.* Lib. III, Tract V De Septimo praecepto decalogi. No. 565 (ex
            typographia). Vaticana, Romeae.
DePhilippis, D., and D.S. Metzger
    1993   Needle Acquisition Difficulty Is Associated with Needle-Sharing Not Drug Use.
            Presentation at the Conference of the American Psychological Society, Chicago.
Donoghoe, M.C., K.A. Dolan, and G.V. Stimson
    1992   Life-style factors and social circumstances of syringe sharing in injecting drug
            users. *British Journal of Addiction* 87:993-1003.
Ellis-Hagler, E.
    1993   Community Perspectives on Needle Availability. Speech delivered before the
            Dimensions of HIV Prevention: Needle Exchange Forum, Henry J. Kaiser Family
            Foundation.
Elovich, R., and R. Sorge
    1991   Toward a community-based needle exchange for New York City. *AIDS and Pub-
            lic Policy Journal* 6:165-174.
Eskenazi, S.
    1989   Poll gives support to needle exchange. *News Tribune*, February 6.
Feldman, H.W., and P. Biernacki
    1988   The ethnography of needle sharing among intravenous drug users and implications
            for public policies and intervention strategies. Pp. 28-39 in *Needle Sharing Among
            Intravenous Drug Abusers: National and International Perspectives*, R.J. Battjes
            and R.W. Pickens, eds. Rockville, MD: National Institute on Drug Abuse.
Fuller, J.D.
    1993   Reflections of a Clinical Bystander. Plenary presentation for the 3rd North Ameri-
            can Syringe Exchange Convention, Boston, MA.
Gerstein, D.R., and H.J. Harwood, eds.
    1990   *Treating Drug Problems, Volume 1: A Study of the Evolution, Effectiveness, and
            Financing of Public and Private Drug Treatment Systems.* Washington, DC: Na-
            tional Academy Press.
Glanz, A., C. Byrne, and P. Jackson
    1989   Role of community pharmacies in prevention of AIDS among injecting drug misusers:
            Findings of a survey in England and Wales. *British Medical Journal* 299:1076-
            1079.
Groseclose, S.L., B. Weinstein, T.S. Jones, L.A. Valleroy, L.J. Fehrs, and W.J. Kassler
    in press Impact of increased legal access to needles and syringes on practices of injecting-
            drug users and police officers—Connecticut, 1992-1993. *Journal of Acquired
            Immune Deficiency Syndromes.*

Hart, P.D.
1994   Memorandum: Survey Among 1,001 Americans to Explore Attitudes Toward the
          Drug Problem and Drug Policy. Peter D. Hart Research Associates, Inc., Wash-
          ington, D.C.
Heimer, R., E.H. Kaplan, K. Khoshnood, B. Jariwala, and E.D. Cadman
1993   Needle exchange decreases the prevalence of HIV-1 proviral DNA in returned
          syringes in New Haven, Connecticut. *American Journal of Medicine* 95(2):214-
          220.
Hollander, Cohen, McBride Associates
1985   Maryland Telephone Survey (unpublished material), November.
Hubbard, R.L., M.E. Marsden, J.V. Rachal, H.J. Harwood, E.R. Cavanaugh, and H.M. Ginzburg
1989   *Drug Abuse Treatment: A National Study of Effectiveness.* Chapel Hill, NC:
          University of North Carolina Press.
Jakobovits, I.
1959   Pp. 45-58 in *Jewish Medical Ethics.* New York, NY: Block Publishing Company.
Jones, J.
1981   *Bad Blood: The Tuskegee Syphilis Experiment—A Tragedy of Race and Medicine.*
          New York, NY: The Free Press.
Joseph, S.C.
1989   A bridge to treatment: The needle exchange pilot program in New York City.
          AIDS Education and Prevention 1:340-345.
Karpen, M.
1990   A comprehensive world overview of needle exchange programs. *AIDS Patient
          Care* 4:26-28.
Kirp, D.L., and R. Bayer
1993   AIDS and race. *Atlantic* July:38-39 and 40.
Latino Commission on AIDS
1994   Press Release, December 19.
Lavrakas, P.J.
1990   Chicagoans' Knowledge About and Attitudes Towards AIDS. Northwestern Uni-
          versity Survey Laboratory, March.
Lawrence, M., W. Atkinson, G. Risi, and A. Lauro
1991   Needle-sharing among intravenous drug users in New Orleans. *Journal of the
          Louisiana State Medical Society* 143:18-21.
Lincoln, C., and L. Mamiya
1990   *The Black Church in the African American Experience.* Durham, NC: Duke
          University Press.
Longshore, D., S. Hsieh, B. Danila, and M.D. Anglin
1993   Methadone maintenance and needle/syringe sharing. *The International Journal of
          the Addictions* 28:983-996.
Lurie, P., and D. Chen
1993   A review of programs in North America. Pp. 11-34 in *Dimensions of HIV Preven-
          tion: Needle Exchange,* J. Stryker and M.D. Smith, eds. Menlo Park, CA: The
          Henry J. Kaiser Family Foundation.
Lurie, P., A.L. Reingold, B. Bowser, D. Chen, J. Foley, J. Guydish, J.G. Kahn, S. Lane, J.
Sorensen, P. DeCarlo, N. Harris, and T.S. Jones
1993   *The Public Health Impact of Needle Exchange Programs in the United States and
          Abroad: Volume 1.* San Francisco, CA: University of California.
Magura, S., J.I. Grossman, D.S. Lipton, et al.
1989   Determinants of needle sharing among intravenous drug users. *American Journal
          of Public Health* 79:459-462.

Malone, C.
    1994   Presentation at informal workshop convened by the Panel on Needle Exchange and
                Bleach Distribution Programs, Irvine, California, January 5.
McLellan, A.T., D. Metzger, A.I. Alterman, J. Cornish, and H. Urschel
    1992   How effective is substance abuse treatment? Compared to what? In *Advances in
                Understanding the Addictive States*, C.P. O'Brien and J. Jaffe, eds. New York,
                NY: Raven Press.
McLellan, A.T., A.I. Alterman, G.E. Woody, and D. Metzger
    1993   Are psychosocial services necessary in substance abuse treatment? A dose-rang-
                ing study of psychosocial services. *Journal of the American Medical Association*
                296:1953-1959.
Media General/Associated Press
    1989   National Telephone Survey (unpublished material), May 13.
Metzger, D., and D. DePhilippis
    1994   Treatment Community Views on Needle Exchange and Bleach Distribution Pro-
                grams. Paper commissioned by the Panel on Needle Exchange and Bleach Distri-
                bution Programs, National Research Council and Institute of Medicine.
Metzger, D., G. Woody, D. DePhilippis, T. McLellan, C.P. O'Brien, and J.J. Platt
    1991   Risk factors for needle sharing among methadone treated patients. *American Journal
                of Psychiatry* 148:636-640.
Metzger, D.S., G.E. Woody, A.T. McLellan, C.P. O'Brien, P. Druley, H. Navaline, D. DePhilippis,
P. Stolley, and E. Abrutyn
    1993   Human immunodeficiency virus seroconversion among in- and out-of-treatment
                intravenous drug users: An 18-month prospective follow-up. *Journal of Acquired
                Immune Deficiency Syndromes* 6:1049-1056.
Murphy, S.
    1987   Intravenous drug use and AIDS: Notes on the social economy of needle sharing.
                Contemporary Drug Problems Fall:373-395.
Newsday
    1989   New York City Telephone Survey (unpublished material), February 19.
Normand, J., R.O. Lempert, and C.P. O'Brien, eds.
    1994   *Under the Influence? Drugs and the American Work Force*. Washington, DC:
                National Academy Press.
Northeast Research
    1989   Connecticut Telephone Survey (unpublished material), May.
Novick, D.M., H. Joseph, T.S. Croxson, E.A. Salsitz, G. Wang, B.L. Richman, L. Poretsky,
J.B. Keefe, and E. Whimbey
    1990   Absence of antibody to human immunodeficiency virus in long-term, socially re-
                habilitated methadone maintenance patients. *Archives of Internal Medicine* 150(1):97-
                99.
O'Brien, M.
    1989   Needle exchange programs: Ethical and policy issues. *AIDS Public Policy Jour-
                nal* 4:75-82.
Office of National Drug Control Policy
    1992   Needle exchange programs: Are they effective? *ONDCP Bulletin No. 7*. Wash-
                ington, DC: Executive Office of the President.
Pellegrino, E.D.
    1990   Ethics. *Journal of the American Medical Association* 263(19):2641-2642.
Primm, B.
    1990   Needle exchange programs do not solve the problem of HIV transmission. *AIDS
                Patient Care* August:18-20.

1995   Speech delivered before the Sterile Needle Conference, The Johns Hopkins University, Baltimore, Maryland, February 15-16.

Rettig, R.A., and A. Yarmolinsky, eds.
1995   *Federal Regulation of Methadone Treatment.* Washington, DC: National Academy Press.

Rodriguez, S.
1994   Presentation at informal workshop convened by the Panel on Needle Exchange and Bleach Distribution Programs, Irvine, California, January 5.

The Roper Center for Public Opinion Research
1987   Connecticut Telephone Survey (unpublished material), May.

Ross, M.W., A. Stowe, A. Wodak, M.E. Miller, and J. Gold
1993   A comparison of drug use and HIV infection risk behavior between injecting drug users currently in treatment, previously in treatment, and never in treatment. *Journal of Acquired Immune Deficiency Syndromes* 6:518-528.

Schwartz, R.H.
1993   Syringe and needle exchange programs: Part I. *Southern Medical Journal* 254:614-617.

Selwyn, P.A., C Feiner, C.P. Cox, C. Lipshutz, and R.L. Cohen
1987   Knowledge about AIDS and high-risk behavior among intravenous drug users in New York City. *AIDS* 1:247-254.

Shipp, E., and M. Navarro
1991   Reluctantly, Black churches confront AIDS. *New York Times*, November 18.

Siegal, H.A., R.G. Carlson, R.S. Falck, and J. Wang
1995   Drug abuse treatment experience and HIV risk behaviors among active drug injectors in Ohio. *American Journal of Public Health* 85(1):105-108.

Singer, M., R. Irizarry, and J.J. Schensul
1991   Needle access as an AIDS prevention strategy for IV drug users: A research perspective. *Human Organization* 50(2):142-153.

Stryker, J.
1989   IV drug use and AIDS: Public policies and dirty needles. *Journal of Health Policy, Politics and Law* 14:719-740.

Talmey-Drake Research Strategy, Inc.
1991   Denver Telephone Survey (unpublished material), June.

Thomas, S.B., and S.C. Quinn
1991   The Tuskegee Syphilis Study, 1932 to 1972: Implications for HIV education and AIDS risk education programs in the Black community. *American Journal of Public Health* 81(11):1498-1505.

1993   The burdens of race and history on Black Americans' attitudes toward needle exchange policy to prevent HIV disease. *Journal of Public Health Policy* Autumn:320-347.

1994   Community Response to the Implementation of Needle Exchange and Bleach Distribution Programs. Paper commissioned by the Panel on Needle Exchange and Bleach Distribution Programs.

Tsai, R., E.H. Hog, P. Webeck, and J. Mullins
1988   Prevention of human immunodeficiency virus infection among intravenous drug users in New South Wales, Australia: The needles and syringes distribution programme through retail pharmacies. *Asia-Pacific Journal of Public Health* 2:245-251.

University of Utah
1989   Utah Telephone Survey (unpublished material). Survey Research Center, May.

U.S. General Accounting Office
1993   *Needle Exchange Programs: Research Suggests Promise as an AIDS Prevention Strategy.* Washington, DC: U.S. Government Printing Office.

Washington State Department of Health
   1991   *General Population KAP Survey Report*, October. HIV/AIDS Program.
Watters, J.K., M.J. Estilo, G.L. Clark, and J. Lorvick
   1994   Syringe and needle exchange as HIV/AIDS prevention for injection drug users. *Journal of the American Medical Association* 271(2):115-120.
Weiner, T.
   1993   Anti-drug unit of C.I.A. sent ton of cocaine to U.S. in 1990. *New York Times*, November 20, p. 1.
Wolk, J., A. Wodak, J.J. Guinan, P. Macaskill, and J.M. Simpson
   1990   The effect of a needle and syringe exchange on a methadone maintenance unit. *British Journal of Addiction* 85:1445-1450.

5

The Legal Environment

This chapter considers the effects on needle-sharing behavior among injection drug users that arise from various legal structures. We begin with a brief historical review of U.S. drug control policies to provide a better understanding of why various legislative bodies of government (federal, state, and local) have enacted laws that directly contribute to the scarcity of injection equipment.

U.S. DRUG CONTROL POLICY

The involvement of the U.S. government in matters of drug control policy has gone through various distinct phases during this century (Courtwright, 1992). As with other individual behaviors that deviate from the social norms of the time and are perceived by most as threatening the well-being of the majority, the breadth of government interventions has varied with the perceived magnitude of the problem. The perceived magnitude of the drug abuse problem in the United States is not driven exclusively by the incidence or prevalence of drug use, but is closely tied to the demographics and behavioral characteristics of the drug-using population.

Early in this century, the federal government became progressively more involved through a series of laws and judicial rulings that criminalized and regulated nonmedical drug use. The 1906 Pure Food and Drug Act helped slow the spread of medical addictions, which resulted mainly from the liberal narcotic prescription practices of physicians at the time. The Harrison

Narcotic Act of 1914, which regulated the sale, distribution, and possession of narcotics, was later strengthened by the Narcotic Drug Import and Export Act of 1922.

As discussed by Courtwright (1992), the period from the 1920s through the mid-1960s was characterized by a rigid, strict, and punitive approach toward dealers and users. The drug control policy of that era was, in many ways, a reflection of the drug addiction philosophy of Harry Jacob Anslinger, who was commissioner of the Bureau of Narcotics from its creation in 1930 until 1962. It was during this period that various states passed legislation to regulate the sale, distribution, and possession of drug paraphernalia (Pascal, 1988). These statutes generally prohibited the possession of any paraphernalia intended for the use of any narcotic drugs, and some required a prescription for the purchase of syringes. The primary difference between these two types of laws was that paraphernalia laws required a demonstration of criminal intent, whereas prescription laws did not—a distinction that still is reflected in the latest versions of those statutes.

The mid-1960s through late 1970s were characterized by a relaxation of the strict policing of the drug user and the pursuit of new treatment avenues (e.g., methadone maintenance). During the Reagan and Bush administrations, there was a resurgence of the strict law enforcement approach to drug control strategy, with a strong emphasis on supply reduction rather than demand reduction. The get-tough approach of the time is evident from the language contained in two antidrug bills (1986 and 1988) passed by Congress, which contained substantial civil penalties for personal use and possession. Public statements from Robert Martinez, President Bush's director of the Office of National Drug Control Policy, also reflect the strict and punitive approach of that administration (Office of National Drug Control Policy, 1992).

Although this nation has gone through different periods of government involvement and control over drug use, the dominant approach during the twentieth century clearly has been that of restrictive drug control policies, which has resulted in a substantial number of federal, state, and local laws that attempt to restrict the sale, distribution, and possession of drugs. Moreover, in their attempt to regulate and curtail illicit drug use, legislators have enacted statutes whose goals are to restrict indirectly the use of illicit drugs. That is, they have passed criminal laws restricting the sale, distribution, and possession of drug paraphernalia.

The primary intent of these criminal laws seems to have been to impact drug use by restricting and limiting the purchase of drug instrumentation and devices that facilitate drug use itself. For example, concerns regarding the sale of marijuana and other cannabinoids paraphernalia in "head shops" led to the enactment of many local and state drug paraphernalia laws (American Civil Liberties Union, 1994). An obvious secondary intent was to prevent merchants from profiting from the drug trade. It would seem that the underlying premise or rationale for the forceful involvement in drug control by governments is to protect the health and well-being of members of society by engaging police power to eliminate the drug trade and to free society from the negative health consequences and deviant behaviors that have been associated with drug abuse.

At the core of U.S. drug control policy is the belief that a scarcity of drugs and drug paraphernalia, coupled with harsh punishments for dealers and users, will cause a reduction in drug abuse and undesirable behaviors that are often tied to such drug abuse. (For a detailed treatment and analysis of the history of drug policy in the United States, the reader is referred to the following publications: Courtwright, 1982, 1992; Morgan, 1981; Musto, 1987, 1991; and Reuter, 1992.)

Legislative/Statutory Environment

Two categories of laws have been enacted that directly impact the availability of sterile syringes and other injection drug use paraphernalia: *drug paraphernalia laws* and *prescription laws.*

Drug paraphernalia laws prohibit the manufacture, sale, distribution, and possession of equipment and materials intended for use with narcotics (Gostin, 1993). Under these laws, over-the-counter sale of hypodermic syringes and needles is technically allowed. A valid medical prescription for the purchase of syringes or needles is not required. In 45 states and the District of Columbia (see Figure 5.1) such laws are in effect (Valleroy et al., in press). The most recent versions of these state and local laws (late 1970s and early 1980s) are based on the Model Drug Paraphernalia Act (art. 2), which was formulated by the Drug Enforcement Administration in 1979 as an amendment to the Uniform Controlled Substances Act (9 U.L.A., Part II, 1988). Under that model act, drug paraphernalia are broadly defined and specifically include hypodermic syringes, needles, and other objects used to inject controlled substances into the body.

In the midst of the AIDS epidemic, the federal government enacted a federal statute to further limit the sale, distribution, and possession of drug paraphernalia. In 1986, the federal government joined the regulation and control arena of drug paraphernalia by enacting the Mail Order Drug Paraphernalia Control Act (21 U.S.C. § 857, 1986) as section 1821-1823 of the Anti-Drug Paraphernalia Act (P.L. 99-570). This statute encompasses any activity involving drug paraphernalia (broadly defined) crossing interstate lines. The significance of this act is that it establishes federal jurisdiction over matters regulating drug paraphernalia that, until then, had been the territory of state and local governments.

Prescription laws are distinctly different from drug paraphernalia laws.

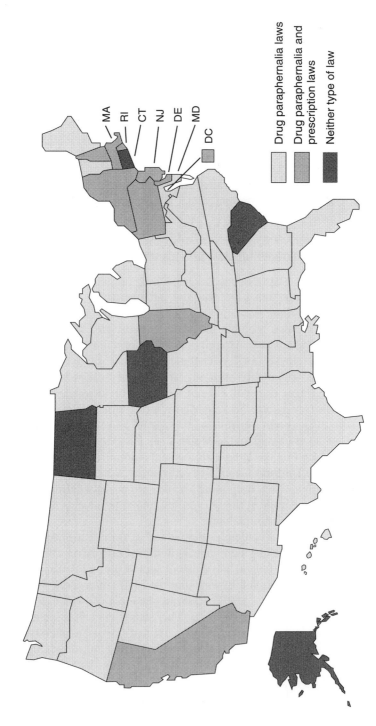

FIGURE 5.1 Drug paraphernalia and prescription laws by state. SOURCE: Valleroy et al., in press:Figure 1.

In contrast with paraphernalia laws, prescription laws do prohibit the sale, distribution, and possession of hypodermic syringes or needles without a valid medical prescription regardless of knowledge of intended use. Prescription laws are in effect in nine states (see Figure 5.1), the District of Columbia (Valleroy et al., in press), and Puerto Rico. (The nine states are California, Delaware, Illinois, Massachusetts, New Hampshire, New Jersey, New York, Pennsylvania, and Rhode Island.) In those jurisdictions, it is a criminal offense to sell or possess syringes or needles without a valid medical prescription. Connecticut and Maine have recently modified their prescription laws to allow syringes and needles to be sold over the counter. Typical prescription statutes also attempt to set certain limitations on the physician's discretion to dispense such valid prescriptions. That is, not only do these statutes require a valid medical prescription, but they also place some legal constraints on physicians by requiring that prescriptions be issued only in cases with a legitimate medical purpose (Gostin, 1993). As depicted in Figure 5.1, all states with prescription laws also have paraphernalia laws, and only five states (i.e., Alaska, Connecticut, Iowa, North Dakota, and South Carolina) have laws permitting both the purchase and the possession of syringes without a medical prescription.

Judicial Rulings

Constitutionality

In examining legislation pertaining to the regulation of drug paraphernalia, an important consideration is the recognized broad authority of the states to regulate the manufacture, sale, prescription, and use of drugs by exercising their police powers. The constitutionality of this broad authority has been acknowledged by the Supreme Court as far back as 1921 (Minnesota ex re. Whipple v. Martinson, 256 U.S. 41) and was reiterated by the Court in more recent cases (Robinson v. State of California, 1962). Moreover, in subsequent years, unsuccessful challenges to the authority of state and local laws to regulate drug paraphernalia (in contrast to drug use itself) have been made (Wheeler v. United States, 276 A.2d 722, D.C.1971; Village of Hoffman Estates v. Flipside, Hoffman Estates, Inc., 455 U.S. 489, reh'g denied, 456 U.S. 950, 1982). In these cases, the Supreme Court has made it clear that state and local government authority to enact laws aimed at controlling drug use also extends to their authority to control the instruments of drug use. Thus, state and local government authority to restrict individuals from manufacturing, selling, or using drug paraphernalia appears to be on firm constitutional footing.

The prescription laws have also withstood constitutional challenges (People v. Bellfield, 33 Misc. 2d 712, 230 N.Y.S.2d 79 [1961], aff'd, 11 N.Y.2d

947, 183 N.E.2d 230 [1962]). Moreover, the Federal Mail Order Paraphernalia Act of 1986 has also survived constitutional scrutiny (United States v. Main Street Distributing Inc., 700 F. Supp. 655, E.D.N.Y., 1988).

State and Local Litigation

Needle exchange programs have operated in what may fairly be called ambiguous legal circumstances. Arrests are sometimes made. Most prosecutions to date have involved needle exchange workers arrested for violating state or local drug paraphernalia or prescription laws (see American Civil Liberties Union, 1994, for a list of recent cases). The *necessity defense* has been the strategy most frequently used by attorneys arguing these cases. This defense strategy rests on the legal doctrine that an individual should not be held liable for an offense if the individual has engaged in a criminal activity in order to avoid a greater imminent harm, that is, to save lives (i.e., by preventing HIV transmission). Although this defense has been used repeatedly and successfully to obtain acquittals in the courts, it has serious limitations. For example, such favorable decisions:

• do not create any legal or judicial precedent for future cases—for example, an individual could be required to stand trial following an acquittal if he or she is arrested for repeating criminal actions subsequent to the earlier trial;

• can be invoked only in situations that satisfy stringent criteria (e.g., no adequate alternative to avert the harm was available; see Gostin, 1993:53); and

• may not be a viable defense for the clients of needle exchange programs, i.e., injection drug users.

The authority of public health officials to sanction needle exchange programs has sometimes been challenged. Many cities and states have provisions in their public health codes that may under certain circumstances allow public health laws to take precedence over criminal laws to protect community health. (In a critical judicial opinion, the Washington Supreme Court unanimously declared that in the narrow circumstances of the case, the State of Washington's needle exchange program was lawful.)

When legal exemptions are granted under the general public health authority, regulations and reporting requirements may be imposed, limiting the ability of program staff to adapt their services to the needs of their clients (e.g., spending time labeling needles, limiting the number of syringes exchanged per visit). Specific examples of regulations that may run counter to the intended service provisions of programs are provided in the original New York City and Washington, D.C., case studies presented in Chapter 3.

For a more detailed discussion of the legal environment surrounding needle exchange programs, the reader is referred to the following publications: Gostin (1991a, 1991b, 1993) and Pascal (1988).

DO PARAPHERNALIA AND PRESCRIPTION LAWS CONTRIBUTE TO HIV TRANSMISSION?

Contaminated needles and syringes are a primary mechanism for transmitting HIV among injection drug users. According to some researchers, "it would be difficult to design a system better suited to promote the transmission of a blood-borne infection" (Friedland and Klein, 1987). The causal role of sharing[1] used injection equipment in transmitting diseases has been well documented for some time (Brecher, 1941; Louria, 1967; Cherubin, 1967; Centers for Disease Control and Prevention, 1993) and for a variety of blood-borne diseases, such as hepatitis and bacterial endocarditis (Selwyn and Alcabes, 1994). Sharing contaminated injection equipment has also been shown to be the primary mechanism of HIV transmission among injection drug users (Chaisson et al., 1987; Chitwood et. al., 1990; Marmor et al., 1987; Schoenbaum et al., 1989; Friedland et al., 1985; Vlahov et al., 1990).

Given the clear risk of transmission of HIV infection when used drug equipment is shared, why do injection drug users engage in this activity? Various investigators have attempted to shed light on that important question. The sharing of drug paraphernalia is a dynamic behavioral process that is a function of multiple factors and their interactions:

- demographic factors, such as age, gender, maturity of drug career, and treatment history;
- paraphernalia availability, both in the community at large and at the time of injection;
- perception of risk of arrest and of HIV infection and other diseases;
- situational/contextual variables, such as the use of shooting galleries;
- group norms and social networks, involving the cohesion of groups; and
- drug of choice (e.g., cocaine, heroin, amphetamine, polydrug use), which is also related to intensity of use (i.e., frequency of injection).

Needle Scarcity and Sharing

Early reports focused on the psychological and cultural factors involved in sharing (e.g., Des Jarlais et al., 1986; Howard and Borges, 1972), often describing the sharing activity as a ritual engaged in by injection drug users to bond with each other. However, with the emergence of AIDS, several ethnographers have reexamined the relative importance of such factors in relation to other more pragmatic factors, such as needle scarcity (Carlson, 1991; Kane and Mason, 1992; Koester, 1992). For example, researchers have established that legal restrictions play an important role in the scarcity of needles and syringes within the injection drug user community (Des Jarlais and Friedman, 1992; Feldman and Biernacki, 1988; Koester, 1989; Murphy, 1987). These findings are consistent with empirical findings of a large-scale longitudinal study (Mandell et al., 1994). An analysis of baseline data on 2,524 injection drug users indicates that sharing behavior is related to economic and legal considerations as well as to the frequency of injection and drug class.

Koester (1994) recently provided a detailed description and explanation of how the scarcity of sterile needles caused by these legal constraints has contributed to the sizable amount of sharing among injection drug users. At first glance, it would appear that, given the misdemeanor offenses associated with conviction on paraphernalia possession in many states, such convictions would not constitute a serious deterrent to having injection drug users purchase sterile needles from pharmacies (it is legal to purchase them without a prescription in most states) to ensure that they have access to sterile equipment when they need to inject drugs. Koester's data indicate that most of his study participants did, in fact, frequently purchase needles from pharmacies. Nonetheless, these same individuals also stated that the imminent fear of arrest for possession of paraphernalia (which deterred them from carrying sterile needles) was greater than the distant threat of AIDS. Several researchers have reported that knowledge about the risk of infection associated with sharing is insufficient to affect behavior change (Inciardi, 1990; Friedman et al., 1992; Page et al., 1990a). In a study of out-of-treatment injection drug users (Celentano et al., 1991), 98 percent of active injection drug users reported that they were aware that HIV was transmitted through sharing contaminated needles and syringes, yet 70 percent reported sharing. Such findings were also observed with in-treatment injection drug users (Magura et al., 1989). These researchers reported that 40 percent of their sample reported sharing in the last month and that knowledge of AIDS risk was not empirically associated with that behavior.

Although fear of AIDS is often not a decisive motivation, it does bring about some meaningful behavioral changes among injection drug users. Since the early years of the AIDS epidemic, studies have reported significant risk reduction among injection drug users (Des Jarlais and Hopkins, 1985; Des Jarlais et al., 1985, 1988; Hopkins, 1988; Kleinman et al., 1990; Selwyn et al., 1987). They reported an expansion of the street black market of injection equipment in New York City; the demand for sterile injection equipment was strong enough to lead to a noticeable increase in the illicit sales of such devices. An important point raised by Koester is that the fear of being caught carrying needles or syringes appears to vary across cities with similar prescription and paraphernalia laws, depending on the extent to which laws are enforced. Therefore, in cities in which these laws are consistently not enforced, injection drug users may be more likely to regularly carry sterile equipment, which reduces their need to share. Koester's findings show that drug paraphernalia laws, at least in Denver, play a significant role in explaining the high-risk sharing behaviors among certain segments of the injection drug user community. In addition to Koester's ethnographic data, empirically derived descriptive data from large-scale studies provide indirect support for the negative impact of these laws on sharing behaviors (Des Jarlais and Friedman, 1992; Nelson et al., 1991) as well as on HIV seroincidence among injection drug users (Friedman et al., 1994). For example, in a natural experiment in Baltimore, Nelson et al. (1991) were able to document lower transmission rates of HIV among injection drug users who are diabetic (i.e., with unrestricted legal access to sterile needles and syringes) compared with nondiabetic injection drug users.

Recent analyses (Metzger and DePhilippis, 1994) of data from a prospective study on the efficacy of methadone treatment in Philadelphia (Metzger et al., 1991) have elucidated the relationship between the difficulty of needle acquisition among injection drug users and their rate of needle sharing and drug use. A total of 12 months after the inception of this study, 202 of the original cohort of 325 study participants reported injection drug use in the last 6 months and formed the basis of the analyses. There was no significant difference between the needle-sharing rates of subjects who reported easier needle access at the 12-month follow-up and those who did not report easier needle access. Of those who reported *increased difficulty* of needle acquisition, 70 percent reported sharing needles at follow-up, compared with 8 percent of the subjects who did not report greater difficulty. Finally, these researchers found that changes in difficulty of needle acquisition were not associated with either increased or decreased use of any drugs (i.e., heroin, cocaine, amphetamines, benzodiazepines, marijuana).

These studies provide some evidence that existing statutes do affect the availability of sterile needles and syringes, are related to equipment sharing, and, as a consequence, can adversely affect the rate of transmission of HIV infection.

Changes in the Laws in Connecticut

Clearly, it is plausible that reducing legal strictures on the acquisition and possession of drug paraphernalia should result in less needle sharing, with attendant beneficial reduction in the risk of HIV infection. However, empirical checking of what actually occurs when such laws are changed gives a better reading on the effects of such changes.

The Centers for Disease Control and Prevention (CDC) recently conducted a study to investigate the impact of a new legislation in Connecticut (Valleroy et al., in press; Groseclose et al., in press), which was enacted in May 1992 and became effective in July 1992 (Connecticut General Statutes, Sections 21a-65, 21a-240, 21a-267, 1992). The intent of these new statutes was to increase the availability of sterile injection equipment in an attempt to reduce the use of contaminated needles and syringes among the injection drug user community and, consequently, the rate of HIV transmission in the state. Prior to passage of these new laws, it was illegal in Connecticut to purchase or possess needles or syringes without a valid medical prescription. The new laws permit, but do not require, pharmacists to sell up to 10 needles or syringes per visit to individuals without a prescription and allow individuals to possess up to 10 clean needles or syringes.

CDC's assessment (Centers for Disease Control and Prevention, 1993; Valleroy et al., 1993; Valleroy, 1993; Groseclose, 1993; Valleroy et al., in press; Groseclose et al., in press) of the impact of these new statutes focused on monitoring the pharmacies' sales of nonprescription and prescription needles and syringes, injection drug users' knowledge and behavioral changes, and law enforcement officers' behaviors.

Needle Sales

Pharmacy sales over a period of 1 following the effective date of the new laws (July 1, 1992, to June 30, 1993) were monitored for sentinel pharmacies (five) located in neighborhoods where there was a high prevalence of injection drug use (Hartford) and pharmacies (five) located in neighborhoods with low prevalence of injection drug use (Wethersfield). In addition to this prospective surveillance study in select pharmacies in two communities, the CDC research team also conducted a telephone survey of pharmacy managers using a statewide stratified random sample (stratified by type of location; five largest cities versus other locations) of pharmacies in November 1993. Of the 163 randomly selected pharmacies, 139 participated, with 64 (46 percent) located in the five largest cities and 75 (54 percent) in the other locations.

The results of the prospective surveillance study showed a steady increase in the number of nonprescription needles and syringes sold per month for pharmacies located in Hartford (from 460 in July 1992 to 2,482 by June 1993) compared with a stable number of nonprescription needles and syringes being sold per month in Wethersfield (averaging 210 per month). The number of prescription needles and syringes sold by Hartford pharmacies during that same 1-year period remained stable with an average of 3,775 sold per month. Initial nonprescription sales (July 1992) in these pharmacies (i.e., in neighborhoods with high drug-use prevalence), represented 11 percent of total needles/prescription sales, and by June 1993 nonprescription sales represented 43 percent of total sales. Moreover, we should note that the average number of prescription needles and syringes sold per transaction was 63 (because most prescription sales in Hartford are to diabetics, who typically buy a supply of 100 needles and syringes per transaction at a cost of $25.00), compared with an average of 3 needles and syringes sold per nonprescription transaction (average cost of $0.51 per individual needle and syringe).

Only 10 of the 15 originally sampled pharmacies participated in this 1-year study. In neighborhoods with high drug-use prevalence, three participating pharmacies stopped selling nonprescription needles and syringes because of drug user-related incidents. The first pharmacy dropped out after a used syringe was found on a display shelf, the second stopped selling nonprescription needles and syringes after a drug user disrupted business a few hours after a robbery, and the third pharmacy dropped out after a transvestite drug user hustled an upper-middle-class customer for money to buy a syringe. Two of the original seven pharmacies in Wethersfield never sold nonprescription needles and syringes because they feared incidents with drug users.

Results of the telephone survey showed that pharmacy managers differed across the two strata (i.e., largest cities versus other locations) in terms of their reported estimated prevalence of injection drug use in their respective neighborhoods. That is, 75 percent of the managers in the largest cities reported that there were many injection drug users in their neighborhood, compared with 15 percent of all managers in other locations.

Findings from the survey also indicated that in the five largest cities stratum, 73 percent of the participating pharmacies sold nonprescription syringes in November 1993, compared with 85 percent in all other locations. Although a lower proportion of large-city pharmacies reported selling nonprescription syringes than pharmacies in other locations, a significantly larger number of syringes were sold in these five cities than in the other locations (i.e., 93 per pharmacy per week compared with 12 per pharmacy per week, respectively).

Of the participating pharmacy managers, 19 percent reported that they had experienced one or more negative incidents related to the sale of nonprescription syringes. A content analysis of these incidents revealed that 76 percent of the serious incidents (e.g., being attacked with a syringe by a drug user, a customer injecting drugs inside the pharmacy, used syringes found inside and outside the pharmacy) involved used syringe disposal issues. The authors (Valleroy et al., in press) estimated that by November 1993 (15 months after the laws were enacted), 83 percent of all Connecticut pharmacies were selling nonprescription syringes. These data suggest that the new Connecticut laws increased injection drug user access to sterile syringes, especially in areas with high prevalence of drug use.

Injection Drug Users' Behaviors

The CDC project (Groseclose et al., in press) assessed injecting drug users' knowledge of the new laws, their needle and syringe purchasing practices, and their needle-sharing behaviors, both before and after the new laws were in effect. To do so, the investigators conducted two cross-sectional surveys of active injection drug users employing a structured interview format. The first survey ($n = 124$) occurred shortly after the new laws were in effect (between August and November 1992) and the second cross-sectional survey ($n = 134$) was carried out between March and June 1993. In the initial survey, injection drug users were asked to describe their practices and behaviors in June 1992 (30 days before the laws were enacted). The second cross-sectional survey assessed injection drug user practices and behaviors after the new laws were implemented by asking participants to describe their behaviors during the 30 days preceding the interview. Findings concerning injection drug users' knowledge of the new laws (i.e., that it is legal to purchase and possess up to 10 needles and syringes) show that the percentage of active injectors who said they knew that they could both buy and possess clean needles and syringes increased significantly from 55 to 68 percent between the two time periods. At the second survey period, fewer than 8 percent did not know that either purchase or possession of needles was newly legally authorized, down from 22 percent interviewed during the baseline survey. These results reflect that drug users became aware of the changes in the laws.

In investigating active injectors' supply sources, the study compared purchasing sources during the month preceding the new laws with purchasing sources at the time of the second survey (9 to 12 months after the laws were enacted). Results clearly show a shift in most frequently reported source of needles and syringes from the street before the laws were enacted to pharmacies 9 to 12 months after the laws were enacted. That is, 74 percent of the injection drug users interviewed reported they had purchased syringes on the street before the new laws, compared with 28 percent after the laws were enacted. Moreover, 78 percent of the study participants reported they had purchased syringes from a pharmacy after the new laws compared with 19 percent before the laws were enacted.

The study also found a decline in sharing between the first and second surveys. In the earlier survey, which was done before the law went into effect, 52 percent of those active injectors who had ever shared reported some sharing in the previous month; in the later survey, this dropped to 31 percent. This finding reinforces the expectation that eased legal access to syringes results in less sharing.

One finding that appeared peculiar at first was that there was no significant increase observed in the percentage of active injectors who reported that they always carried needles and syringes with them on the street after the new laws were enacted (26 percent before compared with 34 percent after the new laws). The research team compared the percentage of active injectors who reported having been harassed by police at least once during the 6-month period before (13 percent) and the 6-month period after the new laws were in effect (14 percent). They found that approximately the same percentage of participants in both cross-sectional surveys (13 and 14 percent, respectively) reported having been harassed at least once in both of these periods. Therefore, the unchanged level of always carrying needles corresponds to the unchanged level of de facto police activity rather than the de jure legal change.

In an attempt to assess whether police officers were at higher risk of needlesticks due to the increase in needles in circulation resulting from these new laws, researchers reviewed Occupational Safety and Health Administration records for reported needlestick incidents and found no significant changes in the number of needlestick injuries among Hartford police (i.e., six injuries in 1,007 drug-related arrests for the 6-month period before the new laws, compared with two in 1,032 arrests for the 6-month period after the new laws were enacted).

SHOULD THE LAWS BE CHANGED?

CDC's evaluation of the Connecticut experience indicates that needle scarcity can be reduced by repealing existing legal hurdles (paraphernalia and prescription laws) as they relate to injection equipment. Moreover, CDC's monitoring of police harassment of injection drug users for possession of paraphernalia seems to reinforce the concern, voiced by participants at the panel's workshop (see Chapter 4), that law enforcement officers need to be educated about the health effects and other ramifications of the laws. Pharmacists and law enforcement officers can play a pivotal role in increasing the availability of sterile needles and syringes. Street officers need to be made aware of the severe health consequences associated with needle scarcity and of the significant role they can play in reducing the spread of

HIV in the general population. Merely changing the laws and obtaining the approval and endorsement of police department heads may not be sufficient.

A similar principle applies to pharmacists (Koester, 1994; Compton et al., 1992). Although it is legal to purchase needles and syringes in most states in this country, many pharmacists refuse to sell to injection drug users. There is a clear need to address the concerns of pharmacists and pharmacy owners and law enforcement officers, as well as to make them realize how critical their collaboration is in the nation's fight against AIDS. Furthermore, CDC's study disclosed the importance of educating injection drug users about any changes in laws that impact their ability to purchase or carry injection equipment.

Changing the Laws

As briefly discussed above, in their attempt to curtail the use and sale of illicit drugs and the harmful consequences that often accompany drug abuse, legislators have enacted statutes that indirectly address drug use (paraphernalia and prescription laws). Moreover, the judicial system appears to have recognized the timebound merit of drug paraphernalia and prescription laws as they pertain to injection equipment (Gostin, 1993). However, the fact remains that this is a matter that the legislature—not the courts—must address and resolve. As the epidemiologic data on HIV presented in Chapter 1 suggest, the prominent—and increasingly critical—role of injection drug use in transmitting HIV, within both the injecting drug user and, subsequently, the general population (heterosexual and perinatal), requires immediate action to protect public health.

In view of the hindering effects of paraphernalia and prescription laws on the prevention of HIV transmission, the panel urges that state prescription laws be repealed and that all paraphernalia laws be amended to allow for the possession of drug injection equipment. It should be noted that this recommendation has already been made in major policy reports by other groups (Institute of Medicine of the National Academy of Sciences, 1986; National Commission on Acquired Immune Deficiency Syndrome, 1991).

The panel is cognizant that any legislative changes would inevitably require some form of government regulation (Des Jarlais et al., 1994) and proposes that public health agencies and the research community (i.e., National Institutes of Health, Centers for Disease Control and Prevention) appoint a task force to delineate the details of these regulations—for example, eligibility requirements for program participation, type of exchange of needles allowable (one-for-one or otherwise), maximum number of needles a participant is allowed to exchange per visit—to ensure that they meet health needs and concerns regarding the spread of HIV. Regulatory guidelines must address such issues as the disposal of used needles and syringes, who can distribute injection equipment, the maximum number of needles and syringes an individual can purchase or possess, and many other issues.

Consequences

The experiences of other industrialized countries (Porter and Gostin, 1991) that have no paraphernalia or prescription laws (e.g., Netherlands, Italy) point out that merely amending these statutes to alleviate the scarcity of sterile injection equipment should not be expected to eliminate syringes and needles as a important route of HIV transmission. In that regard, it seems important to distinguish between two levels of syringe and needle availability (T. Stephen Jones, Centers for Disease Control and Prevention, February 1994, personal communication): the first, *community availability*, is a necessary condition for the second level, *time of injection availability*, to be met. However, it is not a sufficient condition for ensuring that the second level will be attained. That is, amending paraphernalia and prescription laws would increase the availability of syringes and needles within a community but would not necessarily ensure that injection drug users have a sufficient supply of sterile equipment for each injection. Availability at the time of injection is more difficult to achieve (Bruneau, 1994).

Countries in which community availability is no longer a problem (e.g., Netherlands, Australia, Canada, France) still observe the sharing of syringes and needles at the time of injection. This is in part due to the fact that time of injection availability is a function of multiple factors, including drug purchasing, preparing, and distributing norms and practices among injectors and environmental factors (e.g., police harassment and community availability). It is important to realize that increasing community availability will not completely eliminate sharing behavior.

In the United States, nine states have prescription laws. These nine states are located in a region with high concentrations of injection drug users (the Northeast). In these states, injection drug users (who typically have limited contact with medical services) have to visit a physician to obtain a prescription. Elimination of this barrier would increase the availabililty of sterile injection equipment to injection drug users whose access is currently quite limited. Finally, repeal of the prescription laws in the nine states that have them would increase availability.

Although needle exchange programs tend to reduce the discarding of used syringes (for they are assets, when exchangeable), augmenting the pharmacy sales of needles will tend to increase the number of needles that reach users and pose a potential increase in the total number of discarded needles. Alternatives for dealing with these issues have already been put forth in the United States and other countries. For example, in an attempt to minimize the improper disposal of used needles, some countries (e.g.,

Australia) make available special containers that allow for proper disposal of used syringes in the needle exchange programs and pharmacies. Systematic evaluation of this issue should begin promptly and must take into account the concerns of community groups presented in Chapter 4 of this report.

CONCLUSIONS

The panel concludes that:

• Any marked increase in the supply of sterile needles to injection drug users above current levels through pharmacy sales is likely to call for new measures to ensure the safe disposal of used needles. Whereas this problem has been solved in other countries (e.g., Australia provides special containers in public places that allow for proper disposal of used syringes, as well as individual returnable containers for used syringes), it is important to design good solutions to the disposal issue in the United States now.

• Laws that make it a criminal offense to possess injection equipment (paraphernalia laws) were designed to decrease the prevalence of injection drug abuse, but they also inhibit users from carrying their own supply of needles and syringes and thus unwittingly contribute to the sharing of contaminated ones.

• Laws requiring a prescription for the purchase of new needles and syringes (prescription laws) constrain the availability of sterile injection equipment and thus promote the sharing of contaminated equipment.

RECOMMENDATIONS

The panel recommends that:

• The Assistant Secretary for Health should cause the disposal issue to be studied and appropriate means of needle disposal to be developed. A task force should be appointed and should include health safety specialists, infectious disease specialists, injection drug use researchers, and community representatives/civic leaders.

• Legislative bodies should remove legal sanctions for the possession of injection paraphernalia.

• Appropriate legislative bodies should repeal laws in the nine states that require a prescription in order to purchase injection equipment.

NOTE

1. *Sharing* is a term that has been coined by the research community. More accurate terminology used by injection drug users has been described in Koester (1994); Carlson et al. (in press); Kane and Mason (1992); Murphy (1987); Page et al. (1990b). But, for the sake of consistency, we will continue to use the term in this document to refer to any of the following behaviors: borrowing, lending, renting, needle transfer, etc.

REFERENCES

American Civil Liberties Union
1994   *Briefing Book: Needle Exchange, Harm Reduction, and HIV Prevention in the Second Decade*, R. Harlow and R. Sorge, eds. New York, NY: ACLU AIDS Project.

Brecher, E.M.
1941   The case of the missing mosquitoes. *Reader's Digest* February.

Bruneau, J.
1994   Presentation at informal workshop convened by Panel on Needle Exchange and Bleach Distribution Programs, National Research Council and Institute of Medicine. January 5.

Carlson, R.G.
1991   HIV Needle Risk Behavior Among IDUs in West Central Ohio: An Ethnographic Overview. Invited paper presented at the Conference on AIDS and Anthropology in the United States, Atlanta, Georgia, October 16-17.

Celentano, D.D., D. Vlahov, S. Cohn, J.C. Anthony, L. Solomon, and K.E. Nelson
1991   Risk factors for shooting gallery use and cessation among intravenous drug users. *American Journal of Public Health* 81(10):1291-1295.

Centers for Disease Control and Prevention
1993   *Morbidity and Mortality Weekly Report*, March 5, Vol. 42, No. 8.

Chaisson, R.E., A.R. Moss, R. Onishi, D. Osmond, and J.R. Carlson
1987   Human immunodeficiency virus infection in heterosexual intravenous drug users in San Francisco. *American Journal of Public Health* 77(2):169-172.

Cherubin, C.
1967   The medical sequelae of narcotic addiction. *Annals of Internal Medicine* 67:23-33.

Chitwood, D.D., C.B. McCoy, J.A. Inciardi, D.C. McBride, M. Comerford, E. Trapido, H.V. McCoy, J.B. Page, J. Griffin, M.A. Fletcher, et al.
1990   HIV seropositivity of needles from shooting galleries in South Florida. *American Journal of Public Health* 80:150-152.

Compton III, W.M., L.B. Cottler, and S.H. Decker
1992   Legal needle buying in St. Louis. *American Journal of Public Health* 82:595-596.

Courtwright, D.
1982   *Dark Paradise: Opiate Addiction in America Before 1940.* Boston, MA: Harvard University Press.
1992   A century of American narcotic policy. Pp. 1-61 in D.R. Gerstein and H.J. Harwood, eds., *Treating Drug Problems (Volume 2).* Institute of Medicine. Washington, DC: National Academy Press.

Des Jarlais, D.C., and S.R. Friedman
1992   AIDS and legal access to sterile drug injection equipment. *Drug Abuse: Linking*

Policy and Research, E.D. Wish, ed. *Annals, American Academy of Political and Social Science* 521:42-65.

Des Jarlais, D.C., and W. Hopkins
1985   "Free" needles for intravenous drug users at risk for AIDS: Current developments in New York City. *New England Journal of Medicine* 313(23):1476.

Des Jarlais, D.C., S. Friedman, and W. Hopkins
1985   Risk reduction for acquired immune deficiency syndrome among intravenous drug users. *Annals of Internal Medicine* 103:755.

Des Jarlais, D.C., S. Friedman, and D. Strug
1986   AIDS and needle sharing within the IV drug use subculture. Pp. 141-160 in *The Social Dimensions of AIDS: Methods and Theory*, D. Feldman and T. Johnson, eds. New York, NY: Praeger.

Des Jarlais, D.C., S.R. Friedman, and R. Stoneburner
1988   HIV infection and intravenous drug use: Critical issues in transmission dynamics, infection outcomes, and prevention. *Review of Infectious Diseases* 10(1):151-158.

Des Jarlais, D.C., D. Paone, S.R.Friedman, N. Peyser, and R.G. Newman
1994   Regulating syringe exchange programs: A cautionary note. *Journal of the American Medical Association* 272(6):431-432.

Feldman, H.W., and P. Biernacki
1988   The ethnography of needle sharing among intravenous drug users and implications for public policies and intervention strategies. Pp. 28-39 in *Sharing Among Intravenous Drug Abusers: National and International Perspectives*, R.J. Battjes and R.W. Pickens, eds. Research Monograph 80, National Institute on Drug Abuse.

Friedland, G., and R. Klein
1987   Transmission of human immunodeficiency virus. *New England Journal of Medicine* 317:1125-1135.

Friedland, G.H., C. Harris, C. Butkus-Small, D. Shine, B. Moll, W. Darrow, and R.S. Klein
1985   Intravenous drug abusers and the acquired immune deficiency syndrome (AIDS): Demographic, drug use, and needle-sharing patterns. *Annals of Internal Medicine* 145(8):1413-1417.

Friedman, S., A. Neaigus, D.C. Des Jarlais, J.L. Sotheran, J. Woods, M. Sufian, B. Stepherson, and C. Sterk
1992   Social intervention against AIDS among injecting drug users. *British Journal of Addiction* 87(3):393-404.

Friedman, S.R., M.C. Doherty, D. Paone, and B. Jose
1994   Notes on Research on the Etiology of Drug Injection. Paper commissioned by the Panel on Needle Exchange and Bleach Distribution Programs, National Research Council and Institute of Medicine.

Gostin, L.
1991a   The interconnected epidemics of drug dependency and AIDS. *Harvard Civil Rights-Civil Liberties Law Review* 26:113-184.
1991b   The needle-borne HIV epidemic: Causes and public health responses. *Behavioral Sciences and the Law* 9:287-304.
1993   Law and policy. Pp. 35-61 in *Dimensions of HIV Prevention: Needle Exchange*, J. Stryker and M.D. Smith, eds. Menlo Park, CA: The Henry J. Kaiser Family Foundation.

Groseclose, S.L.
1993   Legislative Changes, The Connecticut Experience: Survey of Injecting Drug Users. Presentation at Workshop on Needle Exchange and Bleach Distribution Programs, Panel on Needle Exchange and Bleach Distribution Programs, National Research Council and Institute of Medicine. Baltimore, MD, September 28.

Groseclose, S.L., B. Weinstein, T. S. Jones, L.A. Valleroy, L.J. Fehrs, and W.J. Kassler
in press   Impact of increased legal access to needles and syringes on practices of injecting-
            drug users and police officers—Connecticut, 1992-1993. *Journal of Acquired
            Immune Deficiency Syndromes.*
Hopkins, W.
1988   Needle sharing and street behavior in response to AIDS in New York City. In
            *Needle Sharing Among Intravenous Drug Abusers: National and International
            Perspectives*, R. Battjes and R. Pickens, eds. Rockville, MD: National Institute
            on Drug Abuse.
Howard, J., and P. Borges
1972   Needle sharing in the Haight: Some social and psychological functions. Pp. 125-
            136 in *It's So Good, Don't Even Try It Once*, D. Smith and G. Gay, eds. New
            Jersey: Prentice Hall.
Inciardi, J.
1990   HIV, AIDS and intravenous drug use: Some considerations. *Journal of Drug
            Issues* 20(2):181-194.
Institute of Medicine and National Academy of Sciences
1986   *Confronting AIDS: Directions for Public Health, Health Care, and Research.*
            Washington, DC: National Academy Press.
Kane, S., and T. Mason
1992   The limits of epidemiological categories and the ethnography of risk. Pp. 199-224
            in *The Time of AIDS*, G. Herdt and S. Lindenbaum, eds. Newbury Park, CA: Sage
            Publications.
Kleinman, P.H., D.S. Goldsmith, S.R. Friedman, W. Hopkins, and D.C. Des Jarlais
1990   Knowledge about and behaviors affecting the spread of AIDS: A street survey of
            intravenous drug users and their associates in New York City. *International Jour-
            nal of the Addictions* 25(4):345-361.
Koester, S.K.
1989   When Push Comes to Shove: Poverty, Law Enforcement and High Risk Behavior.
            Paper presented at the Annual Meeting of the Society for Applied Anthropology,
            Santa Fe, New Mexico.
1992   Ethnography and High Risk Drug Use. Paper presented at the Fifty Fourth Annual
            Meeting of the College on the Problems of Drug Dependence, Keystone, Colorado,
            June 23.
1994   Copping, running and paraphernalia laws: Contextual variables and needle risk
            behavior among injection drug users in Denver. Forthcoming in *Human Organiza-
            tion* 53(3).
Koester, S.K., and L. Hoffer
1994   Indirect sharing: Additional HIV risks associated with drug injection. *AIDS &
            Public Policy Journal* Summer:100-105.
Louria, D.B., T. Hensle, and J. Rose
1967   The major medical complications of narcotic addiction. *Annals of Internal Medi-
            cine* 67:1-32.
Magura, S.J., I. Grossman, D.S. Lipton, et al.
1989   Determinants of needle sharing among intravenous drug users. *American Journal
            of Public Health* 79(4):459-462.
Mandell, W., D. Vlahov, C. Latkin, M. Oziemkwska, and S. Cohn
1994   Correlates of needle sharing among injection drug users. *American Journal of
            Public Health* 84(6):920-923.

Marmor, M., D.C. Des Jarlais, H. Cohen, S.R. Friedman, S.T. Beatrice, N. Dubin, W. el-Sadr, D. Mildvan, S. Yancovitz, U. Mathur, et al.
1987   Risk factors for infection with human immunodeficiency virus among intravenous drug abusers in New York City. *AIDS* 1(1):39-44.

Metzger, D., G. Woody, D. DePhilippis, T. McLellan, C.P. O'Brien, and J.J. Platt
1991   Risk factors for needle sharing among methadone treated patients. *American Journal of Psychiatry* 148:636-640.

Morgan, H.W.
1981   *Drugs in America: A Social History, 1800-1980.* Syracuse, NY: Syracuse University Press.

Murphy, S.
1987   Intravenous drug use and AIDS: Notes on the social economy of needle sharing. *Contemporary Drug Problems* Fall:373-395.

Musto, D.F.
1987   *The American Disease: Origins of Narcotic Control.* Expanded Edition. Oxford, Eng.: Oxford University Press.
1991   Opium, cocaine and marijuana in American history. *Scientific American* July:40-47.

National Commission on Acquired Immune Deficiency Syndrome
1991   *Report: The Twin Epidemics of Substance Use and HIV.* Washington, DC: National Commission on Acquired Immune Deficiency Syndrome.

Nelson, K.E., D. Vlahov, S. Cohn, A. Lindsay, L. Solomon, and J.C. Anthony
1991   Human immunodeficiency virus infection in diabetic intravenous drug users. *Journal of the American Medical Association* 266:2259-2261.

Office of National Drug Control Policy
1992   Needle exchange programs: Are they effective? *ONDCP Bulletin No. 7.* Washington, DC: Executive Office of the President.

Page, J.B., P.C. Smith, and N. Kane
1990a   Shooting galleries, their proprietors, and implications for prevention of AIDS. *Drugs and Society* 51(1):69-85.

Page, J.B., D. Chitwood, P. Smith, N. Kane, and D. McBride
1990b   Intravenous drug use and HIV infection in Miami. *Medical Anthropology Quarterly* 4(4):56-71.

Pascal, C.B.
1988   Intravenous drug abuse and AIDS transmission: Federal and state laws regulating needle availability. Pp. 119-136 in *Needle Sharing Among Intravenous Drug Abusers: National and International Perspectives,* R.J. Battjes and R. Pickens, eds. Research Monograph 80, National Institute on Drug Abuse.

Porter, L., and L. Gostin
1991   Legal Environment Surrounding the Availability of Sterile Needles and Syringes to Injecting Drug Users. Unpublished manuscript.

Reuter, P.
1992   Hawks ascendant: The punitive trend of American drug policy. *Daedalus: Journal of the American Academy of Arts and Sciences* 121(3):15-52.

Schoenbaum, E.E., D. Hartel, P.A. Selwyn, R.S. Klein, K. Davenny, M. Rogers, C. Feiner, and G. Friedland
1989   Risk factors for human immunodeficiency virus infection in intravenous drug users. *New England Journal of Medicine* 321(13):874-879.

Selwyn, P.A., and P. Alcabes
1994   The Potential Impact of Needle Exchange Programs on Health Outcomes Other Than HIV and Drug Use. Paper prepared for the Panel on Needle Exchange and

Bleach Distribution Programs, National Research Council and Institute of Medicine.

Selwyn, P.A., C. Feiner, C.P. Cox, C. Lipshutz, and R.L. Cohen
1987   Knowledge about AIDS and high-risk behavior among intravenous drug users in New York City. *AIDS* 1(4):247-254.

Valleroy, L.A.
1993   Legislative Changes, The Connecticut Experience, Pharmacies. Presentation at Workshop on Needle Exchange and Bleach Distribution Programs, Baltimore, MD, September 28. Panel on Needle Exchange and Bleach Distribution Programs, National Research Council and Institute of Medicine.

Valleroy, L.A., B. Weinstein, S. Groseclose, W. Kassler, T.S. Jones, and R. Rolfs
1993   Evaluating the Impact of a New Needle/Syringe Law: Surveillance of Needle/Syringe Sales at Connecticut Pharmacies. Poster C24-3189. IXth International Conference on AIDS, Berlin, Germany, June 6-11.

Valleroy, L.A., B. Weinstein, T.S. Jones, S.L. Groseclose, R.T. Rolfs, and W.J. Kassler
in press   Impact of increased legal access to needles and syringes on community pharmacies' needle and syringe sales—Connecticut, 1992-1993. *Journal of Acquired Immune Deficiency Syndromes.*

Vlahov, D., A. Muñoz, S. Cohn, D.D. Celentano, J.C. Anthony, and K.E. Nelson
1990   Association of drug injection patterns with antibody to human immunodeficiency virus type 1(HIV-1) among intravenous drug users in Baltimore. *American Journal of Epidemiology* 132:847-856.

Part 2
The Impact of Needle Exchange and Bleach Distribution Programs

6

The Effectiveness of Bleach as a Disinfectant of Injection Drug Equipment

The needles and syringes used by injection drug users are produced for the delivery of legal drugs or biologics that require intravenous, intramuscular, intradermal, or subcutaneous delivery. They are manufactured according to exacting standards to ensure sterility and are intended for use by a single individual for a single injection on only a single occasion. As detailed in Chapter 5, the limited availability of adequate numbers of sterile needles and syringes results in their frequent reuse and sharing by injection drug users. The repeated use of needles and syringes necessarily compromises their sterility and safety. The sharing of injection equipment by

Note: a significant portion of the discussion in this chapter is based on Alice Gleghorn's (1994) paper commissioned by the panel, *Practical Issues of Needle and Syringe Disinfection Programs.* It reviews the history of bleach distribution programs and includes descriptions of these programs in San Francisco, Chicago, New York, and the various locations involved in the National AIDS Demonstration Research Project. Method variation in bleach use by injection drug users, encompassing substances and techniques used, comparisons of injection drug users who disinfect and those who do not, and problems with bleach disinfection are also discussed, as well as provisional federal regulations and the extension of bleach distribution programs. Information was also obtained from another commissioned paper, *Inactivation of HIV: Application to Injecting Drug Use Equipment,* by Linda Martin, Walter Bond, T. Stephen Jones, and Martin Favero (1994). This paper reviews the processes and biological aspects of disinfection and inactivation of the human immunodeficiency virus and discusses the applications of these studies to the cleaning and disinfection of syringes and needles reused by injection drug users.

injection drug users is particularly hazardous because it provides an efficient means for transmission of a number of blood-borne infectious diseases, including the HIV, hepatitis B (HBV), and hepatitis C viruses and the human T-cell leukemia viruses (HTLV-I and HTLV-II).

With the advent of the AIDS epidemic, the recognition of the rapid dissemination of HIV infection within injection drug user communities, and legal constraints associated with access to injection equipment (see Chapter 5), the use of bleach to clean and disinfect previously used needles and syringes has been encouraged by outreach workers in an attempt to improve the safety of the inherently unsafe practice of sharing needles and syringes among injection drug users. This chapter reviews the scientific literature on the efficacy of bleach as a disinfectant and the effectiveness of bleach distribution programs on reducing the potential harmful effects associated with injection drug use—risk behaviors and HIV transmission.

TRANSMISSION OF HIV AMONG INJECTION DRUG USERS

HIV is clearly a blood-borne pathogen. However, it is not yet known what proportion of HIV transmission between individuals results from the transfer of free infectious virus present in the plasma fraction of the blood of an infected individual, in the HIV-infected peripheral blood cells, or both. The sharing of needles and syringes by injection drug users can result in the transmission of pathogens spread as free virus (such as HBV) or via the transfer of infected cells (such as HTLV-I and HTLV-II). Resolution of the vehicle for HIV transmission may prove to be important, since HIV present within infected cells or as free virus may be differentially susceptible to the various available disinfection methods.

The actual amount (infectious dose) of HIV necessary to transfer the infection from one person to another is not known. In the absence of this information, attempts to model the effectiveness of any virus disinfection strategy are difficult because the level of inactivation needed to prevent transfer of the infection is unclear. Ideally, a disinfectant strategy will completely eliminate the infectivity of all HIV contaminating a surface. However, to be effective at limiting the transmission of HIV between individuals, such a strategy need only reduce the level of infectivity below the minimal infectious dose.

At present, the process of evaluating the effectiveness of various disinfection strategies relies on tissue culture models, in which virus inactivation is measured by the ability to isolate infectious virus following disinfectant treatment. Unfortunately, it is not known whether the available tissue culture-based HIV isolation methods are sensitive enough to detect the minimum infectious dose of virus responsible for transferring HIV infection between individuals. If virus isolation methods are not sensitive enough, a preparation of HIV that was completely inactivated in the laboratory might still be able to transmit infection in vivo.

The amount of both free HIV and virus-infected cells present in the blood of infected individuals varies with the stage of the infection (see Chapter 1). During the acute infection stage, newly infected persons have extremely high levels of HIV present in circulating peripheral blood cells and in the plasma. When a host antiviral immune response is generated, typically within 1 to 3 months of initial infection, the levels of infected cells and plasma virus fall dramatically. HIV replication continues throughout the asymptomatic phase of the disease, primarily within the lymphoid organs of infected persons. During this period, recirculating HIV-infected lymphocytes and cell-free virus can be detected in the peripheral bloodstream. As a result, HIV-infected injection drug users are likely to be able to transmit the virus to others by sharing injection equipment throughout the entire course of their infection. Increasing levels of HIV and HIV-infected cells appear in the blood of infected persons as immune containment of virus replication fails and clinical disease becomes manifest.

Although epidemiologic evidence obtained from studies of heterosexual and perinatal transmission of HIV infection suggests that individuals who are in the acute or advanced stages of HIV infection may be more infectious than those in the early stages of the infection, no information concerning this issue has been reported in injection drug users (see Chapter 1). It seems reasonable to expect, however, that not all HIV-positive injection drug users are equally infectious. From the perspective of disinfection strategies for needles and syringes, effective methods need to be able to inactivate the viral burden present in contaminating blood derived from even the most highly infectious individuals.

Although it is commonly assumed that HIV transmission among injection drug users results from sharing contaminated needles and syringes, there are a number of additional factors that may account for virus spread. For example, HIV contamination of other materials used by injection drug users, including the paraphernalia used to mix and prepare drugs for injection ("cookers") and the water used to dissolve the drugs or rinse the needles and syringes between their use by different individuals, can potentially serve to transmit HIV. The relative roles of these different materials and processes in spreading HIV among injection drug users are not known.

BLEACH AS A DISINFECTANT

Definition of Terms

Although the terms *sterilization* and *disinfection* are widely employed, they are often misused (Block, 1983). *Sterilization* is the use of physical or chemical procedures to destroy *all* forms of microbial life, including highly resistant bacterial endospores. Sterilization is frequently accomplished using high-pressure steam autoclaving, ethylene oxide gas, or prolonged exposure to dry heat. *Disinfection* is the elimination of all vegetative microorganisms and pathogenic viruses, but not bacterial or fungal spores, from an inanimate object. As such, disinfection processes lack the margin of safety achieved through sterilization procedures. Furthermore, the effectiveness of a disinfection procedure is influenced significantly by a number of factors, including the nature and number of contaminating microorganisms, the type and condition of the materials to be disinfected, and the amount of organic matter (such as blood) present (Klein and Deforest, 1965a; Rhame, 1986; Rutala and Weber, 1987; Rutala, 1987; Van Houton and Hayre, 1991).

A *germicide* is an agent that destroys microorganisms, especially pathogens, on either living or inanimate objects. Disinfectants can be categorized into high-, medium-, and low-level agents based on their potency of germicidal action. Disinfectants that are widely used at present include alcohols, hypochlorites (such as bleach) and other chlorine-containing compounds, formaldehyde, glutaraldehyde, hydrogen peroxide, iodophors, phenolics, and quaternary ammonium compounds. The level of contamination with organic matter of objects to be disinfected is referred to as the *bioburden*, and it is of particular importance in the disinfection of surfaces contaminated with blood that harbors infectious pathogens. *Contact time* is defined as the length of time that a contaminated object or surface is exposed to a disinfectant. *Cleaning* is the removal of foreign (especially organic) material. *Decontamination* is the removal of pathogenic microorganisms from objects so they are safe to handle.

The Role of Cleaning in Disinfection

Thorough cleaning must always precede chemical disinfection of any equipment (Klein and Deforest, 1965a; Rhame, 1986; Rutala and Weber, 1987; Rutala, 1987; Van Houton and Hayre, 1991). The mechanical action of cleaning can itself remove a large proportion of the microorganisms present. Cleaning also removes organic material that can inactivate or diminish the potency of the germicide used. The presence of blood on or in equipment being processed for reuse, including needles and syringes, can contribute to the failure of a given disinfection or sterilization procedure in three ways. First, organic material may contain large and/or diverse microbial populations. Second, it may trap microorganisms and prevent effective penetration of chemical germicides. Third, it may directly and rapidly inactivate certain germicidal chemicals, including bleach and other chlorine-containing solutions, iodine-based disinfectants, and quaternary ammonium-based compounds. Physical cleaning is often the most important step in a disinfection process, and even a rigorous disinfection procedure may not inactivate contaminating bacteria or viruses if these are protected by organic material, such as blood.

Bleach is a solution of sodium hypochlorite, and it exerts rapid and broad-spectrum disinfecting action (Hugo and Russell, 1982; Ingraham, 1992; Klein and Deforest, 1965a, 1965b; Rutala and Cole, 1984; Rutala, 1990; Van Houton and Hayre, 1991). Sodium hypochlorite solutions in concentrations of 0.05 to 0.5 percent (500-5,000 milligrams per milliliter) free and available chlorine are generally considered to be intermediate-level disinfectants and are among the most effective, most convenient, and least expensive germicides. The precise mechanism through which bleach exerts its germicidal action is not known, but it is believed to be mediated by the ability of free chlorine to denature proteins, inactivate sulfhydryl-containing enzymes, and damage nucleic acids (RNA and DNA).

Household bleach manufactured in the United States contains approximately 5 percent sodium hypochlorite (50,000 milligrams per milliliter chlorine [Cl_2]). Bleach solutions exhibit sporicidal activity, are tuberculocidal, inactivate vegetative bacteria, and are fungicidal and virucidal. Klein and Deforest (1963) reported that 25 viruses tested, including picornaviruses, were inactivated within 10 minutes by as little as 0.02 percent (200 milligrams per milliliter) available chlorine.

The efficacy of a bleach solution to act as a disinfectant is determined by the concentration of free and available chlorine present in the solution (Klein and Deforest, 1965a, 1965b; Rutala and Cole, 1984; Rutala, 1990; Van Houton and Hayre, 1991). *Chlorine demand* is a term used to describe the amount of chlorine that is expended in the course of reaction with inorganic and organic materials. After this demand is met, any remaining chlorine is referred to as *available chlorine*. The level of available chlorine present to effect disinfection is influenced by a number of variables, including the amount of organic material in the infectious material and the temperature, pH, and hardness of the water used to dilute the bleach solution. Serum proteins and other organic material in blood will reduce the chlorine in bleach available for microbial inactivation (Favero and Bond, 1991; Klein and Deforest, 1965a; Rutala and Cole, 1984; Rutala, 1987). In practice in the health care setting, it is thus recommended that blood-contaminated surfaces first be cleaned to remove as much visible blood as possible prior to treatment with bleach.

The disinfectant potential of a bleach solution is not constant; rather, it decreases with time because of the relative instability of the active chlorine component. Bleach solutions lose potency at an accelerated rate when exposed to sunlight, oxygen, and heat. Bleach solutions prepared with tap water at pH 8 or greater are stable for about one month when stored at room temperature in a closed, opaque container.

Susceptibility of HIV to Disinfection

Microorganisms vary widely in their level of resistance to chemical germicides (Favero and Bond, 1991; Hugo and Russell, 1982; Rutala and Weber, 1987; Klein and Deforest, 1965a). The types of microorganisms present can have a significant effect on the contact time and the concentration of germicide necessary to ensure the sterilization or disinfection of a contaminated object. Among pathogenic microorganisms, bacterial spores are the most resistant to sterilization and disinfection. In general, the presence of lipid in a virus is associated with a high degree of susceptibility to all germicides. The blood-borne pathogens HIV and HBV both are surrounded by lipid-containing membranes and thus are expected to be among the microorganisms least resistant to disinfection and sterilization. In principle, and in practice in the laboratory and the health care environment, there is no reason to believe that HIV is resistant to disinfection (Conte, 1986; Centers for Disease Control [CDC], 1987).

The identification of HIV as the cause of AIDS and the availability of tissue culture models to study virus infectivity permitted the laboratory evaluation of methods to disinfect HIV present on surfaces. The primary goal of the initial studies of disinfection methods was to determine the optimal approaches to disinfect reusable medical devices and to safely clean surfaces contaminated with blood from HIV-infected patients. Although varying in their precise protocols, all early studies were performed using HIV obtained from the supernatants of virus-infected tissue culture cell lines (Spire et al., 1984; Resnick et al., 1986; Martin et al., 1985). The virus present in such supernatants is not associated with infected cells, and this is referred to as *cell-free virus*. The infectious titer of cell-free HIV found in tissue culture supernatants ranges from 10^4 to 10^6 tissue culture infectious doses (TCID) per milliliter volume; these titers are several orders of magnitude higher than those typically present in the blood of HIV-infected individuals (Pantaleo et al., 1993). In addition, the amounts of proteins and other organic materials present in tissue culture fluids are usually less than those found in blood.

It is important to emphasize that preparations of cell-free HIV may demonstrate significantly different levels of susceptibility to disinfecting agents than samples of virus-infected cells, particularly as they may be found in blood specimens that are rich in cellular and extracellular (plasma) protein content. Cell-free HIV derived from supernatants of tissue culture cells is most susceptible to disinfection, whereas infected cells (and possibly cell-free virus present in the plasma) contained within blood specimens are more difficult to inactivate (Flynn et al., 1994; Shapshak et al., 1994). The role that the HIV contained in clotted blood present within needles and syringes may play in virus transmission is not known. Should HIV trapped in clotted blood remain infectious, it may be more difficult to inactivate by disinfectant treatment because of the substantial increase in contact time that may be needed (see special issue of *the Journal of Acquired Immune Deficiency Syndromes* 7:7, 1994).

To date, no satisfactory approaches to measure the infectivity of HIV present in clotted blood or model the efficiency of inactivation of the virus contained in clotted blood specimens have been devised. For these reasons, the experimental methods that have been used to monitor HIV inactivation by disinfectants have (to various degrees) approximated, but not reproduced, the circumstances through which HIV transmission occurs between injection drug users sharing contaminated injection equipment.

Laboratory Studies

Laboratory-based HIV inactivation studies commonly have been performed by mixing high-titer preparations of cell-free HIV with various dilutions of disinfectants for varying periods of time. Following designated time(s) of exposure, serial dilutions of each virus-disinfectant mixture are then added to $CD4^+$ T-cells (that are susceptible to HIV infection) in tissue culture. The cultures are then monitored for evidence of active replication of HIV, as evidenced by increasing levels of virus-specific antigens (the p24 core antigen) or enzymatic activities (reverse transcriptase). Increasing levels of HIV p24 or reverse transcriptase activity in the tissue culture supernatants from cells exposed to disinfectant-treated virus preparations is indicative of the failure of disinfection. The absence of HIV p24 antigen or reverse transcriptase in test culture provides evidence that the concentration and exposure time of disinfectant used successfully inactivated the amount of HIV present in the original inoculum. Because of the inherent toxicity of disinfectants, it is essential that appropriate controls be performed to determine if the test disinfectant killed the indicator $CD4^+$ T-cells used to propagate the virus; such toxicity can undermine the sensitivity of the virus isolation procedure and lead to overestimating the effectiveness of the disinfectant at inactivating the virus itself.

Studies performed to date have usually employed laboratory-adapted strains of HIV and immortalized T-lymphocyte cell lines. Although there is no known reason to expect differences between the laboratory strains of HIV and primary virus isolates with respect to their intrinsic susceptibility to disinfection, this issue has not been addressed by researchers in the field. Similarly, most experimental evaluations of HIV disinfection methods have used immortalized $CD4^+$ T-cell lines as indicator cells rather than primary cultures of T lymphocytes or macrophages for HIV isolation. The impact of the choice of indicator cells on the sensitivity of virus detection following disinfection is not known.

Spire and colleagues (1984), using an assay for the presence of HIV reverse transcriptase activity (and not the residual infectivity of the virus preparation itself), examined the inactivation of cell-free HIV by commonly used disinfectants. Their results suggested that 25 percent ethanol or 1 percent glutaraldehyde should be sufficient to disinfect medical instruments, and that 0.2 percent sodium hypochlorite should be sufficient to disinfect contaminated environmental surfaces. They also reported that HIV was inactivated by a 1:400 dilution of beta-propiolactone or 30 millimolar sodium hydroxide, but that formalin 0.1 percent required 48 hours to render reverse transcriptase activity undetectable.

Resnick and colleagues (1986) pointed out that assays for reverse transcriptase activity are not reliable alternatives to tests for infectious virus. These authors, using concentrated preparations of cell-free HIV, found that infectious virus could be recovered from dried material for 3 to 7 days. In an aqueous environment, cell-free HIV retained its infectivity for more than 2 weeks at room temperature. However, HIV infectivity was completely eliminated following 1 minute of exposure to sodium hypochlorite 0.5 percent (a 10 percent solution of household bleach), alcohol 70 percent, or a 0.5 percent solution of the detergent NP-40.

Martin and colleagues (1985), using antigen detection methods to monitor virus replication in tissue culture, reported that cell-free HIV could be inactivated by a variety of disinfectants at concentrations well below those commonly employed. They reported that HIV infectivity was efficiently inactivated by 0.3 percent hydrogen peroxide, 50 percent ethanol, 0.5 percent paraformaldehyde, 0.5 percent Lysol (a proprietary mixture of phenolics and surfactants), and a 1/1,000 dilution of household bleach (approximately 50 milligram per milliliter chlorine). Since that time, many laboratories have performed HIV inactivation studies with various compounds. The results of many of these studies have been reviewed by Sattar and Springthorpe (1991) and confirm the predicted susceptibility of HIV to inactivation by a wide variety of chemical disinfectants.

CDC Recommendations

Based on the results of these early studies, recommendations were formulated by the Centers for Disease Control for the sterilization, disinfection, and housekeeping procedures in health care settings (Centers for Disease Control, 1987). These guidelines continue to serve effectively and have not been modified. An example of an effective disinfection procedure used in the health care environment relevant to the consideration of inactivation of HIV present on blood-contaminated surfaces is provided by the example of the disinfection of hemodialysis machines. Patients infected with HIV who are undergoing hemodialysis do not require isolation from other dialysis patients. Although the dialyzer itself is disposable, the recommendations for disinfecting the dialysis fluid pathways of the hemodialysis machine (exposure to 500 to 750 milligrams per liter of sodium hypochlorite for 30 to 40 minutes)—originally intended for controlling bacterial contamination—are also effective in inactivating HIV (Centers for Disease Control, 1986; Conte, 1986).

In sum, when used appropriately, there is no doubt that bleach can effectively disinfect surfaces contaminated by HIV-infected blood.

BLEACH DISTRIBUTION PROGRAMS

In the mid-1980s, the recognition of an impending epidemic in the spread of HIV infection in injection drug users led to discussion among health care professionals and providers concerning potential intervention strategies to limit virus transmission. Although HIV infection had entered the injection drug user population in San Francisco by 1985, it had not yet assumed the high level of prevalence that was seen among injection drug users in the New York metropolitan area. A San Francisco group of community health outreach workers that came to be known as the Mid-City Consortium to Combat AIDS proposed that the types of education and behavior change efforts that had been successfully conducted among homosexual and bisexual men in the area (Becker and Joseph, 1988) might also attenuate the transmission of HIV among injection drug users (Newmeyer, 1988). However, the opportunities for public health interventions were limited.

California's paraphernalia and prescription laws made the prospects for legally authorized needle exchange remote. The most effective risk reduction behavior, cessation of drug use, was not a realistic option for many injection drug users because of the nature of the addictive process and limited treatment resources (Murphy, 1987). Social norms for sharing injection equipment among injection drug users, as well as legal and economic constraints, all placed restrictions on an individual's ability and motivation to keep a needle and syringe set for personal use only (Des Jarlais et al., 1986; Hopkins, 1988; Feldman and Biernacki, 1988). Therefore, the option of disinfecting needles and syringes seemed to hold the greatest promise for realistic interventions to limit HIV transmission among injection drug users.

Ethnographic studies were conducted in San Francisco to determine characteristics that would make a disinfection strategy acceptable to injection drug users (Newmeyer, 1988). Newmeyer listed five essential features of a disinfection technique as follows: "(1) it should be quick, preferably taking less than 60 seconds; (2) it should be inexpensive; (3) it should use materials conveniently available; (4) it should be safe to the user and his/ her injection equipment; and (5) it should be effective at neutralizing viruses" (Newmeyer, 1988:160). In determining an appropriate disinfectant, published studies available at the time—particularly those of Martin et al. (1985) and Resnick and colleagues (1986)—were the primary sources of information regarding the efficacy of various disinfectants for inactivation of HIV under laboratory conditions.

Based on these studies, several disinfectants were considered, including bleach, hydrogen peroxide, and isopropyl alcohol. According to Newmeyer (1988), hydrogen peroxide was rejected due to its limited shelf life and sensitivity to light exposure; the potential for isopropyl alcohol to be confused with other readily available sources of alcohol in beer, wine, and hard liquors eliminated it from consideration. Boiling syringes in water for 15 minutes was another strategy considered; however, this strategy was deemed impractical due to the length of time required, the facilities needed, and the fact that boiling melted the syringe (Murphy, 1987). As a result of these considerations, household bleach (approximately 5 percent sodium hypochlorite) was determined to be the most feasible. Bleach met the criteria for cost and availability, and reviews of the available literature (Becker et al., 1974; Froner et al., 1987) suggested that accidental injection of bleach would not produce great harm to injection drug users. Aside from fading the numbers inscribed on the syringe barrel (Newmeyer, 1988) and corrosion of the rubber stopper of the plunger of the syringe, bleach did not seem to have excessive deleterious effects on the injection equipment.

Following the selection of bleach as the disinfectant of choice, community health outreach workers in San Francisco began a campaign of bleach distribution and provided simple, graphic instructions for its use in disinfecting needles and syringes (Watters, 1987). The initial bleach distribution efforts were part of a broader education program to decrease the risk of HIV infection among injection drug users that included condom distribution and voluntary HIV counseling and testing. The educational message delivered was: "The best protection is to stop using drugs; if you can't stop using, don't inject; if you can't stop injecting, at least keep your own outfit and don't share it with anyone; if you do share, use bleach to reduce your risk." The recommended protocol for bleach disinfection was to fill needles and syringes twice with bleach, followed by two water rinses (Newmeyer, 1988; Froner et al., 1987; Watters, 1987). These initial disinfection guidelines recommended the use of full-strength bleach, which was believed by the San Francisco community health outreach workers to provide a more potent and convenient disinfectant than the diluted bleach preparations used in the early laboratory studies.

Program Evaluation

Prior to 1993, the instructions for bleach use disseminated across the country were relatively consistent with the methods developed by the Mid-City Consortium in San Francisco (Gleghorn, 1993). With few exceptions (Flynn et al., 1994), bleach has been exclusively promoted as the disinfectant of choice for injection equipment. As a result, awareness of bleach disinfection strategies among injection drug users is high (Meyers et al., 1990). Therefore, a review of the studies that have evaluated cleaning techniques used by injection drug users provides indications concerning user compliance with the recommended bleach techniques.

The bleach distribution program in San Francisco was well accepted by injection drug users. Among those interviewed in neighborhoods with high drug use, Watters (1987, 1994) reported that prior to initiation of the outreach program, only 3 percent of the sample used bleach to clean their equipment. In contrast, 9 months after beginning the community health outreach worker (CHOW) intervention, 76 percent of injection drug users interviewed reported bleach use. In addition, prior to program initiation, *regular* cleaning of needles and syringes was reported by only 21 percent of those who reported any cleaning attempts. In the follow-up interview, injection drug users who used bleach reported doing so 90 percent of the time. Although other reports (Chaisson et al., 1987) from San Francisco reported less dramatic (approximately fivefold) increases in bleach use, they noted important additional effects of outreach efforts that included bleach distribution on other HIV-related risk behaviors, including decreases in needle sharing and increases in condom use (Chaisson et al., 1987; Sorenson et al., 1989).

Moreover, in these early studies of the adoption of bleach disinfection by injection drug users, a significant positive relationship was observed between access to community health outreach workers and reported use of bleach disinfection (Watters, 1987). Another important variable in the success of bleach education programs appears to be the direct provision of bleach to injection drug users. For example, the AIDS Outreach Program (AOP) provided street-level education on bleach use but did not actually *distribute* bleach (Neaigus et al., 1990). Evaluation of the impact of this program found that only low levels of regular bleach use were noted both at baseline and during follow-up interviews (16 and 18 percent, respectively). In interpreting these results, Neaigus and colleagues (1990) suggested that outreach efforts aimed at increasing bleach use should include distribution of bleach.

Following the lead of San Francisco, bleach distribution programs proliferated rapidly in cities across the United States. Using techniques adopted from medical epidemiology and community ethnography, workers in Chicago (Wiebel, 1990, 1993a) initiated an active program of education, intervention, and research, employing a field staff with extensive knowledge of and familiarity with the local community of injection drug users. In an evaluation of this approach (Wiebel et al., 1990), active injecting drug users were queried about their use of bleach disinfection at baseline and at 6 months following the initiation of the educational program. Bleach use as a disinfection strategy was adopted by many injection drug users. Two-thirds of the study participants who initially used bleach "less than always" reported an increase in bleach use, with one-third of the follow-up sample reporting "always" using bleach.

Similarly, researchers in New York (Friedman et al., 1990) helped form an organization of injection drug users in an effort to decrease HIV risk behaviors. Injection drug users in recovery provided HIV risk-reduction education for active users. These groups encouraged the adoption of safe sexual and drug-related behaviors and offered AIDS education, individual counseling, and HIV testing. In an evaluation of this program, follow-up comparisons were made between injection drug users who participated in the education and organizing effort and those who did not. Although use of new needles and condoms increased in both groups, only the organized injection drug users showed an increase in consistent bleach use.

Additional studies sponsored by the National Institute on Drug Abuse (NIDA) evaluated AIDS risk behaviors and trends in HIV infection in injection drug users in methadone treatment programs (Battjes and Pickens, 1992, 1993). Reported trends over the five-year period included increased use of bleach and alcohol by injection drug users to clean injection equipment in four of the seven cities studied: New York; Asbury Park, N.J.; Trenton, N.J.; Baltimore, Md.; Chicago, Ill.; San Antonio, Tex.; and Los Angeles. Additional studies conducted in Indianapolis and Los Angeles County have reported increased rates of bleach use (McKee et al., 1992; Longshore et al., 1993). These changes appear to reflect the increasing awareness and acceptance of bleach as an HIV prevention strategy.

In a survey of nearly 3,000 injection drug users in Baltimore conducted in 1988 and 1989, Latkin and colleagues (1992) reported that a variety of substances, including water, bleach, and alcohol, were used by injection drug users to clean contaminated needles and syringes. In addition to the use of various agents, the methods reportedly used by injection drug users for syringe disinfection were often imprecise and variable. Gleghorn and colleagues (Gleghorn et al., 1994; Gleghorn, 1994) studied cleaning practices used by injection drug users via videotaping mock needle and syringe cleaning sessions. They found that more than 80 percent of the 161 subjects studied used bleach for less than 30 seconds, although they reported cleaning for longer periods of time.

McCoy and colleagues (1992, 1994) studied injection drug users in Miami who had been taught a bleach disinfection procedure consisting of two complete fillings of the syringe with bleach, followed by two complete fillings with rinse water, and discarding of the used cleaning solutions. Study participants were then evaluated for proper disinfection technique 6 to 12 months following initial training. At follow-up, a substantial proportion of the injection drug users did not perform all of the previously taught steps, and less than half completely filled the syringe with bleach or rinsed the syringe twice with bleach. These investigators also reported that compliance with disinfection methods decreased as the number of steps required increased.

Several behavioral characteristics of injection drug users have been found to be associated with use or nonuse of needle and syringe disinfection (Brown and Beschner, 1993; Latkin et al., 1992; Gleghorn et al., 1994; Edlin et al., 1993). Injection drug users who use shooting galleries, or who share needles and syringes with more than one partner, may be more likely to use bleach or alcohol for disinfection (Latkin et al., 1992). Neither injection frequency nor cocaine injection has been found to be associated with disinfectant use (Latkin et al., 1992). Injection drug users who also smoke crack cocaine report a lower rate of cleaning needles and syringes prior to injecting than nonsmokers, even though they inject less frequently (Edlin et al., 1993). Crack cocaine-smoking injection drug users are also more likely to use unsafe needles and to share rinse water, cookers, and cotton (Edlin et al., 1993).

Injection drug users who disinfect their injection equipment with bleach or alcohol are also more likely to be acquainted with other HIV risk reduction behaviors (Celentano et al., 1991). Knowledge of bleach effectiveness, condom effectiveness, and several other HIV transmission risks is higher among injection drug users with a history of bleach or alcohol disinfection. Further studies of beliefs and attitudes that differentiate bleach users from nonusers or that predict bleach use are needed to increase the adoption of effective cleaning strategies.

The National AIDS Demonstration Research (NADR) program represents a large-scale multisite prevention effort supported by the National Institute on Drug Abuse (National Institute on Drug Abuse, 1994). A total of 28 sites participated in this aspect of the NIDA initiative. This undertaking has produced what is probably the largest single database on out-of-treatment injection drug users with evaluative data on outreach program effectiveness. Brown (1994) describes the NADR "standard" intervention as typically involving at least: (1) the provision of information about and distribution of condoms and bleach by outreach and counseling staffs; (2) one session of individual educational counseling regarding AIDS transmission and strategies for AIDS risk reduction; (3) an offer to make available HIV testing; (4) posttest counseling for those accepting HIV testing;

and (5) prior to counseling, the administration of a structured interview schedule. In addition, 18 sites developed "enhanced" interventions involving didactic training sessions and other additional initiatives, including: (1) individual and group counseling on behavior change strategies; (2) couples counseling; (3) cognitive skills training; (4) peer networks; and (5) social skills training. As described in Chapter 3, it is apparent that these outreach programs are multicomponent AIDS prevention programs that do not rely exclusively on distributing bleach bottles in their attempt to reduce HIV risk behaviors and the transmission of HIV infection.

The NADR report (National Institute on Drug Abuse, 1994) indicates that these 28 sites assessed 33,407 injection drug users at intake. However, only those participants whose initial and follow-up data could be linked (13,475) formed the basis of the program evaluation component of this project. As such, these data represent a fraction of the total number of injection drug users who were served (or at least assessed) by the NADR projects (a 40 percent follow-up rate). For sex partners, 6,216 were assessed and 1,637 (26 percent) were followed.[1] As reflected by the substantial variation in follow-up rates[2] across sites, the quality of data provided by individual sites varied considerably. Given the considerable potential problems associated with attempting to integrate these data, the following section summarizes the evaluation results of one specific NADR site that has provided detailed information on program delivery and comprehensive longitudinal data on meaningful outcome measures (risk behaviors and HIV seroconversion).

The Chicago Experience

Chicago's NADR program (which is now supported by local funding) collected longitudinal data over a 4-year period in an attempt to assess program impact on risk behaviors and HIV seroconversion (Wiebel et al., 1993b, 1994). This program was similar to the other NADR sites in its focus on out-of-treatment injectors and use of street outreach workers as HIV prevention educators; however, it had unique elements as well. The project's prevention activities has six key features:

1. The intervention is carried out by street outreach workers who are *former injectors*.

2. Outreach staff identify and target *social networks* of injectors, rather than isolated individuals.

3. Outreach staff educate network members about HIV and AIDS and work with them to *realistically assess their own risks* for HIV infection. Complete *confidentiality* is stressed throughout.

4. Staff then offer *multiple options* for coping with identified risks.

Options may include referral to treatment to stop injecting altogether, social strategies to avoid sharing injection equipment, and, for those who still share, instruction on how to clean injection equipment with bleach and water to reduce the risk of HIV transmission. Outreach workers carry supplies of bleach, water, cotton, condoms, and information pamphlets at all times and distribute materials as needed in all encounters.

5. In *repeated encounters* with injection drug users, outreach workers *support and reinforce behavioral change.*

6. The intervention's impact is further extended by *promoting prevention advocacy within injection drug user social networks* for HIV risk reduction.

Chicago's program represents the more intensive end of the range of NADR outreach programs in the frequency and duration of contacts that take place between street outreach workers and networks of injection drug users. As stated above, this program cannot be considered simply a bleach distribution program, although it uses bleach and other injection supplies as tools to facilitate interaction with street addicts and to reduce injection harm. It focuses on total risk awareness, education, and reduction, rather than solely on distributing bleach and providing instruction in bleach use.

To monitor trends in risk behavior and HIV incidence, a panel of injection drug users was recruited for study and followed over a 4-year period. The results of seven waves (baseline and six follow-ups) of interview and serologic data collection from 1988 through 1992 were analyzed.

The sample was recruited from the three Chicago neighborhoods in which the outreach was conducted: the mostly African American South Side, the ethnically mixed North Side, and the largely Puerto Rican Northwest Side. These neighborhoods were selected for their high concentration of injection drug activity, the variety of injectable drugs represented in the areas, and the broad demographic mix of user characteristics known to exist in Chicago. Recruitment targeted injectors in the three outreach areas in community settings such as street corners, copping (drug sales) areas, and shooting galleries. Injectors were identified on the basis of street outreach workers' knowledge of them and injectors' identification of others in their injection networks (targeted sampling).

Between March and August 1988, baseline interviews and blood specimens were collected from a cohort of 850 injection drug users. Of this initial cohort, 209 (24.6 percent) were HIV seropositive at their first serologic evaluation. Those injection drug users initially HIV seronegative and thus at risk for infection ($n = 641$) were the focus of the evaluation.

Subsequent to the 1988 baseline assessment, six waves of follow-up interviews and blood specimen collections were performed through fall 1992. The questionnaires used at the baseline and follow-up waves assessed the demographic characteristics, medical and drug treatment history, and recent drug-use and sexual behavior of respondents. Serologic screening for HIV-1 antibodies used venous specimens. Specimens repeatedly reactive in whole-virus lysate enzyme-linked immunosorbent assays (ELISA) were confirmed by Western blot.

The sample of 641 seronegative injection drug users was primarily male (76 percent); about two-thirds were age 40 or younger; somewhat more than half were African American, 26 percent white, and 18 percent Hispanic; and almost half reported injecting twice a day or more at recruitment. As of September 1992—4 years after the program began—the status of the cohort was 83 (13 percent) observed to have seroconverted, 42 (7 percent) had died and were seronegative at last serologic evaluation, 208 (32 percent) were seronegative at last evaluation and were lost to follow-up, and 308 (48 percent) were seronegative at the end of the study period. The cohort had second measures on 88 percent (513 of 641) of the baseline sample, and over-time follow-up response rates were 85, 84, 82, 78, and 68 percent, respectively, of the base sample in each of the successive waves.

Figure 6.1 shows the rate of HIV seroconversions per 100 person years (py). A decline in seroincidence was observed, from 8.4 per hundred py at the first follow-up wave to approximately 2.0 per hundred py after 1990.

Table 6.1 presents the percentages of the cohort reporting that they had engaged in HIV-related risk behavior since their last interview. The denominator for each wave is the number observed at each wave at risk of seroconverting (i.e., prior seroconverters are eliminated). The gender-specific prevalence of sexual risk behavior is nearly identical at each wave.

Survival analysis (i.e., Cox proportional hazard survival model) of HIV seroconversion incorporated the two behavioral risk variables, injecting risk and sexual risk, that varied over interviewing waves, as well as gender, age, race, and site/neighborhood. The only variable found to be associated with HIV seroconversion was the time-dependent behavioral risk variable "injecting risk" (RR = 9.8, $p < .001$). The time-dependent sexual risk variable and all demographic variables were not found to be associated with seroconverting.

Risky injection behavior was reported by 100 percent of the study cohort at baseline (1988) and only 14 percent at wave six (1992). (Neither risk behavior nor HIV status was an initial recruitment factor.) The observed decline in seroincidence in this cohort appears to have resulted from changes in drug-use risk behaviors attributable, at least in part, to the intervention.

This study design obviously cannot completely rule out alternative explanations for the observed decline in seroconversion in the studied cohort. One such alternative explanation could be that the findings were the result of other prevention efforts, especially given the increased amount of media attention directed at HIV risk reduction and other community efforts occur-

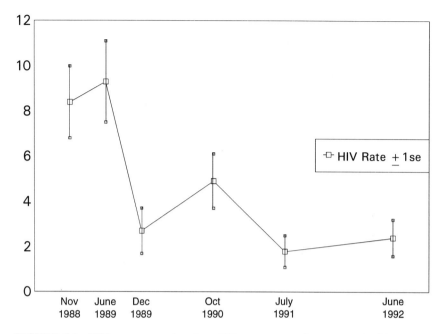

FIGURE 6.1 HIV seroconversion (per 100 person years) among out-of-treatment injection drug users in Chicago 1988-1992. SOURCE: *Prevention of New HIV Infections Among Out-of-Treatment Injection Drug Users: A Four Year Prospective Study* (Wiebel et al., 1994).

ring during that period. However, two independent data sets do provide support for the potential causal program effect on the observed findings.

During the sixth reinterview wave, the researchers recruited from nearby neighborhoods 248 previously unsurveyed street injection drug users. The prevalence of drug-use risk behavior among those who were seronegative was 50 percent for those with no reported outreach program contact. In addition, NIDA's surveys of drug treatment entrants in Chicago over a number of years include questions about needle sharing. The prevalence of self-reported needle sharing among 500 injection drug user treatment entrants surveyed in 1992 was 67 percent. The higher rates of risky injections found in these independent samples of injection drug users in the same communities lend some credence to the potential causal effect of the intervention on the observed decline in injection drug-use risk behaviors and HIV seroconversion. Nonetheless, it should be noted that these two separate data sets reflect substantially lower levels of drug-use risk behaviors than were observed at baseline among members of the intervention group (i.e., 100 percent). This implies that one cannot completely rule out some

TABLE 6.1 Percentage of Those at Risk of Converting (HIV Negative) Engaging in Sex Risk and Injecting Risk Behaviors

Midpoint	May 1988	November 1988	June 1989	December 1989	October 1990	July 1991	June 1992
Sexual risk	71	66	60	61	—	55	45
Injecting risk	100	54	46	37	27	19	14

SOURCE: *Prevention of New HIV Infections Among Out-of-Treatment Injection Drug Users: A Four Year Prospective Study* (Wiebel et al., 1994).

partial secular trend effect on the intervention group's observed drug-use risk behavior change.

There are a number of other possible uncontrolled factors that could account for the observed reduction in the injection drug-use risk behaviors and HIV seroconversion. Although participants were not "selected" for services on the basis of their measured level of risk, it is possible that they agreed to become a participant when their needle risk was at an abnormally high level. Due to maturation or instability in their levels of use, we would expect that on subsequent assessment, these clients would reveal a lower level of risk behavior (i.e., they would regress toward the population mean). Without a control group, it is not possible to assess the extent to which trait instability or maturation is at work.

Saturation of the at-risk pool of injectors (which happens when most of the susceptible injectors have already been infected) is yet another possible alternative explanation for the result depicted in Figure 6.1. Although the Chicago researchers contend that saturation could not account for the reported decline in seroincidence, because HIV seroprevalence remained constant in their cohort at 32 percent throughout their prospective study, it is still possible that saturation did impact on their findings. That is, saturation among those who remained susceptible (susceptibility being defined on the basis of risk of exposure through drug-use risk behavior) may have occurred, given that a substantil proportion of the cohort removed their risk of exposure (i.e., their drug-use risk behavior) and were no longer in the pool of susceptibles (assuming no risk of exposure through sexual-risk behavior).

Nonetheless, the data tend to suggest that there was a decrease in risky drug-use behavior over time, with an attendant decrease in new HIV infection in the cohort as originally assembled (irrespective of other risk behaviors).[3] It also highlights that bleach distribution occurs in the context of street outreach, making it difficult to disentangle bleach effect per se from the outreach worker effect. Moreover, the corresponding decline in self-report drug-use risk behavior and HIV incidence does also provide supporting evidence for the construct validity of self-report data.

The null results of epidemiologic studies reviewed earlier in conjunction with the program evaluation results reviewed above reveal the potential critical role of outreach activities in achieving meaningful behavioral change. In fact, these investigators (Wiebel et al., 1994) reported that injection drug users in the study group most frequently reduced risk *not* by always using bleach to clean injection equipment, but, rather, by eliminating the sharing of syringes and other injection equipment altogether. These changes in injection practices occurred over a time when there was no syringe exchange in Chicago, nor were there local laws permitting the possession of nonprescription needles, which suggests a high level of motivation on the part of cohort members to avoid HIV infection.

Therefore, in light of these findings, it would be misleading to consider the outreach efforts undertaken solely as bleach distribution programs.

Limitations of Bleach Disinfection

Although bleach, when properly used, provides an effective disinfectant in the health care setting, a number of variables may limit its effectiveness when used by injection drug users to disinfect contaminated needles and syringes. The physical and biological parameters that govern the effectiveness of any disinfectant (discussed earlier in this chapter) are critically important factors in determining whether the cleaning and disinfectant method used by a given injection drug user will result in effective disinfection of their injection equipment. Needles and syringes are not designed for reuse and are difficult to completely clean and disinfect. The presence of organic matter in the residual blood, either liquid or dried, remaining in the contaminated injection equipment decreases the potency of bleach as a disinfectant. The presence of blood in a previously used syringe necessitates thorough rinsing with water prior to bleach treatment. Residual, potentially infectious HIV present within clotted blood may be even more resistant to elimination by cleaning and disinfection methods. Furthermore, the infectivity of HIV-infected cells found within the blood remaining in used needles and syringes may be more resistant to disinfection than the cell-free or cell-associated HIV preparations studied in laboratory settings.

Reports by Shapshak and colleagues (Shapshak et al., 1993, 1994; McCoy et al., 1994) indicate that complete inactivation of preparations of cell-free HIV that had been concentrated ("pelleted") by centrifugation required prolonged (greater than 30 second) exposure to undiluted bleach. Although the laboratory model used in this study does not directly approximate the real-life circumstances of bleach disinfection of contaminated injection equipment, these reports resulted in significant concern and confusion about the validity of previous recommendations concerning bleach disinfection methods.

Another factor that may limit the effectiveness of disinfection efforts is that needles and syringes may become recontaminated if other drug injection paraphernalia, such as the cooker or the cotton used, are not cleaned or replaced (Koester et al., 1990). However, two studies (Marmor et al., 1987; Samuels et al., 1991) have found no association between shared cookers and HIV seroprevalence. Sharing water for mixing drugs or for rinsing the syringe after bleach use is another source of contamination (Koester et al., 1990; Inciardi and Page, 1991). Various methods of dividing drugs for sharing purposes also hold the potential for contamination (see Chapter 1).

These practices include *frontloading* (removing the needle from one syringe and filling that syringe by inserting the needle from another drug-filled syringe directly into the barrel), and *backloading* (removing the plunger from the back of the syringe and filling that syringe through the back with drugs from a second syringe). Studies of these factors have to date yielded conflicting results, with a report from New York finding a positive association between frontloading and HIV seroprevalence (Jose et al., 1992), and a study in Baltimore (Samuels et al., 1991) reporting similar seroprevalence rates for injection drug users who did and did not practice frontloading. Samuels and colleagues noted, however, that these results do *not* mean "that the behaviors are without risk of HIV infection among [injection drug users] . . . (but) that the associated risks are probably low relative to other (HIV risk) behaviors."

Impact of Bleach Disinfection on HIV Transmission

If disinfection of injection equipment is an effective means of preventing HIV infection, then HIV seroconversion rates would be expected to be lower among injection drug users who consistently disinfect their injection equipment. Prior to the initiation of the original CHOW program in San Francisco, Chaisson and colleagues (1987) found no protective effect for those injection drug users who reported cleaning their needles and syringes with boiling water or alcohol. Later, Moss and Chaisson (1988) reported that there was no relationship found between behavior change, including reported bleach use, and seroprevalence. In contrast, Watters (1994) reported that, although the seroprevalence rate among heterosexual injection drug users in San Francisco nearly doubled between 1986 and 1987, there was a stabilization of seroprevalence following the introduction of the bleach distribution and other HIV prevention programs. However, seroprevalent infections for which the date of onset of infection is unknown are not the optimal endpoint from which to measure effectiveness of an intervention, since other risk reduction factors, such as decreased needle sharing, were operating simultaneously. In such circumstances, any change in seroprevalence cannot be attributed solely to the bleach distribution programs.

More recently, Vlahov and colleagues have studied the relationship between the reported injection equipment disinfection practices of injection drug users and rates of HIV seroconversion. Their initial report (Vlahov et al., 1991) described a small nested case-control study of HIV seroconverters and HIV-seronegative injection drug users by their self-report frequency of using disinfectants all the time, less than all the time, and no use of disinfectants. Although no statistically significant protective effect was detected, the results of this study suggested a possible modest protective effect of bleach or alcohol disinfection among injection drug users who reported always using disinfectants. A follow-up study by these investigators reexamined this result (Vlahov et al., 1994), using a larger sample size and examining the influence of potentially confounding variables on the study outcome, including the effect of drug-use variables, the possibility of sexual acquisition of HIV infection (Solomon et al., 1993), and the potential for study participants to provide socially desirable responses to the investigator's questions concerning disinfection practices (Latkin et al., 1993). Nevertheless, similar null results were obtained, with injection drug users who reported using disinfectants all the time compared with those who reported no use of disinfectants (Vlahov et al., 1994). Thus, bleach use, as practiced in Baltimore in the early 1990s, did not eliminate or substantially reduce the risk of HIV seroconversion among injection drug users who reported using it all the time.

Similar findings were subsequently found in New York (Titus et al., 1994), in a case-control study. After adjusting for possible confounders, no evidence that bleach use protected against incident HIV infection was reported. Another study of HIV seroconversion among injection drug users in San Francisco showed no protective effect with bleach disinfection (Moss et al., 1994). It remains to be established whether these disappointing results derive from exaggerated reporting of injection drug users about their actual disinfection practices, the use of inadequate disinfection methods, contamination of water or ancillary injection paraphernalia with HIV, or the inability of bleach or alcohol to effectively disinfect contaminated needles and syringes within the context of their actual use by injection drug users.

Responding to concerns arising from laboratory studies about prevailing methods for bleach inactivation of HIV and epidemiologic studies that suggest little, if any, protective effect of needle and syringe disinfection efforts, the Centers for Disease Control, the National Institute on Drug Abuse, and the Center for Substance Abuse Treatment (CSAT) sponsored a meeting in February 1993 at which the current status of bleach outreach and research was reviewed. Discussions from this meeting provided the basis for the publication of provisional guidelines on bleach disinfection (Curran et al., 1993). These published guidelines included the following recommendations:

- Cleaning should be done twice—once immediately after use and again just before reuse of needles and syringes.
- Before using bleach, wash out the needle and syringe by filling them several times with clean water. (This will reduce the amount of blood and other debris in the syringe. Blood reduces the effectiveness of bleach.)
- Then, use full-strength liquid household bleach (not diluted bleach).
- Completely fill the needle and syringe with bleach several times. (Some suggest filling the syringe at least three times.)

• The longer the syringe is completely full of bleach, the more likely HIV will be inactivated. (Some suggest the syringe should be full of bleach for at least 30 seconds.)

• After using bleach, rinse the syringe and needle by filling several times with clean water. *Don't reuse water* used for initial prebleach washing; it may be contaminated.

• For every filling of the needle and syringe with prebleach wash water, bleach, and rinse water, fill the syringe completely ("to the top").

• Shaking and tapping the syringe are recommended when the syringe is filled with prebleach wash water, bleach, and rinse water. Shaking the syringe should improve the effectiveness of all steps.

• Taking the syringe apart (removing the plunger) may improve the cleaning/disinfection of parts (e.g., behind the plunger) that might not be reached by solutions in the syringe.

Although the intent of these guidelines was to provide clear recommendations to be used by outreach workers in risk reduction programs in the injection drug user community and to attempt to maximize the effectiveness of bleach disinfection methods, responses to this revision have been mixed. Some, including researchers as well as injection drug users and outreach workers, have interpreted the revised guidelines to mean that bleach is ineffective and have called for using bleach only as a last resort (Donoghoe and Power, 1993). Other outreach workers have expressed concern that changing the guidelines undermines their credibility with injection drug users (Haverkos and Jones, 1994). Whereas implementing these recommendations is likely to increase the effectiveness of bleach disinfection of needles and syringes, the lack of adequate laboratory models of injection equipment disinfection makes this difficult to document. Given the importance of limiting HIV transmission among injection drug users, the margin of safety in disinfection methods is desirable. However, should recommended disinfection strategies prove too complex or cumbersome, they may be less likely to be followed.

At least one report indicates that injection drug users accept the majority of the guidelines (Corby, 1993). In the 5 months following publication of the guidelines, 17 focus groups were held in eight cities across the country to gauge injection drug users' acceptance of the new guidelines. Two of the eight recommended practices were judged as unlikely to be adopted: cleaning both before and after injection and disassembling the syringe. Many injection drug users felt that the first was unnecessary and the second would damage the equipment or would be too difficult to do.

SUMMARY

The reuse of needles and syringes that are intended for use by a single individual on a single occasion is an inherently unsafe practice. The repeated use of needles and syringes commonly violates their sterility and predisposes the user to life-threatening infections from a wide variety of bacterial and viral pathogens. The sharing of injection equipment by injection drug users provides an efficient means of transmitting HIV, hepatitis B and C viruses, and the human T-cell leukemia viruses (HTLV-I and HTLV-II). The only reliable ways to limit the transmission of HIV and other viral infections among injection drug users are either to refrain from injecting drugs or not to share injection equipment with other users. If an injection drug user is unable or unwilling to refrain from using injection drugs, the use of a sterile, disposable needle and syringe for each injection represents the next best alternative. However, in circumstances in which supplies of sterile needles and syringes are inadequate or unavailable, disinfection strategies provide another means to decrease the risk of transmission of HIV and other infectious agents between injection drug users who are compelled to share injection equipment.

Bleach disinfection of contaminated needles and syringes is the most commonly used and familiar strategy employed by injection drug users, and, if used according to current recommendations made by the Centers for Disease Control and Prevention, the National Institute on Drug Abuse, and the Center for Substance Abuse Treatment, is likely to be effective in disinfecting contaminated injection equipment. Definition of the precise efficacy of bleach as a disinfectant of HIV-contaminated needles and syringes has been hampered by the lack of a laboratory model that faithfully recapitulates the real-life circumstances of injection drug use. Unfortunately, too little attention and too few resources have been devoted to studies to define the simplest, most effective disinfection methods for injection equipment used by injection drug users.

The inability of initial epidemiologic studies to demonstrate a significant protective effect of disinfection practice against HIV infection of injection drug users is disconcerting. Unfortunately, evaluation and epidemiologic studies performed to date do not clearly identify the reasons for the similar rates of incident HIV infections reported between those who always clean their needles and syringes and those who never do. It is not yet known whether this results from inadequate disinfection techniques used by injection drug users who become infected, their overestimation of the frequency of their use of needle and syringe disinfection in interviews with researchers, or physical or biological factors that compromise the ability of bleach, a potent disinfectant in other circumstances, to effectively disinfect contaminated injection equipment. Certainly, a number of observational studies indicate that injection drug users may use variable, and often clearly inadequate, disinfection strategies. Furthermore, adherence to recommended disinfection protocols after training may decrease with time. Increasingly complex disinfection strategies may be less likely to be retained or adopted by injection drug users.

Additional research is needed to identify approaches that most effectively transmit to injection drug users the importance of disinfection of contaminated injection equipment and that ensure maximal compliance with recommended procedures. In the interim, promotion of a clear, consistent method of disinfection procedures, such as those recommended in the recent CDC/NIDA/CSAT publication, is essential to help decrease the risk of HIV infection for injection drug users who continue to share needles and syringes.

Bleach can be an effective and potentially life-saving intervention for injection drug users who share needles and syringes. Bleach distribution programs have been a popular and effective component of community health outreach efforts to decrease HIV risk behaviors among injection drug users. Continued advocacy of bleach disinfection will be necessary even if sterile needles and syringes become more widely available through exchange programs or the relaxation of prescription laws.

Research efforts to better model the efficacy of disinfection strategies for blood-contaminated needles and syringes should be actively encouraged. Emphasis should be placed on models that are relevant to the typical practices and circumstances of injection drug use behaviors. Additional field research studies are needed to further evaluate the effectiveness of bleach disinfection in decreasing the risk of HIV infection among injection drug users. A better understanding of the reasons for the limited protective impact of needle and syringe disinfection practices documented to date is essential. Research to identify effective education strategies to maximize injection drug user familiarity with and practice of effective bleach disinfection methods is needed.

Conclusions

The panel concludes that:

- Bleach, *if used according to the recommendations of the Centers for Disease Control and Prevention, the National Institute on Drug Abuse, and the Center for Substance Abuse Treatment*, is likely to be an effective HIV prevention strategy for injection drug users who share needles and syringes.
- Concerted efforts are essential to increase the awareness of injec-

tion drug users of the importance of disinfecting shared injection equipment and the importance of following the appropriate procedures.

Recommendations

The panel recommends that:

• Health research funding agencies (e.g., the National Institutes of Health, the Centers for Disease Control and Prevention, and the Agency for Health Care Policy and Research) should support research directed toward identifying the simplest to use and most effective disinfection strategies, employing agents that are readily available to injection drug users.

• Health research funding agencies (e.g., the National Institutes of Health, the Centers for Disease Control and Prevention) should support development of effective education strategies for familiarizing injection drug users with methods of effective bleach disinfection.

NOTES

1. The disparity between the number of follow-up and the number of individuals included in the analyses (in particular, the sex partners) is not discussed in the final report.

2. The follow-up rates per site were not reported for all sites. Of those reported, the rates ranged from a low of 2 percent to a high of 74 percent.

3. The Chicago study was completed before the needle exchange evaluation study reviewed in Appendix A. As the reader will note, this cohort of injection drug users (which represented a sizable proportion of the needle exchange sample) had experienced substantial reductions in drug-use risk behavior and HIV incidence prior to the needle exchange evaluation study. This provides an historical context for reviewing the needle exchange evaluation project presented in Appendix A.

REFERENCES

Battjes, R., and R. Pickens
  1992   Trends in HIV Infection and AIDS Risk Behaviors Among Intravenous Drug Users in Selected U.S. Cities. Abstract No. PoC 4247. *International Conference on AIDS* 8(2):C286.
  1993   Trends in HIV Infection and AIDS Risk Behaviors Among Intravenous Drug Users in Selected U.S. Cities. Abstract No. PO-C15-2950. *International Conference on AIDS* 9(2):709.
Becker, M.H., and J.G. Joseph
  1988   AIDS and behavioral change to reduce risk: A review. *American Journal of Public Health* 78(4):394-410.
Becker, G.L., S. Cohen, and R. Borer
  1974   The sequelae of accidentally injecting sodium hypochlorite beyond the root apex. *Oral Surgery* 38(4):633-638.

Block, S.S., ed.
1983   Definition of terms. Pp. 877-881 in *Disinfection, Sterilization and Preservation*, 3rd edition. Philadelphia, PA: Lea & Febiger.
Brown, B.S.
1994   Review of the Effects of Bleach Distribution Programs. Paper commissioned by the Panel on Needle Exchange and Bleach Distribution Programs.
Brown, B.S., and G.M. Beschner, eds.
1993   *Handbook on Risk of AIDS—Injection Drug Users and Sexual Partners*. Westport, CT: Greenwood Press.
Celentano, D.D., D. Vlahov, A.S. Menon, and B.F. Polk
1991   HIV knowledge and attitudes among intravenous drug users: Comparison to the U.S. population and by drug use behaviors. *Journal of Drug Issues* 21(3):635-649.
Centers for Disease Control
1986   Recommendations for providing dialysis treatment to patients infected with human T-lymphotropic virus type III/lymphadenopathy-associated virus. *Morbidity and Mortality Weekly Report* 35(23):376-378, 383.
1987   Recommendations for prevention of HIV transmission in health-care settings. *Morbidity and Mortality Weekly Report* 1S-18S.
Chaisson, R.E., A.R. Moss, R. Onishi, D. Osmond, and J.R. Carlson
1987   Human immunodeficiency virus infection in heterosexual intravenous drug users in San Francisco. *American Journal of Public Health* 77(2):169-172.
Conte, J.E., Jr.
1986   Infection with human immunodeficiency virus in the hospital. Epidemiology, infection control, and biosafety considerations. *Annals of Internal Medicine* 105(5):730-736.
Corby, N.
1993   Injection Drug Users Willingness to Adopt New Bleaching Recommendations. A paper presented at the 6th Annual AIDS Update in San Francisco, California.
Curran, J.W., L.W. Scheckel, and R.A. Millstein
1993   *HIV/AIDS Prevention Bulletin*, April 19. Washington, DC: Department of Health and Human Services, Public Health Service, and Centers for Disease Control and Prevention.
Des Jarlais, D.C., S.R. Friedman, and D. Strug
1986   AIDS and needle sharing within the IV-drug use subculture. Pp. 111-125 in *The Social Dimensions of AIDS: Methods and Theory*, D. Feldman and T. Johnson, eds. New York, NY: Preager.
Donoghoe, M.D., and R. Power
1993   Household bleach as disinfectant for use by injecting drug users. *Lancet* 341(8861):1658.
Edlin, B.R, K. Irwin, Y. Serrano, P. Evans, and C. McCoy
1993   The Impact of Cocaine Smoking on Injection Practices of Street-Recruited Drug Injectors. Abstract No. PO-C15-2952. *International Conference on AIDS* 9(2):709.
Favero, M.S., and W.W. Bond
1991   Disinfection, sterilization and preservation. In *Chemical Disinfection of Medical and Surgical Materials*. Philadelphia, PA: Lea & Febiger.
Feldman, H.W., and P. Biernacki
1988   The ethnography of needle sharing among IVDUs and implications for public policies and intervention strategies. In *Needle Sharing Among IVDUs: National and International Perspectives*, R.J. Battjes and R.W. Pickens, eds. NIDA Research Monograph No. 80:28-39. Washington, DC: National Institute on Drug Abuse.

Flynn, N., S. Jain, E.M. Keddie, J.R. Carlson, M.B. Jennings, H.W. Haverkos, N. Nassar, R. Anderson, S. Cohen, and D. Goldberg
1994   In vitro activity of readily available household materials against HIV-1: Is bleach enough? *Journal of Acquired Immune Deficiency Syndromes* 7(7):747-753.

Friedman, S.R., M. Sufian, A. Neaigus, B. Stepherson, et al.
1990   Organizing Drug Users Against AIDS: A Comparison With Outreach for Producing Risk Reduction. Abstract No. S.C. 733. *International Conference on AIDS* 6(3):272.

Froner, G.A., G.W. Rutherford, and M. Rokeach
1987   Injection of sodium hypochlorite by intravenous drug users [letter]. *Journal of the American Medical Association* 258(3):325.

Gleghorn, A.A.
1993   Limitations of Bleach Use. A paper presented at the 6th Annual AIDS Update, San Francisco, California.
1994   Use of bleach by injection drug users. Pp. 294-302 in *Proceedings, Workshop on Needle Exchange and Bleach Distribution Programs*. Washington, DC: National Academy Press.

Gleghorn, A.A., M.C. Doherty, D. Vlahov, D.D. Celentano, and T.S. Jones
1994   Inadequate bleach contact times during syringe cleaning among injection drug users. *Journal of Acquired Immune Deficiency Syndromes* 7(7):767-772.

Haverkos, H.W., and T.S. Jones
1994   HIV, drug-use paraphernalia, and bleach. *Journal of Acquired Immune Deficiency Syndromes* 7(7):741-742.

Hopkins, W.
1988   Needle sharing and street behavior in response to AIDS in New York City. In *Needle Sharing Among IVDUs: National and International Perspectives*, R.J. Battjes and R.W. Pickens, eds. NIDA Research Monograph No. 80:18-27. Washington, DC: National Institute on Drug Abuse.

Hugo, W.B., and A.D. Russell
1982   Types of antimicrobial agents. Pp. 8-106 in *Principles and Practice Disinfection, Preservation and Sterilization*, W.B. Hugo and G.A. Ayliffe, eds. Oxford, England: Blackwell.

Inciardi, J.A., and J.B. Page
1991   Drug sharing among intravenous drug users. *AIDS* 5(6):772-773.

Ingraham, A.S.
1992   The chemistry of disinfectants and sterilants. *Contemporary Topics* 31:18-23.

Jose, B., S.R. Friedman, A. Neaigus, R. Curtis, and D.C. Des Jarlais
1992   "Frontloading" Is Associated With HIV Infection Among Drug Injectors in New York City. Abstract No. ThC1551. *International Conference on AIDS* Th76.

Klein, M. and A. Deforest
1963   Antiviral action of germicides. *Soap Chemistry Specialist* 39:70-72, 95-97.
1965a   Principles of viral inactivation. Pp. 422-434 in *Disinfection, Sterilization, and Preservation*, S.S. Block, ed. Philadelphia, PA: Lea & Febiger.
1965b   The chemical inactivation of viruses. *Federation Proceedings* 24:319.

Koester, S., R. Booth, and W. Wiebel
1990   The risk of HIV transmission from sharing water, drug-mixing containers and cotton filters among intravenous drug users. *International Journal of Drug Policy* 1(6):28-30.

Latkin, C.A., D. Vlahov, J.C. Anthony, S. Cohn, and W. Mandell
1992   Needle-cleaning practices among intravenous drug users who share injection equipment in Baltimore, Maryland. *International Journal of the Addictions* 27(6):717-725.

Latkin, C.A., D. Vlahov, and J.C. Anthony
1993   Socially desirable responding and self-reported HIV infection risk behaviors among intravenous drug users. *Addiction* 88:517-526.

Longshore, D., M.D. Anglin, K. Annon, and S. Hsieh
1993   Trends in self-reported HIV risk behavior: Injection drug users in Los Angeles. *Journal of Acquired Immune Deficiency Syndromes* 6(1):82-90.

Marmor, M., D.C. Des Jarlais, H. Cohen, S.R. Friedman, S.T. Beatrice, N. Dubin, W. el-Sadr, D. Mildvan, S. Yancovitz, U. Mathor, et al.
1987   Risk factors for HIV infection with human immunodeficiency virus among intravenous drug users in New York City. *AIDS* 1(1):39-44.

Martin, L.S., J.S. McDougal, and S.L. Lokoski
1985   Disinfection and inactivation of the human T-lymphotrophic virus type-III/lymphadenopathy-associated virus. *Journal of Infectious Diseases* 152(2):400-403.

McCoy, C.B., H.V. McCoy, P. Shapshak, N. Weatherby, et al.
1992   HIV Intervention Strategies Based on Field and Laboratory Studies. Abstract No. PoC 4292. *International Conference on AIDS* 8(2):C293.

McCoy, C.B., J.E. Rivers, H.V. McCoy, P. Shapshak, N.L. Weatherby, D.D. Chitwood, J.B. Page, J.A. Inciardi, and D.C. McBride
1994a   Compliance to bleach disinfection protocols among injecting drug users in Miami. *Journal of Acquired Immune Deficiency Syndromes* 7(7):773-776.

McCoy, C.B., P. Shapshak, S.M. Shah, H.V. McCoy, J.E. Rivers, J.B. Page, D.D. Chitwood, N.L. Weatherby, J.A. Inciardi, D.C. McBride, D.C. Mash, and J.K. Watters
1994b   HIV-1 prevention: Interdisciplinary studies and reviews on efficacy of bleach and compliance to bleach prevention protocols. Pp. 255-283 in *Proceedings, Workshop on Needle Exchange and Bleach Distribution Programs*. Washington, DC: National Academy Press.

McKee, M.M., V.A. Caine, and L.M. Bryson
1992   Promoting Safe Injection Technique and Condom Usage Among Injection Drug Users in Indianapolis, IN. Abstract No. PoD 5085. *International Conference on AIDS* 8(2):D401.

Meyers, M., R. Nemeth-Coslett, F. Snyder, and P. Young
1990   Needle Cleaning Methods Reported by Intravenous Drug Users Who Are Not in Drug Treatment. Abstract No. S.C. 743. *International Conference on AIDS* 6(3):274.

Moss, A.R., and R.E. Chaisson
1988   AIDS and intravenous drug use in San Francisco. *AIDS and Public Policy Journal* 3:37-41.

Moss, A.R., K. Vranizan, R. Gorter, P. Bacchetti, J. Watters, and D. Osmond
1994   HIV seroconversion in intravenous drug users in San Francisco, 1985-1990. *AIDS* 8:223-231.

Murphy, S.
1987   Intravenous drug use and AIDS: Notes on the social economy of needle sharing. *Contemporary Drug Problems* Fall:373-395.

National Institute on Drug Abuse
1994   *Outreach/Risk Reduction Strategies for Changing HIV-Related Risk Behaviors Among Injection Drug Users: The National AIDS Demonstration Research (NADR) Project.* NIH Publication No. 94-3726. Bethesda, MD: National Institutes of Health.

Neaigus, A., M. Sufian, S.R. Friedman, D.S. Goldsmith, B. Stepherson, P. Mota, J. Pascal, and D.C. Des Jarlais
1990   Effects of outreach intervention on risk reduction among intravenous drug users. *AIDS Education and Prevention* 2(4):253-271.

Newmeyer, J.A.
1988   Why bleach? Fighting AIDS contagion among intravenous drug users: The San Francisco experience. *Journal of Psychoactive Drugs* 20(2):159-163.

Pantaleo, G., C. Graziosi, and A.S. Fauci
1993   New concepts in the immunopathogenesis of human immunodeficiency virus infection. *New England Journal of Medicine* 328(5):327-335.

Resnick, L., K. Veren, Z. Salahudin, S. Tondreau, and P.D. Markham
1986   Stability and inactivation of HTLV-III/LAV under clinical and laboratory environments. *Journal of the American Medical Association* 255(14):1887-1891.

Rhame, F.S.
1986   The inanimate environment. Pp. 233-249 in *Hospital Infections*, J.V. Bennett and P.S. Brachmann, eds. Boston, MA: Little, Brown and Co.

Rutala, W.A.
1987   Disinfection, sterilization, and waste disposal. Pp. 257-282 in *Prevention and Control of Nosocomial Infections*, R.P. Wenzel, ed. Baltimore, MD: Williams and Wilkins.
1990   APIC guideline for selection and use of disinfectants. *American Journal of Infection Control* 18(2):99-117.

Rutala, W.A., and E.C. Cole
1984   Antiseptics and disinfectants—Safe and effective? *Infection Control* 5(5):215-218.

Rutala, W.A., and D.J. Weber
1987   Environmental issues and nosocomial infections. Pp. 131-171 in *Clinics and Critical Care Medicine: Infection Control in Intensive Care*. New York, NY: Churchill Livingston.

Samuels, J.F., D. Vlahov, J.C. Anthony, L. Solomon, and D.D. Celentano
1991   The practice of "frontloading" among intravenous drug users: Association with HIV-antibody [letter]. *AIDS* 5(3):343.

Sattar, S.A., and V.S. Springthorpe
1991   Survival and disinfectant inactivation of the human immunodeficiency virus: A critical review. *Reviews of Infectious Diseases* 13(3):430-447.

Shapshak, P., C.B. McCoy, J.E. Rivers, D.D. Chitwood, D.C. Mash, N.L. Weatherby, J.A. Inciardi, S.M. Shah, and B.S. Brown
1993   Inactivation of human immunodeficiency virus-1 at short time intervals using undiluted bleach [letter]. *Journal of Acquired Immune Deficiency Syndromes* 6(2):218-219.

Shapshak, P., C.B. McCoy, S.M. Shah, J. B. Page, J.E. Rivers, N.L. Weatherby, D.D. Chitwood, and D.C. Mash
1994   Preliminary laboratory studies of inactivation of HIV-1 in needles and syringes containing infected blood using undiluted household bleach. *Journal of Acquired Immune Deficiency Syndromes* 7(7):754-759.

Solomon, L., J. Astemborski, D. Warren, A. Muñoz, S. Cohn, D. Vlahov, and K.E. Nelson
1993   Difference in risk factors for human immunodeficiency virus type 1 seroconversion among male and female intravenous drug users. *American Journal of Epidemiology* 137:892-898.

Sorenson, J.L., J. Guydish, M. Costantini, and S.L. Batki
1989   Changes in needle sharing and syringe cleaning among San Francisco drug abusers. *New England Journal of Medicine* 320(12):807.

Spire, B., F. Barré-Sinoussi, L. Montagnier, and J.C. Chermann
1984   Inactivation of lymphadenopathy associated virus by chemical disinfectants. *Lancet* 2(8408):899-901.

Titus, S., M. Marmor, D. Des Jarlais, M. Kim, H. Wolfe, and S. Beatrice
1994   Bleach use and HIV seroconversion among New York City injection drug users. *Journal of Acquired Immune Deficiency Syndromes* 7(7):700-704.

Van Houton, J., and M.D. Hayre
1991   Disinfectants and sterilants: Their chemistry, use and evaluation. *AALAS Bulletin* 30:24-27.

Vlahov, D., A. Muñoz, D.D. Celentano, S. Cohn, J.C. Anthony, H. Chilcoat, and K.E. Nelson
1991   HIV seroconversion and disinfection of injection equipment among intravenous drug users, Baltimore, Maryland. *Epidemiology* 2(6):444-446.

Vlahov, D., J. Astemborski, L. Solomon, and K.E. Nelson
1994   Field effectiveness of needle disinfection among injection drug users. *Journal of Acquired Immune Deficiency Syndromes* 7(7):760-766.

Watters, J.
1987   A street-based outreach model of AIDS prevention for intravenous drug users: Preliminary evaluation. *Contemporary Drug Problems* Fall:411-423.
1994   Historical perspective on the use of bleach in HIV/AIDS prevention. *Journal of Acquired Immune Deficiency Syndromes* 7(7):743-746.

Wiebel, W.W.
1990   Identifying and gaining access to hidden populations. In *The Collection and Interpretation of Data from Hidden Populations*, E.Y. Lambert, ed. NIDA Research Monograph No. 98:4-11. Washington, DC: National Institute on Drug Abuse.
1993   *The Indigenous Leader Outreach Model, Intervention Manual*. National Institute on Drug Abuse, Department of Health and Human Services Publication no. 93-3581.

Wiebel, W.W., D. Chene, and W. Johnson
1990   Adoption of Bleach Use in a Cohort of Street Intravenous Drug Users in Chicago. Abstract No. S.C. 742. *International Conference on AIDS* 6(3):274.

Wiebel, W.A., Jimenez, N. Johnson, L. Ouellet, L. Lampinen, J. Murray, B. Jovanovic, and M.U. O'Brien
1993   Positive Effect on HIV Seroconversion of Street Outreach Intervention with IDU in Chicago: 1988-1992. Presented at the Ninth International Conference on AIDS, June 6-11, Berlin.

Wiebel, W.W., W. Johnson, B. Jovanovic, and J. Murray
1994   Prevention of New HIV Infections Among Out-of-Treatment Injection Drug Users: A Four Year Prospective Study. Draft paper.

7

The Effects of Needle Exchange Programs

This chapter assesses the effects of needle exchange programs on HIV infections and drug use behaviors. Five major sources provide the evidentiary basis for the panel's assessment: (1) a 1991 review carried out by congressional request of the effectiveness of needle exchange programs (U.S. General Accounting Office, 1993), (2) a second comprehensive evaluation carried out by University of California researchers for the Centers for Disease Control and Prevention (Lurie et al., 1993), (3) selected studies published since the two 1993 literature reviews, (4) detailed examination of a set of recent studies in New Haven, Connecticut, and (5) detailed examination of a set of recent studies in Tacoma, Washington. This chapter concludes with the panel's conclusions and recommendations, which are based on the evidence presented in the chapter and throughout the report.

Evaluations of needle exchange programs have been published by Stimson et al. (1988), Des Jarlais (1985), the U.S. General Accounting Office (GAO) (1993), and the University of California (Lurie et al., 1993). We highlight the findings of the latter two reports, which were commissioned specifically by the federal government as evaluations of needle exchange programs. Both were published in 1993 and deal with needle exchange programs as they existed up to that time.

Needle exchange programs operate in a rapidly changing environment, and the panel reviews a number of studies that were published subsequent to the major reviews by GAO and the University of California.

Two strong lines of evidence emerged from the panel's examination of recent research on the effects of needle exchange programs on the spread of

HIV infection: studies from New Haven and Tacoma. These two sets of studies were selected on the basis of the wealth of published information available about the programs they analyze. That is, not only do they provide a sizable amount of information on various endpoints of interest (i.e., incident infection and risk behaviors), but they also have carefully addressed potential alternative explanations for their reported findings.

POTENTIAL OUTCOMES

At the outset, it is important to recognize that the effects of needle exchange programs can be viewed from a number of different perspectives. Some of these perspectives involve outcomes relevant to improving the health status of injection drug users, and others reflect community-level concerns regarding potential negative effects that may be associated with the implementation of such programs. The following section identifies the outcome domains that are relevant to those distinct perspectives and are most germane to the panel's task of assessing the effects of needle exchange programs.

Possible Positive Outcomes

Needle exchanges are established in order to: (1) increase the availability of sterile injection equipment and (2) at the same time, remove contaminated needles from circulation among the program participants. Operation of the exchange, then, is expected to result in a supply of needles with reduced potential for infecting program participants with HIV and also to reduce sharing between individuals because of easier access to clean needles for any program participant. Typical exchanges also maintain such services as education concerning risk behaviors, referral to drug treatment programs (a step toward eliminating the route for all infection), and distribution of condoms. These measures offer independent prospects for reducing the spread of HIV. Appraisal of the success of a needle exchange program may involve measuring, for example, the numbers of needles exchanged; the cleanliness of circulating needles; the prevalence and incidence of HIV and other needle-borne diseases; referrals to drug treatment programs; enrollments in treatment programs; and changes in the risk behaviors of needle exchange participants. An observed pattern of favorable outcomes would reflect health benefits from the operation of the program.

Possible Negative Outcomes

The possibility of negative results from needle exchange program operations also demands attention. One possible negative outcome is an in-

TABLE 7.1 Possible Outcomes and Expectations of Successful Needle Exchange Programs

Possible Positive Outcomes:	PossibleNegative Outcomes:
Reduction in pool of infected needles	Increase in drug use among needle exchange program clients
Reduction in drug-related risk behavior	Increase in new initiates to injection drug use
Reduction in sexual risk behavior	Increase in drug use in wider community
Increase in referrals to drug abuse treatment	Increase in number of contaminated needles unsafely discarded (e.g., on street)
Reduction in new infections among client population	

crease in the number of improperly discarded used needles. Another possibility is that the issuance of injection equipment, condoned by government, will "send a message" undercutting efforts at combatting illegal drug use and will promote more drug use (with more attendant HIV incidence). A third possible negative outcome is that needle exchanges will lower the perception of risk of injection drug use and thus attract more users to inject drugs and to other forms of illegal drug use.

Appraisal of the success of a needle exchange program, then, should also attend to measures of these possible negative outcomes. An observed pattern of negative outcomes would weigh against the idea that needle exchange programs are beneficial.

Assessment of the effects of needle exchanges involves the simultaneous consideration of a number of intended positive and unintended negative outcomes (Table 7.1). Ideally, a successful exchange program would reduce the risk of new infection among injection drug users without increasing drug use and health risks to the public.

THE PANEL'S APPROACH TO THE EVIDENCE

The purpose of this section is to clearly explain the panel's perspective in assessing the effectiveness of needle exchange programs. We first briefly review the basis for the traditional review procedures. We then outline the argument for a different approach—one that examines the patterns of evidence in order to assess effectiveness.

The Traditional Approach:
Considering the Preponderance of the Evidence

Traditional reviews of experimental analysis search for studies with well-controlled research designs. By well-controlled designs, we mean ones that can substantially protect against the introduction of systematic influences (i.e., bias) other than the intervention condition under consideration. High ratings on credibility are usually given to comparative designs that involve: (1) random assignment of participants to conditions (i.e., needle exchange program versus "usual services"); (2) minimal attrition of participants from being measured; (3) measurement procedures that minimize the role of response biases; and (4) sufficient statistical sensitivity (i.e., statistical power).

It is unlikely that evaluations of needle exchange programs will ever be carried out with ideal controls that warrant high confidence in the conclusions that can be drawn from a single definitive study. There are at least two broad reasons for this: (1) multiple actions generally are initiated in a given community setting, making it difficult to separate the effects of a needle exchange program from those of other prevention efforts by studying time trends and (2) the development of a comparative research design that relies on random assignment of individuals to receive needle exchange program services (or not) has technical, ethical, and logistical difficulties. Given these limitations, it seems reasonable to explore alternative means of assessing the credibility of the evidence's underlying claims about the effectiveness of needle exchange programs. Before doing so, however, it is useful to examine how previous research reviews have attempted to incorporate the traditional emphasis on design-induced control.

Two reviews were commissioned by the federal government and published in 1993: one by the U.S. General Accounting Office (1993) and one by the University of California at San Francisco (Lurie et al., 1993). Prior to 1993, a number of other studies were published (Des Jarlais et al., 1985; Stimson et al., 1988).

A close examination of the manner in which these studies were conducted strongly suggests their reliance on the quality of the evidence in individual studies, which is based on the strength of their research designs. The language of the assessments also reflects the expectation that, when they are taken as a collective across studies, even though the designs are less than ideal, the *preponderance of evidence* will weigh in favor of or against a definitive conclusion about needle exchange programs.

Taken together, these studies tend to suggest that needle exchange programs are either neutral or positive in terms of potential positive effects and that they do not demonstrate any potential negative effects. However, each study's conclusions are often less than firm because of its methodological limitations.

An Alternative Approach: Looking at the Patterns of Evidence

When the designs of a group of studies are limited, little inferential clarity is gained by looking at the preponderance of evidence, even if it converges across all available studies. At a minimum, there must be a sufficient number of higher-quality (i.e., high-credibility) studies within the pool of studies to assess whether the evidence from the lower-quality studies is biased in a particular fashion.

Rationale

For well-designed interventions with well-designed experimental assessment procedures, examining each outcome one at a time is obviously justifiable on statistical and logical grounds. However, in light of the fact that most studies that have attempted to assess the effectiveness of needle exchange programs have limited study designs and that there are serious practical constraints associated with conducting a randomized control trial, some may conclude that it is impossible to ever determine whether needle exchange programs are effective. In the panel's view, however, such a conclusion is both poor scientific judgment and bad public health policy. Indeed, to adopt the position that evidence short of a randomized trial is useless amounts to denying the possibility of learning from experience— which, though often difficult, is not impossible.

In many areas of social sciences and public health research, the so-called definitive study—a randomized control experiment (that is, a randomized double-blind placebo controlled trial)—is an ideal that cannot be implemented. For example, it is unethical to consider use of a clinical trial design to show that smoking causes lung cancer (Hill, 1965). Scientific judgment develops instead through a series of studies using cross-sectional retrospective and prospective designs, in which later research avoids the flaws of earlier work but may introduce problems of its own. The improbability of being able to carry out the definitive study of the effects of certain HIV and AIDS prevention programs, including needle exchange programs, does not necessarily preclude the possibility of making confident scientific judgments about the effects of such prevention programs. As A. Bradford Hill (1965:300), one of this century's foremost biostatisticians, commented three decades ago:

> All scientific work is incomplete—whether it be observational or experimental. All scientific work is liable to be upset or modified by advancing knowledge. That does not confer upon us a freedom to ignore the knowledge we already have, or to postpone the action that it appears to demand at a given time.

Sooner or later there comes a time for decision on the basis of evidence in hand. In the case of the efficacy of needle exchange programs, urgency is added because the disease in question—AIDS—is fatal, is contagious, and has been seen to spread rapidly in various settings. Previous assessments of individual studies (as well as the panel's own) did not rate them as highly conclusive, because none of them used the gold standard of randomized controlled research designs. The panel therefore elected to rely on an approach that assesses the *pattern of evidence* in determining the effects of these HIV and AIDS prevention programs rather than relying on a preponderance of evidence approach.

In this approach to assessing the effects of needle exchange programs and the credibility of evidence surrounding a needle exchange program, we look at the *consistency* of the pattern of evidence that is available from multiple data sources about the same program. Taking this approach greatly expands the depth and breadth of the evidentiary base, because we try to understand the relationships among the parts of the intervention model, the process, and their outcomes. Rather than interpreting the effects of the intervention on individual outcomes, in isolation, the pattern of evidence approach considers interrelated conditions, such as intermediate outcomes (Cordray, 1986).

For example, consider the evaluation of a needle exchange program that reveals a reduction in new HIV infections over time among injection drug users who used the program. By traditional standards, this design would be classified as relatively weak because there is no control or comparison condition. Without further information, it is not possible to confidently conclude that the introduction of the needle exchange program is responsible for the observed decline on the basis of this one piece of·evidence (the observed decline) alone.

Ruling In Plausibility

By examining whether certain required conditions were present, it is possible to probe the plausibility that the needle exchange program was responsible, at least in part, for the reduction. This type of assessment requires the specification of a series of if-then propositions. That is, if there is a real connection between the introduction of the needle exchange program and the observed decline in new infections, then a series of conditions must be present in order to increase confidence in the conclusion that the program is at least partially responsible for the observed outcome. The conclusion that the needle exchange program is plausibly connected to the decrease in new HIV infections is more credible if there is evidence that, as the putative causal agent, it was actually present in the community. This means that there must be an empirical pattern of evidence that, in effect, *rules in* its plausibility. Programmatically, the pattern of evidence might include:

- information that the needle exchange program was established;

- data that it exchanged a sufficient number of needles;
- data that it provided needles to a substantial enough portion of the injection drug users in the community;
- data that those who used the needle exchange reduced their level of drug-use risk behaviors (e.g., sharing, use of bleach); and
- data that those who used the needle exchange most intensively show a greater level of risk reduction.

The argument that undergirds this approach is that programs have a structure and mechanisms that establish a logical pattern of expectations that can be tested empirically. To the extent that the empirical evidence supports these propositions, the plausibility that the needle exchange program was responsible for the observed change should increase. *That is, the plausibility increases through repeated assessments.* As a simple example, if there is a reduction in HIV incidence but the needle exchange program failed to exchange a single needle, it is not reasonable to conclude that the needle exchange program was responsible for the decline, regardless of the strength of the design underlying the HIV incidence data. However, through multiple assessments, involving a logical network of evidence, it may be possible to derive a portrait of the plausibility that the needle exchange program is implicated in the change process.

Ruling in the plausibility that the needle exchange program is a causal agent, through empirical assessment, is only half the story. It is still possible that other features of the program or research process contain biases that affect the HIV incidence. In traditional discussions of causal analysis, the notion of excluding (or rendering implausible) rival explanations has been the hallmark of competent experimental analysis. To the extent that repeated efforts to probe the results fail to disconfirm the plausibility that the intervention was at least partially responsible, its plausibility should be enhanced. Therefore, an assessment of the pattern of evidence not only entails ruling in the plausibility that the needle exchange program is a causal agent, but also requires *ruling out plausible alternative explanations.*

The Panel's Synthesis

The panel analyzed the patterns of evidence from five sources: two evaluations of the reseach published before 1993, the findings of studies published since 1993, and two sets of studies that provide the best available *detailed* account of how needle exchange programs impact risk behaviors and viral infections—one on New Haven, the other on Tacoma.

The process of selecting studies for detailed examination involved a comprehensive analysis of the research findings of individual needle exchange and bleach distribution projects. The panel generated a list of published papers and presentations on needle exchange evaluation projects in the United States, Canada, and Europe. A meeting was held to judge which reports included data that might be used in a review. The projects were subsequently grouped by city and divided among panel members so that each city project had two independent reviewers. The studies from each city were reviewed, annotated on a formal evaluation form, and then discussed with the full panel at a subsequent meeting. Following this review, at a separate meeting, the panel decided to limit itself to studies conducted in the United States, because the legal and cultural environments of other countries are sufficiently different to raise questions about whether data are applicable to the United States. Two U.S. cities, New Haven and Tacoma, were found to have a sufficient number of data published from a variety of perspectives (e.g., incident infection, behavioral risk) to warrant inclusion in this review.

Various criteria were used in deciding to pursue the New Haven and Tacoma sets of studies. Consistent with the logic of the patterns of evidence approach, the first criterion applied in selecting studies was that the site or project had to have been comprehensively studied. That is, there had to be empirical evidence establishing that the needle exchange program was operational, that the mechanisms of the exchange process had been studied, and that there was an estimate of HIV incidence or, as in the case of New Haven, a proxy measure.

The level of activity in the prevention environment can make it difficult to isolate the influence of the needle exchange program. A second criterion was that, in the sites and projects selected, the needle exchange program had to be the predominant (if not the only) intervention ongoing at the time of the assessment. This criterion implies a selection process that focuses on high-contrast sites (i.e., the needle exchange program intervention dominates prevention activities in the area), thus yielding estimated effects of needle exchange that cannot readily be attributed to other prevention activities reaching the program participants.

U.S. GENERAL ACCOUNTING OFFICE REVIEW

In late 1991, the House Select Committee on Narcotics Abuse and Control requested that the U.S. General Accounting Office carry out a review of the effectiveness of needle exchange programs.[1]

Procedure

GAO researchers carried out an extensive review of the literature to identify empirical evaluation studies that had appeared in refereed or peer-reviewed journals. They conducted site visits to programs located in Tacoma, Washington, and New Haven, Connecticut. Their review identified a total of 20 published studies and 21 abstracts on evaluations of needle exchange programs originating from nine distinct research projects, all but one of which (the Tacoma study) involved programs outside the United States. Among the nine research projects were one from Australia, one from Canada, two from the Netherlands, one from Sweden, and three from the United Kingdom.

The GAO team developed a list of eight relevant outcome measures: (1) rate of needle sharing; (2) prevalence of injection drug use; (3) frequency of injection; (4) rate of new HIV infections; (5) rate of new entrants to injection drug use; (6) incidence rate of other blood-borne infections; (7) rate of other HIV risk behaviors; and (8) risk to the public's health. They also identified three methodological criteria that had to be satisfied before findings could be considered: (1) the findings had to have been *published* in a scientific journal or government research monograph; (2) they had to have reached *statistical significance*; and (3) the reported effects of the needle exchange program could *not* have been *attributed* by the authors *to any other source*. Of the eight listed outcome measures, only three outcomes met the methodological standard of evidence set by the GAO team: (1) rate of needle sharing, (2) prevalence of injection drug use, and (3) frequency of injection. The GAO team summarized descriptive information, whenever it was available, on the ability of needle exchange programs to reach out to injection drug users and refer them to drug treatment and other health services.

Results

Tables 7.2 and 7.3 summarize the GAO findings. Regarding the potential positive outcomes, of the nine research projects reviewed, two reported a reduction in needle sharing, and a third reported an increase. It should be noted that the increase in sharing by needle exchange participants resulted from their passing on more used injection equipment (Klee et al., 1991); this finding was not replicated in a follow-up report by the same investigator (Klee and Morris, 1994). The earlier finding from that study appears to have been a transient effect that occurred before the needle exchange programs in the area reached full operation; that is, needle exchange participants were being used as a source of needles among their respective networks of injection drug users (Klee and Morris, 1994). The researchers concluded, moreover, based on the data available from six of the nine projects, that the needle exchange programs were successful in reaching injection drug users and providing a link to drug treatment and other health services.

Regarding potential negative outcomes of needle exchange programs,

TABLE 7.2   GAO Review: Results of Needle Exchange Program Study
Projects

Project Number by Country	Needle Sharing	Prevalence of Injection	Frequency of Injection Drug Use
Australia			
1		[a]	
Canada			
2			
Netherlands			
3			[a]
4	Reduction		Reduction
Sweden			
5			
United Kingdom			
6			
7			Reduction
8	Increase		
United States			
9	Reduction		[a]

[a]GAO reported these as showing no increase; however, a review of the original studies indicates that no statistically significant findings were reported for the outcome measure assessed.

SOURCE: Adapted from *Needle Exchange Programs: Research Suggests Promise as an AIDS Prevention Strategy* (U.S. General Accounting Office, 1993:7).

all five projects that reported findings on injection drug use by program participants—four on frequency of injection and one on prevalence of use—found that use did not increase. (Note that three of these findings did not reach statistical significance.) This led GAO to conclude that "some research suggests programs may reduce AIDS-related risk behavior" (p. 6) and "most projects suggest that programs do not increase injection drug use" (p. 8). GAO reported that there was sufficient evidence to suggest that needle exchange programs "hold some promise as an AIDS prevention strategy" (p. 4).

In summary, the GAO report, which was the first government report to evaluate needle exchange programs, concluded that such programs hold promise as interventions to limit HIV transmission. The criteria for assessing the validity of the study findings and for including reports in the review were quite stringent. In particular, the criterion of statistical significance means that studies that showed no difference in the frequency of injection or needle sharing were excluded. Therefore, the argument that needle exchange programs cause no harm is not fully characterized because studies

TABLE 7.3 GAO Review: Needle Exchange Program Outcomes
Measured and Reported

Project Number by Country	Attracted Injection Drug Users Not in Treatment	Referred Injection Drug User to Drug Treatment	Referred Injection Drug User to Other Health Services
Australia			
1			
Canada			
2		Yes	Yes
Netherlands			
3			
4	Yes		
Sweden			
5	Yes		Yes
United Kingdom			
6	Yes		
7	Yes	Yes	Yes
8			
United States			
9	Yes	Yes	

SOURCE: Adapted from *Needle Exchange Programs: Research Suggests Promise as an AIDS Prevention Strategy* (U.S. General Accounting Office, 1993:10).

with high level of statistical power that showed no difference were excluded.

UNIVERSITY OF CALIFORNIA REPORT

In September 1993, a second government report, *The Public Health Impact of Needle Exchange Programs in the United States and Abroad*, was published by the University of California for the Centers for Disease Control and Prevention (CDC). This report consists of a summary volume with two supporting volumes and addresses a number of the questions that this panel was asked to address.

Procedure

The University of California report was the work of a team of 12 individuals with expertise in clinical medicine, nursing, psychology, anthropology, sociology, cost-benefit modeling, and epidemiology. None of the team members was identified in published writings as either in favor of or opposed to needle exchange programs. In a process that included discussions with an advisory committee, public health officials, needle exchange program staff members, researchers, experts in drug abuse treatment and injection drug use, and community leaders, a list of 14 research questions was generated: (1) How and why did needle exchange programs develop? (2) How do needle exchange programs operate? (3) Do needle exchange programs act as bridges to public health services? (4) How much does it cost to operate needle exchange programs? (5) Who are the injection drug users who use needle exchange programs? (6) What proportion of all injecting drug users in a community uses the needle exchange program? (7) What are the community responses to needle exchange programs? (8) Do needle exchange programs result in changes in community levels of drug use? (9) Do needle exchange programs affect the number of discarded syringes? (10) Do needle exchange programs affect rates of HIV drug and/or sex risk behaviors? (11) What is the role of studies of syringes in injection drug use research? (12) Do needle exchange programs affect rates of diseases related to injection drug use other than HIV? (13) Do needle exchange programs affect HIV infection rates? and (14) Are needle exchange programs cost-effective in preventing HIV infection?

The investigators conducted a formal review of existing research; made site visits and sent mail surveys to needle exchange programs; formed focus groups with injection drug users; and applied statistical modeling techniques. Data collected from each approach were sorted into 1 of the 14 questions about impact of needle exchange programs. The aim of the literature review was to identify a maximum of written works relating to the effectiveness of needle exchange programs. Computer searches of AIDSline and Medline provided a first cut and were augmented by items from the bibliographies of articles found therein. In addition, the research team reviewed abstracts from the annual International Conference on AIDS from 1988 to 1993 and the annual meetings of the American Public Health Association from 1987 to 1992. To identify unpublished materials, needle exchange program staff were contacted about internal reports, and a search was made for newspaper and magazine clippings, government and institutional reports, and relevant book chapters.

From this effort, 1,972 data sources were identified, which included 475 journal articles, 381 conference abstracts, 236 reports, 159 unpublished materials, 499 newspaper and magazine articles, 94 books or chapters, and 128 personal communications or other sources. All materials were reviewed and coded according to which research question(s) they addressed. Project members were assigned responsibility for synthesizing information for each of the 14 research questions. Each of the studies was assessed using a standardized format and ranked on a scale from 1 to 5:

1. incomplete, inadequate, or not relevant to the research question;
2. unacceptable: contains flaws in design or reporting that make interpretation unreliable;
3. acceptable: provides credible evidence but has limited detail, precision, or generalizability;
4. well done: provides detailed, precise, and persuasive evidence; and
5. excellent: compelling and complete.

The final ranking of an article was determined by agreement of at least two project members. Only studies ranked 3 or higher were used in the synthesis.

In addition to the review of existing research, the University of California team conducted site visits to 15 cities, 10 of which were in the United States, 3 in Canada, and 2 in Europe.[2] The sites were selected on the basis of a published list of programs and reflected the range of existing needle exchange programs with respect to size, legal status, geographical location, injection drug users' HIV seroprevalence, and extent of prior evaluation research. (CDC was consulted during the selection process.) At each site, the research team used multiple data collection methods with multiple iterations, consisting of interviews, focus groups, and observation using a formal qualitative research strategy.

The methodology was codified in a manual. Standardized training of the research staff was provided. In the 15 cities, 33 needle exchange sites were visited and a total of 239 interviews with needle exchange directors and staff, public health officials, injection drug use researchers, community leaders, program participants (11 focus groups), and injection drug users not enrolled in programs (7 focus groups) were completed. Observation guidelines were pretested at two sites and the results were compared qualitatively for interrater reliability before adopting the final guidelines.

Results

Of the nine outcomes and expectations for successful needle exchange programs listed in Table 7.1, the University of California report addressed eight. That is, research findings concerning four of the five possible positive outcome domains were reviewed: reduction in drug-related and sexual risk behaviors, increase in referrals to drug abuse treatment, and reduction in HIV and other infection rates. The report addressed all four possible negative outcomes: increases in (1) drug use by program participants; (2) new initiates to injection drug use; (3) drug use in the community in general; and (4) the number of contaminated needles discarded.

Possible Positive Outcomes

Reduction in High-Risk Behavior

The University of California report reviewed data on reported needle-sharing frequency in studies of needle exchange programs. Of the 26 evaluations addressing behavior change associated with the use of needle exchange programs that were identified, 16 were deemed of acceptable quality (rating 3 or higher). Of the 16 studies, 14 presented data on the frequency of needle sharing; 9 of these had comparison groups reported. As Table 7.4 indicates, 10 of the 14 studies showed a beneficial effect of the needle exchange programs on reported frequency of needle sharing; 4 showed a mixed or neutral effect; and none showed an increased frequency of needle sharing. Regarding sexual risk behavior change, the report concluded that the findings were neutral. That is, four studies reported beneficial effects of needle exchange programs relating to sexual risk associated with number of partners and two reported mixed or neutral effects. When reviewing studies that addressed risk associated with partner choice, three showed beneficial effects and two reported mixed or neutral effects. Finally, beneficial effects of needle exchange programs relating to condom use were observed in one study, mixed or neutral results in another, and adverse effects in three studies.

Increased Referrals to Drug Treatment

The University of California report noted that 17 of 18 U.S. and Canadian programs visited stated that they provide referrals to drug treatment. Of 33 U.S. programs surveyed, 3 reported treatment services on site. The extent to which referrals enter treatment and are retained was described— the 6 programs that collect data on referrals reported 2,208—but was not studied. The report noted (Lurie et al., 1993:236) that the paucity of drug abuse treatment slots in many cities limits the usefulness of needle exchange program referrals to drug abuse treatment. This affects the likelihood that a needle exchange program will refer and that a referral will link a client with treatment.

Reduction in HIV Infection Rates

The University of California report identified 21 studies that were relevant to the issue of whether needle exchange programs impact rates of HIV infection: 2 case studies, 7 serial community cross-sectional studies, 6 serial needle exchange program cross-sectional studies, 1 case-control study,

TABLE 7.4 University of California Report: Studies of Behavior Change
With Quality Rating of Three or Greater

Outcome Measure	Beneficial Needle Exchange Program Effect	Mixed or Neutral Needle Exchange Program Effect	Adverse Needle Exchange Program Effect
Drug risk sharing frequency	Amsterdam[a,b] (Hartgers et al., 1989) London/SW England[a] (Dolan et al., 1991) (Donoghoe et al., 1991) New South Wales (Schwartzkoff, 1989) New York City (Paone et al., 1993) Portland[a] (Oliver et al., 1991) (Oliver et al., 1992) (Des Jarlais and Maynard, 1992) San Francisco[a] (Watters and Cheng, 1991) (Guydish et al., 1989) (Feldman et al., 1989) Tacoma (Hagan et al., 1991b) (Hagan et al., 1992a) Tacoma (Hagan et al., 1993) Wales[a] (Stimson et al., 1991)	Amsterdam[a] (Hartgers et al., 1992) Amsterdam[a] (van Ameijden et al., 1993) England/Scotland[a] (Donoghoe et al., 1989) (Stimson et al., 1988) (Stimson et al., 1989) Manchester[a] (Klee et al., 1991)	
Giving away used needles	London/SW England[a] (Dolan et al., 1991) (Donoghoe et al., 1991) Tacoma (Hagan et al., 1991b) (Hagan et al., 1992a) Tacoma (Hagan et al., 1993)	Amsterdam (van Ameijden et al., 1993)	Manchester[a] (Klee et al., 1991)
Needle cleaning	New South Wales (Schwartzkoff, 1989) Portland[a] (Oliver et al., 1991) (Oliver et al., 1992) (Des Jarlais and Maynard, 1992) Tacoma (Hagan et al., 1993)	Amsterdam (Hartgers et al., 1992)	

TABLE 7.4 Continued

Outcome Measure	Beneficial Needle Exchange Program Effect	Mixed or Neutral Exchange Program Effect	Adverse Needle Exchange Program Effect
Injection frequency	Amsterdam[a],[c] (Hartgers et al., 1989) *Tacoma* (Hagan et al., 1991b) (Hagan et al., 1992a) Wales[a] (Stimson et al., 1991)	New York City (Paone et al., 1993) *San Francisco* (Watters and Cheng, 1991) (Guydish et al., 1989) (Feldman et al., 1989) San Francisco (Guydish et al., 1993) Tacoma (Hagan et al, 1993)	London/SW England[a] (Dolan et al., 1991) (Donoghoe et al., 1991)
Sex risk			
Number of partners	England/Scotland[a] (Donoghoe et al., 1989) (Stimson et al., 1988) (Stimson et al., 1989) New South Wales (Schwartzkoff, 1989)	London/SW England[a] (Dolan et al., 1991) (Donoghoe et al., 1991)	
Partner choice	England/Scotland[a] (Donoghoe et al., 1989) (Stimson et al., 1988) (Stimson et al., 1989)	London/SW England[a] (Dolan et al., 1991) (Donoghoe et al., 1991)	
Condom use	New South Wales (Schwartzkoff, 1989)	Wales[a] (Stimson et al., 1991)	England/Scotland[a] (Donoghoe et al., 1989) (Stimson et al., 1988) (Stimson et al., 1989)

NOTE: SW = southwest.
[a]Compared with control group(s).
[b]Cross-sectional component.
[c]Retrospective component.

SOURCE: *The Public Health Impact of Needle Exchange Programs in the United States and Abroad, Volume 1* (Lurie et al., 1993:414).

and 3 prospective studies. The quality of studies was rated on a 5-point scale ranging from a low of 1 (not valid) to a high of 5 (excellent) and a mid-point of 3 (acceptable). Only two of the studies received a quality rating of 3 or higher, and two others were rated between 2 and 3. None of the studies showed increased prevalence or incidence of HIV infection among needle exchange participants.

Given the quality rating of the studies, it is not surprising that the University of California report concluded that the studies available up to the time of the report (Lurie et al., 1993) do not, and for methodological reasons probably cannot, provide clear evidence that needle exchange programs decrease HIV infection rates. However, needle exchange programs do not appear to be associated with increased rates of infection.

It is intrinsically difficult to measure *effects of intervention* on the incidence of new infections of rare diseases, whose victims ordinarily do not show symptoms at the time of infection. Although most of the early studies used prevalent infection as the outcome measure, the more appropriate measure is incident or new infection. However, a further complication is that incidence is low in most locations, thereby requiring larger study populations to demonstrate program effects. The University of California report noted (Lurie et al., 1993:465) appropriately:

> Well-conducted, sufficiently large case-control studies offer the best combination of scientific rigor and feasibility for assessing the effect of needle exchange programs on HIV rates.

Possible Negative Outcomes

Increase in Program Participant Drug Use

The University of California report noted that eight "acceptable" studies were identified that presented data on the issue of reported injection frequency. As Table 7.4 shows, three studies found reductions in injection associated with needle exchange programs; four found mixed or no effects; and one found an increase in injection compared with controls. This last study also found reduced needle sharing reported among needle exchange participants. This study noted that the apparent increase in injection could be attributed to several other factors, including the differential dropout of low-level injectors. The report also reviewed the methodological limitations of the studies, including the potential for socially acceptable responses by injection drug users. On balance, because of methodological problems, the report drew no strong conclusions about levels of injection drug use.

Increase in New Initiates to Injection Drug Use

The University of California report reviewed a variety of studies and used focus groups to understand whether needle exchange programs could encourage persons to initiate injection drug use. In reviewing the demographic data from the programs, the report noted that the median age of participants across programs ranged from 33 to 41, and the median duration of injection drug use from 7 to 20 years. This suggests that most participants initiated injection drug use prior to using the needle exchange program.

A review of serial cross-sectional studies of injection drug users in San Francisco noted an increase in the mean age of the samples over time from 34 in 1986 to 40 in 1990, suggesting that there was not an increase in young new injectors over time. Researchers in Amsterdam used a capture-recapture method to estimate the number of injection drug users between 1983 and 1988. Despite initiation of a needle exchange program in 1984, no change in the number of injection drug users was reported, and the average age of drug users increased over time. Furthermore, the number of drug users under age 22 decreased from 14 percent in 1983 to 3 percent in 1988. The authors concluded that there was no increase in the number of new initiates into injection drug use.

The report concluded, on the basis of evidence from surveys, that (Lurie et al., 1993:357) "needle exchange programs are not associated with an increase in community levels of injecting."

Focus groups were consulted. Of 10 focus groups from needle exchange programs, comprising 65 injection drug users, 2 individuals thought needle exchange programs could encourage nonparenteral drug users to start injecting. Among seven nonprogram focus groups comprising 47 injection drug users, 2 individuals thought needle exchange programs could encourage nonparenteral drug users to start injecting. The focus group data were viewed as corroborating evidence for the data available from surveys arguing against an effect of needle exchange programs on increasing the community levels of injection drug use.

Increased Drug Use in the Community

The University of California report addressed the potential for increased drug use in the community by reviewing the studies noted in the previous section. Researchers searched for additional data by examining established data sets of drug abuse indicators and answers to additional questions asked of focus groups of injection drug users.

The University of California researchers attempted to relate the presence (or absence) of needle exchange programs to ongoing statistical series like the Drug Abuse Warning Network (DAWN), Drug Use Forecasting (DUF), and Uniformed Crime Reports (UCR), which might reflect altered patterns of drug-related events, such as drug cases in hospital emergency rooms, positive urine drug screens, and drug-related arrests, respectively. The report noted wide variation in these drug-use indicators over time, which suggests inherent lack of precision and limits the manifestation of patterns—if any—relating to needle exchange.

The University of California report also noted that, because needle exchange programs are relatively new, changes in drug use might yet appear with longer follow-up. The report concluded that (Lurie et al., 1993:357) "currently available (national indicator) data provide no evidence of change in overall community levels of drug use associated with needle exchange programs."

The report also noted that the San Francisco and Amsterdam surveys described above provide (Lurie et al., 1993:357) "some evidence that needle exchange programs are not associated with an increase in community levels of injecting or overall drug use."

Increase in Number of Contaminated Needles Unsafely Discarded

The University of California report noted that adverse community responses to needle exchange programs are likely to be centered on the issue of discarded needles and the risk to the public of accidental needlestick injury. However, the report noted that one-for-one exchange rules cannot, in theory, increase the total number of discarded needles, although programs could affect the geographic distribution of discarded syringes. Data on a surveillance project with the Portland, Oregon, needle exchange program noted a decrease in the prevalence of discarded syringes near the program (Lurie et al., 1993:386). Passive surveillance of health or police department reports over time indicated either declines or small increases in needlestick injuries, with the trends due to changes in reporting patterns. The University of California report concluded that needle exchange programs "have not increased the total number of discarded syringes" and, if structured as a one-for-one exchange with no starter needles, "they cannot increase the total number of discarded needles" (Lurie et al., 1993:395).

Summary

Using multiple data sources, the University of California reviewed a number of questions about needle exchange programs. As far as possible positive outcomes are concerned, the report concluded that the data available at the time of the report "do not . . . provide clear evidence that needle exchange programs decrease HIV infection rates," (p. 20) but that "the majority of studies of [program] clients demonstrate decreased risk of HIV drug risk behavior, but not decreased rates of HIV sex risk behavior" (p. 18) In addition, "all but one of the 18 US and Canadian needle exchanges visited . . . stated that they provide referrals to drug abuse treatment" (p. 10) Finally, regarding possible negative outcomes, the report concluded that needle exchange programs have not increased the total number of discarded used needles and syringes (p. 16). The report goes on to state that there is no evidence that drug use among program participants increased, and there is no evidence of change in overall community levels of noninjection or injection drug use (Lurie et al., 1993:15).

EVIDENCE FROM RECENT STUDIES

This section is organized into topical areas that parallel the summaries of the GAO and University of California reports. Study findings are categorized according to the outcomes and expectations of program effects listed in Table 7.1; both possible positive and possible negative effects are reviewed. The information sources for this update comprise: (1) a review of abstracts from the 1994 International Conference on AIDS; (2) the 1994 American Public Health Association conference; (3) papers presented at the National Research Council/Institute of Medicine's Workshop on Needle Exchange and Bleach Distribution Programs (1994); and (4) articles appearing in refereed journals following the release of the University of California report. Since the University of California report was issued, a number of studies on the impact of needle exchange programs have been presented or published. These studies utilize a variety of designs, including an ecological design; a comparison of prevalence rates between injection drug users who use and those who do not use needle exchange programs; HIV incidence rates among needle exchange program attenders; and, using data collected prospectively, a comparison of HIV incidence rates between injection drug users who attend and those who do not attend a needle exchange program.

Possible Positive Outcomes

Reduction in Risk Behavior

Recent publications on needle exchange programs in San Francisco, New York City, and Portland, Oregon, have addressed the issue of the impact of the programs on HIV drug-use risk behaviors and sexual risk behaviors (Watters et al., 1994; Watters, 1994; Lewis and Watters, 1994; Des Jarlais et al., 1994a, 1994b, 1995; Paone et al., 1994a, 1994b; Oliver et al., 1994).

In an ecological study in San Francisco, Watters (1994) examined the trends in risk behaviors and HIV seroprevalence over a 6.5-year period among heterosexual injection drug users over 13 cross-sectional surveys between 1986 and 1992. Interviews (5,956) were conducted with injectors in street settings and drug detoxification clinics. During that time period, multiple prevention efforts targeting injection drug users had been implemented (including outreach, education, voluntary HIV testing and counseling, bleach and condom distribution, and needle exchange programs). Among injection drug users who reported sharing needles, the proportion of those who reported ever using bleach increased from 3 percent in 1986 to 89 percent by 1988 and remained relatively constant at that level through fall 1992.

Sexually active heterosexual male injectors also reported significant changes in condom use (i.e., injection drug users reported using a condom 4.5 percent of the time in 1986, compared with 31 percent of the time in late 1992). However, Lewis and Watters (1994) found that a substantial proportion of sexually active male drug injectors, including heterosexuals, bisexuals, and homosexuals, reported frequently engaging in unprotected sex (i.e., reported condom use was low in all three groups). That is, 56 percent of the heterosexuals who had vaginal sex in the prior 6 months reported no condom use; one-third of the homosexuals who engaged in anal intercourse with male partners reported no condom use; and 41 percent of the bisexual men reported no condom use while engaging in vaginal sex and approximately half (52 percent) reported no condom use while engaging in anal or oral sex with females and/or males.

In another ecological report from New York City, Des Jarlais and colleagues (Des Jarlais et al., 1994a) examined trends in reported risk behaviors and seroprevalence among injection drug users for 1984 and 1990 to 1992 by comparing results of two surveys of injection drug users entering a drug detoxification program. Several trends in drug-use risk behaviors were reported. In 1984, for example, 65 percent of injection drug users reported having used shooting galleries in the preceding 2 years; in the 1990 to 1992 survey, only 3 percent reported injecting in shooting galleries in the preceding 6 months. Substantial reductions in sharing behavior were also observed. Use of potentially contaminated needles declined from 51 to 7 percent of injections. Moreover, an increasing proportion of injection drug users entering the detoxification program reported using the needle exchange programs since they opened in 1990. For the 1990 to 1992 period, results also show that needle exchange participation was associated with a downward trend in the proportion of subjects reporting any injection with needles that had been used by someone else and a reduction in the percentage of study participants reporting having passed on used needles to others. The extent to which the reductions in risk behaviors reported in the two surveys can be attributed to the needle exchange program itself is limited by the fact that the data are ecological trends. Other prevention efforts were occurring in New York City between the two time intervals. Therefore, although the results are consistent with an inference of reduction in risk behaviors following the introduction of a needle exchange program, the study design does not exclude the possibility of contributing or alternate explanations.

In the San Francisco needle exchange program evaluation, Watters (1994) compared frequent needle exchange participants with two comparison groups— injection drug users who used the exchange less frequently and a group who did not use it at all. These researchers found a 47 percent decline (from 66 to 35 percent) in reported sharing behavior among injection drug user study participants between spring 1987 and spring 1992. More refined analyses revealed that frequent needle exchange participants (i.e., used the program more than 25 times in the past year) were less likely to report needle sharing in the past 30 days than study participants who used the needle exchange program less frequently or not at all. In contrast, over the 3-year study period, no change in reported rates of sharing behavior was observed among those not using the program.

In New York City, Paone et al. (1994a) conducted a pre-post analysis that examined the drug-use risk behaviors of 1,752 needle exchange program participants 30 days prior to using the exchange and during their most recent 30 days in the program. Participants reported a two-thirds decline in the proportion of time they injected with previously used needles (12 percent before participating in the needle exchange program, compared with 4 percent in the last 30 days while participating in the program). Similar reductions in renting or buying used needles (73 percent decline) were observed, and similar reductions in the number of participants who reported borrowing used needles were found (59 percent decline). The number of participants who reported using alcohol pads increased from 30 percent before participating in the needle exchange program to 80 percent in the most recent 30 days in the exchange. Although the reduction in high-risk behaviors was based on self-reports of exchange users and no comparison of injection drug users not using the exchange was included in this report, this pattern of reduction in drug-use risk behaviors was found to be relatively stable in recent updates (Des Jarlais et al., 1994b; Des Jarlais et al., 1995; Paone et al., 1994b). These authors also note in their recent updates that minimal changes in sexual risk behaviors were reported. For example, always using a condom with a primary sexual partner increased from 36 percent in the 30 days prior to first using the needle exchange program to 37 percent for the last 30 days while using the program; whereas always using a condom with a casual sexual partner increased from 56 percent in the 30 days prior to first using the exchange program to 60 percent in the last 30 days while using the exchange. However, due to design constraints, it cannot be stated what portion of the reduction in risk behaviors is due to the needle exchange program.

An evaluation of the Portland needle exchange program (Oliver et al., 1994) assessed change in risk behaviors among 753 needle exchange program participants by comparing data collected on each study participant during an intake interview and a 6-month follow-up interview. Significant declines in sharing behaviors (rent needles and syringes: intake = 9 percent compared with 3 percent at follow-up; borrowed needles and syringes: intake = 20 percent compared with 7 percent at follow-up) and increased use of bleach (intake = 51 percent compared with 65 percent at follow-up) were observed. When drug-use risk behaviors of frequent attenders (attended four or more times) were compared with risk behaviors of those who attended three or fewer times, frequent attenders reported greater risk reduction on borrowing and returning used needles to the program. To supplement the pre-post analysis, needle exchange participants were also compared with another group of drug injectors, clients of Portland's National AIDS Demonstration Research (NADR) program (i.e., all received bleach and HIV education and a subset also received counseling). Frequent needle exchange participants were found to be less likely to reuse needles without cleaning or to improperly dispose of used needles than were the NADR clients. The two groups were not found to differ on other risk behaviors assessed. It is worth noting that there was little overlap between the two groups (11 percent). The two interventions apparently are recruiting different participants.

In sum, from the earliest studies of needle exchanges, there has been a dominant trend in the data showing significant and meaningful associations between participation in needle exchange programs and lower levels of drug-use risk behaviors, and small or no change in sexual risk behaviors. The most recent data continue to reflect this trend. Moreover, this pattern of findings has also been observed in foreign cities (Davoli et al., 1995; Hunter et al., 1995).

Reduction in HIV Infection Rates

Two recent ecological studies examined trends in HIV seroprevalence rates among injection drug users, one in New York City and the other in San Francisco (Des Jarlais et al., 1994a; Watters, 1994). Both reported a stabilization of HIV seroprevalence rates that coincided with reductions in high-risk behaviors and the implementation of various prevention programs (including outreach, education, testing and counseling, bleach and condom distribution, and needle exchange programs). Although these ecological studies do not provide direct causal evidence of the effect of such programs, they nonetheless document a pattern in behavioral risk reduction that corresponds with stabilization of seroprevalence rates in distinct populations of injection drug users.

Hagan and colleagues (1994b) reported seroprevalence rates of needle exchange participants and nonparticipants. The cross-sectional sample of needle exchange participants (n = 426) was found to have a 2 percent HIV prevalence rate, compared with an 8 percent rate for the cross-sectional sample of nonparticipants (n = 159). Because the outcome measured in this study was prevalent infection, temporal associations cannot be established with certainty, and the possibility that the results might reflect that the needle exchange program attracts lower-risk injection drug users cannot be dismissed out of hand. However, the results are consistent with the inference that needle exchange programs are associated with a lower risk of infection.

On the basis of recent updates from the 1994 International Conference on AIDS, Des Jarlais (1994; in press) provided descriptive information on HIV incidence among injection drug users who participate in needle exchange programs across 14 different cities (Table 7.5). Some of these incidence rates were measured directly by testing cohorts of needle exchange participants; others were based on self-reports of prior serological tests; still others were derived from statistical modeling techniques (e.g., New Haven).

An examination of the data reveals that, with the exception of data from Montréal, HIV incidence is uniformly low among needle exchange program participants; that is, regardless of whether HIV prevalence is low, moderate, high, or very high among the community of injection drug users in a city, HIV incidence among program participants is consistently low across cities. These findings are consistent with the premise that an AIDS prevention program (e.g., needle exchange program or other outreach intervention) that is able to reach and successfully modify the behavior of injection drug users who are at high risk of becoming infected or of transmitting HIV to others is capable of maintaining a low level of new infections in the population of injection drug users in a community.

The high HIV incidence among needle exchange program participants observed in Montréal is disconcerting. The reader is referred to Appendix A for a detailed discussion of Montréal data. Although the prevalence is moderate and has remained stable, the observed incidence is high among the needle exchange cohort being studied. If the high incidence accurately reflects the rate of new infections in the population of injection drug users in Montréal, an increasing prevalence over time would be expected—it is not possible to think that mortality is as high as the observed incidence. A rational explanation (again, if the prevalence and incidence estimates are unbiased population estimates) could be that Montréal's needle exchange program is attracting a high-risk group of users (selection bias).

TABLE 7.5 HIV Incidence Estimates Among Needle Exchange
Participants in Select Cities

City	HIV Prevalence[a]	Measured HIV Seroconversions[b]	Estimated HIV Seroconversions[c]
Lund, Sweden	Low	0	
Glasgow, Scotland	Low		0-1 (2)
Sydney, Australia	Low		0-1 (2)
Toronto, Canada	Low		1-2 (2)
England and Wales (except London)	Low		0-1 (1)
Kathmandu, Nepal	Low	0	
Tacoma, WA, USA	Low	<1	
Portland, OR, USA	Low	<1	
Montréal, Canada	Moderate	13	
London, England	Moderate		1-2 (4)
Amsterdam, The Netherlands	High	4	
Chicago, IL, USA	High	0	
New York, NY, USA	Very high	2	
New Haven, CT, USA	Very high		0 (3)

[a]Low = 0 to 5 percent; moderate = 6 to 20 percent; high = 21 to 40 percent; very high = 41+ percent.
[b]Cohort study and/or repeated testing of participants in per 100 person years at risk.
[c]Estimated from: (1) stable, very low <2 percent seroprevalence in area; (2) self-reports of previous seronegative test and a current HIV blood/saliva test; (3) HIV testing of syringes collected at exchange per 100 person years at risk; and (4) stable or declining seroprevalence.

SOURCE: Adapted from *Current Findings in Syringe Exchange Research: A Report to the Task Force to Review Services for Drug Misusers* (Des Jarlais, 1994).

Recent reports from Montréal (Hankins et al., 1994; Lamothe et al., 1993; Bruneau et al., 1995) suggest that needle exchange participants still frequently engage in high-risk behaviors, including unsafe cocaine injection and prostitution. The program is located in an area of the city noted for prostitution, and the program operates in the middle of the night, which makes it prone to recruiting high-risk users. Moreover, injection drug users in Montréal who elect to purchase sterile needles in pharmacies can do so without a prescription (further biasing the representation of those who elect to acquire their needles in the middle of the night at the exchange program). Recent epidemiologic data from Montréal (Bruneau et al., 1995) highlight the complex nature of the observed association between sources of sterile needles and HIV seroincidence (see Appendix A). That is, although the risk of seroconversion was found to be higher among needle exchange partici- pants when compared to nonparticipants, injection drug users who used the needle exchange program as their exclusive source of sterile needles were found to be at substantially lower risk than those who used diverse sources of sterile needles. Furthermore, the needle exchange program limit of 15 needles per visit may not be sufficient to properly address drug-use risk behaviors of individuals who inject large amounts of cocaine. There is also a high level of male prostitution among the needle exchange participants.

If the infection rate estimates accurately reflect the population parameters, it would appear that the services offered by the Montréal needle exchange program are insufficient to control HIV transmission in that cohort. Specific ethnographic studies are needed to better understand the primary routes of transmission implicated and their dynamics (e.g., sex, specific drug-use risk behaviors). This would allow the program to better tailor its services (e.g., add new services) and/or the relative intensity of the service delivery according to needs of participants (i.e., primary risks).

The potential ability of needle exchanges to attract injection drug users that are at high risk of seroconversion was also recently reported in the United States by a San Francisco research team (Hahn et al., 1995; see Appendix A for a detailed review of the San Francisco study). Although the disparities in observed seroincidence rates between needle exchange participants and nonparticipants could not be attributed to having been exposed to the needle exchange program, the program appeared to serve a relatively high-risk subset of injection drug users. The authors concluded that the San Francisco program provides a unique setting for intervention because it provides direct access to a population that is at high risk.

Other cities with needle exchange programs that have high seroprevalence data (e.g., New Haven, Chicago, New York) report a low level of HIV seroconversion. The high seroconversion rate in Montréal therefore appears to be the exception, rather than the rule. These data are consistent with the premise that AIDS prevention programs (e.g., needle exchange) are able to stabilize HIV prevalence and very low seroincidence. Obviously, these results are descriptive in nature (there are no comparison groups) and, as a consequence, cannot in themselves provide evidence of the direct causal effect of needle exchange programs on HIV incidence rates. Nonetheless, they do provide valuable insight into HIV incidence rates among needle exchange participants in cities with varying levels of HIV seroprevalence among the local populations of injection drug users.

Other recent reports from New York City (Des Jarlais et al., 1994b, 1995; Paone et al., 1994b) have compared seroconversion rates of various injection drug user groups in the city. The HIV seroconversion rate among high-frequency drug injectors not using the needle exchange programs ranged from 4 to 7 per 100 person years at risk, compared with needle exchange participant groups with seroconversion rates ranging from 1 to 2 per 100 person years at risk. These findings suggest that the use of needle exchange programs has a substantial protective effect for preventing new HIV infections. However, the results need to be interpreted with care. That is, nonequivalence across groups being compared (needle exchange users versus nonusers) precludes making strong causal inferences about the direct effect of the needle exchange on HIV incidence rates. Nonetheless, these data do reflect a significant association between needle exchange participation and HIV infection (Des Jarlais et al., 1994b, 1995).

Possible Negative Outcomes

Program Participant Drug Use

The most recent studies that have examined drug-use behaviors among needle exchange participants show either stable levels of reported drug injection frequency or even slight declines over time among injection drug users who continue to participate in needle exchange programs (Watters et al., 1994; Paone et al., 1994a; Des Jarlais et al., 1994a; Oliver et al., 1994). In the recent New York City study, Paone et al. (1994a) reported a statistically significant decrease in injection frequency among needle exchange participants, from 95 times in the 30 days preceding program participation to 86 times in the 30 days prior to participants' being interviewed.

The only exception to this reported trend comes from an unpublished research manuscript from Chicago researchers (O'Brien et al., 1995a). As noted in the Preface, as the panel was concluding its deliberations, the Assistant Secretary for Health made public statements that a number of unpublished needle exchange evaluation reports had raised doubts in his mind about the effectiveness of these programs. The panel deemed these statements to be significant in the public debate, therefore necessitating appropriate consideration in order for the panel to be fully responsive to its charge. The panel therefore reviewed the unpublished studies, one of which was the aforementioned O'Brien et al. (1995a) Chicago study. As unpublished findings, this research lacks the authority provided by the peer review and publication process. For this reason, the panel gave special attention to scrutinizing and describing in detail results reported by the researchers, as well as appraising their probative value (see Appendix A).

The investigators infer from their findings that those who participate in needle exchange programs spend more money and inject more frequently than nonparticipants as a result of their participation in the program. Their assertion is based on data that, according to these authors, support the contention that program participation is economically driven (i.e., by the cost of needles). The panel's review raised serious concerns about the tenability of their inferences. For instance, a clearly insufficient theoretical and empirical development of the underlying models is used. That is, there are numerous other plausible models that could explain their data. From an economic standpoint, it would seem that individual socioeconomic status may be causally related to both drug abuse and use of the needle exchange program, rather than to the explanation that needle exchange programs cause drug use. Nonetheless, the authors do not test any alternative plausible models to assess the relative fit of their models compared with other viable competing models. Moreover, a weak theoretical justification is provided of their postulated model (e.g., cost of needles is the underlying driving force for using the needle exchange, but that cost is minute compared with other expenses, such as the cost of the drugs themselves).

The empirical information provided on key variables is inadequate. Properties of the distributions of key variables are absent and aggregate summary statistics are used in various models without attention to the possible adverse effect of outliers. The presence of such outliers can severely distort the results and challenges the viability of the inferences drawn by these investigators. Substantial inconsistencies between data on key variables (self-report) presented in the manuscript and information extracted from the needle exchange program records raised serious concerns among panel members. Moreover, as discussed in some detail in Appendix A, the panel had serious reservations about the appropriateness of the modeling techniques as implemented by these researchers.

Although this particular study suffers from serious limitations, the conclusions reached by the authors raise interesting questions and hypotheses that should be subjected to sound empirical testing. These issues should be further studied with adequate designs, measures, and analytical methods. In the meantime, in the panel's opinion, these difficulties are serious enough to preclude making causal inferences about the effect of needle exchange programs.

New Initiates to Injection Drug Use

The concern that having the opportunity to use a needle exchange may lead persons who are not currently injecting to begin injecting demands attention, and some information about this is available.

If the opportunity to participate in needle exchange programs were to lead to an increase in the number of new injection drug users, one would expect to see relatively large numbers of young newer injectors at the needle exchange programs. This has not been observed in any of the earlier studies (e.g., Lurie et al., 1993), or in the most recent publications (Paone et al., 1994a, 1994b; Des Jarlais et al., 1994b; Watters et al., 1994).

Investigators in Amsterdam have recently published data that permit examination of the hypothesis that "mixing" of injecting and noninjecting drug users at needle exchanges will lead noninjectors to begin injecting behavior (van Ameijden et al., 1994). Many of the Amsterdam needle exchanges are operated out of the "low-threshold" methadone programs. These programs provide services to both heroin injectors and heroin smokers and do not require abstinence from illicit drug use as a condition for remaining in the program. Thus, these combined methadone treatment and needle exchange sites do provide frequent opportunities for social interactions between heroin injectors and heroin smokers. Despite this, the proportions of heroin users who smoke and those who inject have remained constant since the exchanges were implemented.

Recent U.S. data also support the conclusion that needle exchange programs do not lead to any detectable increase in drug injection. The recent San Francisco study (Watters, 1994) found an increase in the mean age of injection drug users in the city during the years of operation of the needle exchange programs (i.e., mean age in 1986 was 36 compared with 42 in 1992). Moreover, the author reported that during that 5.5-year period, the median reported frequency of injection declined from 1.9 to 0.7 injection per day and that the percentage of new initiates into injection drug use decreased from 3 to 1 percent. In Portland (Oliver et al., 1994), under 2 percent of program participants had histories of injecting of less than a year. The average duration of injection drug use was 14 years, and more than 75 percent had been injecting for 5 years or more. The presence of a needle exchange program does not appear to cause any increase in the number of new initiates to drug injection. Identifying what factors lead individuals to initiate injection drug use, despite knowing about AIDS, remains an important question for future research.

Discarded Needles and Syringes

Since the University of California report was issued, only one study has dealt with needle exchange programs and improperly discarded needles. Doherty et al.. (1995) conducted a survey of a random sample of city blocks in areas of high drug use in Baltimore before and after implementation of the needle exchange program; their results are consistent with the University of California conclusion that needle exchange programs do not increase the total number of discarded syringes.

THE NEW HAVEN STUDIES

After extended legislative debate, Public Act 90-214 allowed the City of New Haven, Connecticut, to implement—on an experimental basis—a legal needle exchange for injection drug users. On November 13, 1990, the New Haven Needle Exchange Program began operation. This program operated from a van, typically 6 hours a day, 4 days a week, and traveled to specific sites known to involve high levels of drug activity.

The needle exchange program operated on an anonymous basis. Specifically, participants were assigned a fictitious name as a means of identification and tracking. New enrollees who did not have a needle and syringe to exchange at their first encounter with the needle exchange program were provided with a single "rig." After that, exchanges were conducted on a one-for-one basis, with a maximum of five needles and syringes issued on each occasion. Syringes that were distributed were coded to enable tracking and evaluation. The program accepted syringes that had not originated from the program. All returned equipment was placed in a metal canister, and all returned equipment was turned over to an evaluation team at Yale University for assessment. In particular, a sample of returned syringes were assessed for the prevalence of HIV.

In addition to exchanging used sterile equipment, program staff provided AIDS education and information on risk reduction. Condoms and bleach packets were provided to all participants at each encounter. All participants were also provided information on drug treatment and a broad range of other relevant services (e.g., tuberculosis and sexually transmitted disease screening through clinics, HIV testing, maternal and child health services); outreach workers also provided participants with direct assistance in accessing drug treatment and other services.

In July 1992, syringe possession without a prescription was decriminalized. This was followed by a reduction in the monthly volume of exchanges at the program (from about 4,000 to a little more than half that number).

The importance of the evidence from the New Haven studies is twofold. They provide: (1) direct evidence of lower levels of HIV infection among needles in use and (2) indirect, model-based estimates of changes in the incidence of new HIV infections among needle exchange program participants.

The direct evidence involves the impact of the needle exchange program on the critical features of program process. Specifically, the evaluation reveals significant and substantial reductions in the infectivity of the *syringes* exchanged through the needle exchange program. The data also reveal increases in referral to drug treatment and no change in the number of injection drug users.

Prior to the distribution of sterile injection equipment, extremely sensitive DNA analyses using the polymerase chain reaction (PCR) to detect the presence of HIV-infected peripheral blood cells in the returned syringes of existing "street" syringes showed an HIV-positive rate of 0.675; needles from shooting galleries revealed a rate of 0.917; and needles from an underground exchange showed a rate of 0.628. During the first month of the exchange, HIV-positive rate for needles turned into the exchange was 0.639; within 3 months, this rate declined to 0.406 and remained relatively constant (with an increase to 0.485 at the end of the year—November-December 1991). That is, the prevalence of HIV in needles decreased by one-third.

Program Implementation

Measures of syringe infectivity gradually declined over time, with the sharpest decline occurring in the first 3 months after the implementation of the needle exchange program. If the reduction in the infectivity of needles is due to the activities of the program, it is reasonable to expect changes in program operations that parallel the pattern of reductions in needle infectivity. Data about program operations tend to support the plausibility that reductions in infectivity are connected to the activities of the clients of the needle exchange program and the program itself.

In particular, the number of visits increased more rapidly than the number of clients, suggesting that the same clients were exchanging needles more frequently. Specifically, in December 1990 there were about 100 clients and 150 visits. By June 1992 there were 300 clients and 900 visits.

Program data are also consistent with a fundamental concept of the circulation theory advanced by Kaplan—namely, the *law of conservation of needles*. Specifically, there was a close match between the number of inbound and outbound needles, and there was a substantial increase in the volume of exchanges between December 1990 and June 1992. That is, the volume of exchanges increased from less than 500 to over 4,000 in June 1992. (After decriminalization in 1992, the volume of exchanges decreased to between 2,000 and 2,500.) Over the entire study period (November 1990 through June 1993), a total of 80,292 needles were distributed; for the same period, the total number of needles that were returned was 78,067. That is, 97.2 percent of the total number of needles distributed were returned to the needle exchange program. It appears that these figures include the "return" of nonprogram needles. In other papers (e.g., Kaplan and Heimer, 1994), return probabilities of about .7 are shown.

Using estimates of the size of the population of injection drug users in New Haven derived by Kaplan and Soloshatz (1993), it appears that about half of the injection drug users have had contact with the needle exchange program (Lurie et al., 1993).

Central to the circulation theory advanced by Kaplan is the notion that "more frequent exchanging should lead to a reduction in mean needle circulation times" (1994b:226). Data obtained from the syringe tracking system confirm this expectation. In December 1990, the mean circulation time for syrantes was about 7 days. (It should be noted that Kaplan's linear regression results project an estimated preprogram circulation time of 23.5 days; according to the plot in Figure 4 of Kaplan (1994b), the empirically based mean circulation time of 7 days is associated with the third month of operation.) Over the course of the intervention, circulation time declined steadily, to about 3 days in September 1991. Circulation time stabilized between 2 and 3 days thereafter (through June 1992). This appears to be consistent with the linear regression estimates provided in Figure 4 of Kaplan (1994b:248). Kaplan concluded that the needle exchange program "appears to be interrupting the needle circulation process in the manner intended" (1994b:25).

To summarize the empirical results so far, evaluation data reveal: (1) increased exchange rates per injection drug user and (2) increased return of program syringes, resulting in a decrease in mean circulation time for each syringe. Because needles are in circulation for shorter periods, there is a decline in the probability of infection. Taken together, these data indicate that the New Haven needle exchange program, a substantial intervention effort, was a plausible contributor to reductions in the infectivity level of needles.

Estimated Effects on HIV Incidence

Kaplan and colleagues (Kaplan and Heimer, 1992; Kaplan and O'Keefe, 1993) could not directly observe HIV infection in needle exchange program clients (as they could in needles) and, as a consequence, turned to a mathematical modeling approach. They *estimated* the relative effects (the proportionate reduction of incidence per year) and the absolute impact (number of infections prevented per client year) of the New Haven needle exchange program. It was estimated from these models that the project was associated with a relative reduction in HIV incidence of 33 percent.[3]

It was further estimated that between 1 and 3 infections per 100 participant years were prevented annually.[4] A completely different modeling approach (Kaplan and Heimer, 1994b), based on a change point model, yielded a maximum likelihood incidence estimate of zero, with a relatively large confidence interval for that estimated incidence rate (i.e., 0 to 10.2). An update of this rate of new HIV infections among participants yielded a revised maximum likelihood incidence estimate of 1.63 infections per 100 drug injectors per year (Kaplan and Heimer, 1994b, in press), with a 95 percent confidence interval ranging from 0 through 7.2. Moreover, a test of the null hypothesis that no new infections had occurred could not be rejected, providing further support for the efficacy of New Haven's needle exchange program.

Assessment of the Models

Because these assessments are based on mathematical models that, of necessity, must rely on various assumptions, the validity of the resulting estimates hinges critically on the validity of the assumptions that had to be made. Two scientific reviews of the procedures and assumptions embodied in Kaplan's models issued in recent years (U.S. General Accounting Office, 1993; Lurie et al., 1993) provided concordant views regarding Kaplan's models. GAO summarized Kaplan's work as follows (p. 23):

> Both our experts found that the mathematical specifications used in both equations appropriately express the dynamic process of HIV transmission among injection drug users via infected needles. They agree in their assessment that the model is technically sound and incorporates all key parameters.

The University of California review states (p. 478):

> The circulation model is a very significant contribution to NEP [needle exchange program] evaluation efforts. By focusing on how NEP needles alter the characteristics of needles in circulation, the model circumvents reliance on injection drug user self-reports of behavior change. Rather, the model uses syringe tracking and testing data to demonstrate that even if injection drug users made no effort to change behavior (aside from obtaining needles at the NEP), HIV incidence would drop as a result of lower HIV prevalence in the needles. Any additional reduction in risk behavior (such as cessation of sharing or increased bleaching) would reduce HIV incidence even further.

Concerning the numerical estimates, from applying the model to the study data in New Haven, the GAO review concludes (pp. 23-24):

> Our experts agreed that Dr. Kaplan's assumptions serve to underestimate the impact of the New Haven program on the rate of new HIV infections. The expert reviewers strongly believe that 33 percent understates the true percentage reduction in new infections attributable to the program.

> The data used in the model were primarily obtained from three sources: (1) data developed from the program's syringe tracking and testing system, (2) self-reports from injection drug users participating in the program, and (3) data developed from other AIDS research studies. Our experts noted that the data values used from these sources are reasonable and produce a conservative estimate of the program's impact on the rate of new HIV transmissions.

> The model's estimate that the New Haven needle exchange program results in a reduction of new HIV infections among participants over 1 year is defensible as a minimal estimate of the program's impact. The 33 percent difference is strictly attributable to the reduction in levels of infection in

needles due to the shorter length of time that needles are in use (or needle circulation time).

The University of California concludes (p. 484):

> Relative impact would decrease modestly if different values were used for certain model parameters. However, if the model incorporated behavioral risk reductions, relative impact would increase substantially from the 33% published value.

> Absolute impact would probably decrease below the published value of 0.021 infections averted per client-year, because the estimate of non-NEP HIV incidence appears to be too high.

The panel's view is that these models provide important qualitative insight into why needle exchange programs should work. However, conclusions from modeling a complex process can rarely have the force of absolute proof. Kaplan and his colleagues recognize this, offering a range of calculations based on competing assumptions, parameter values, and models. Despite these admirable efforts, it is true that unmodeled features of the needle exchange program process might make the efficacy estimates either too high or too low. For example, the Kaplan model does not take account of changes in the percentage of infected participants that result if disproportionately many dropouts from the program population were infected (or were not infected). Likewise, if new entrants to the needle exchange program population were less infected (or more) that would artificially raise (or lower) the *apparent* effectiveness of the needle exchange program. Therefore, we must regard numerical estimates from these models with some caution.

In summary, the model-based evaluation of the New Haven needle exchange program provides important insights into the dynamics of such programs and useful preliminary estimates of their efficacy. We cannot attach the same level of confidence to these model-based estimates as we could to evaluation programs that included a suitable control group in which individuals were tested (directly) for HIV infection. Unfortunately, such an evaluation program would face formidable obstacles because of concerns about privacy and confidentiality, difficulties ingeniously (and conscientiously) sidestepped by Kaplan's study methods.

Several other outcome variables were also studied at the New Haven needle exchange program, and these are described below.

New Initiates to Injection Drug Use

If needle exchange programs attracted new initiates to injection drug use, a drop in the average age of program participants who enroll over time would be expected to be observed, coupled with a downward shift in the average number of years of injection drug use. Using demographic data obtained from needle exchange program enrollees over the course of the program operation (November 1990 to December 1991), Heimer and colleagues (Heimer et al., 1993) show that the mean age and mean duration of injection did not change over time. Throughout the study period, male and female enrollees were, on average, approximately 33 to 34 years old. Male enrollees reported using injection drugs for about 10 years; female self-reports on duration showed more month-to-month variability (averaging about 5 to 10 years). From this set of indicators, it would appear that the needle exchange program did not increase the number of new initiates.

The authors also provided an additional observation that counters the argument that needle exchange programs encourage the initiation of injection drug use. They argued that, if the presence of a needle exchange program did enhance use, an increase in the number of new initiates to injection drug use would be most prominent following public disclosure of the first report on the effects of the program. But, at the time of the report's release (and publicity), there was "no increase in the percentage of enrolling clients with very short durations of intravenous drug use" (p. 219).

Enrollment in Drug Treatment

Participants requested drug treatment at a nearly constant rate (25 percent) throughout the study period. The percentage entering treatment increased from 15 percent (first 7 months) to 18 percent (end of 1991). Another noteworthy observation is that a substantial proportion of people who visit the program's van are not needle exchange participants but are visiting the van because they are seeking treatment for drug abuse (Heimer, 1994).

Alternative Explanations

As we have noted in our critique of the model-based estimates of HIV incidence, the change in outcomes (especially the infectivity of needles) might possibly be due to changes in the population served. It is possible that the reduction in the infectivity of needles and syringes could be due to changes in the risk characteristics of participants. But little of the available evidence indicates such client population shifts (Kaplan and Heimer, 1994a). The mean age of enrollees and the mean duration of drug use did not change over the course of the program. The percentage of women remained constant at 20 percent over the course of the study (November 1990 to June 1992). Self-reported drug behaviors were not associated with enrollment date. Analyses of changes over time in frequency of injection, use of shooting galleries, injections shared, using cocaine, and risky injection frequency failed to show any statistically significant trends. (More sophisticated, multivariate models were also used, with similar results.)

Although drug behaviors and gender remained statistically constant over time, Kaplan and colleagues (Heimer et al., 1993; Kaplan, 1994a) reported that the racial composition of the study population did change over time; the percentage of white participants steadily increased (from 17 to 39 percent). Because white participants are less at risk, the change in HIV prevalence might be due to the change in the composition of the population served, but, as the authors note, this does not appear to be a viable plausible explanation for the decline in the infectivity of needles. The decline occurred in the first 120 days and then stabilized. The number of white participants steadily increased throughout the duration of the project. The magnitude of the change in composition is also not great enough to explain the reduction in HIV seropositivity. Specifically, the authors state (Heimer et al. 1993:219):[5]

> At the start of the program, 83% of the participants were nonwhite and 67.5% of the syringes were infected. After 7 months, 62% of the clients were nonwhite and 43% of the syringes were infected. If needle exchange were without effect, then 87.3% of the syringes returned by nonwhites ought to test positive, a plausible result. However, –29.2% of the syringes returned by whites would need to test positive, clearly an impossible result.

Also, Heimer et al. (1993) argue that the decrease in prevalence was not the result of reduced needle sharing, because the fraction of syringes assigned to one person but returned by someone else did not change. As noted by the authors, because of the manner in which the exchange operated, it is not possible to know with certainty whether discordant needles (i.e., exchanged by one individual and returned by a different person) had been shared or whether they were simply exchanged by someone else.

Finally, Kaplan and others (Kaplan, 1994a; O'Keefe et al., 1991) report that up to 60 percent of the New Haven needle exchange program participants dropped out. Although the status of those who dropped out was not always clear, as noted above, a small fraction of these participants were known to have entered drug treatment. Kaplan (1994a) argues that even short-term exposure to the needle exchange program could contribute to its aggregate impact.

Summary

The pattern of evidence surrounding the New Haven needle exchange program involves a set of models, driven in large measure by empirical data gathered from participants and the needles they exchanged. Although the estimates of relative and absolute reduction in HIV incidence are based on mathematical models, Kaplan and his colleagues have explored the computational implications of a range of parameter values. These varied models provide estimates that are not dramatically different, lending credibility to the methods. Nevertheless, the models are not infallible.

The most compelling evidence from this set of evaluation studies is the direct evidence from the actual testing of syringes for the presence of HIV positivity. Here the empirical results of monthly assessments show about a one-third reduction in the rates of infected needles. These empirical results are consistent with those produced by the models underlying Kaplan's circulation theory. Furthermore, evidence about the actual operation of the needle exchange program reveals that the mechanisms necessary for change were in place. A substantial number of needles were exchanged (removed from circulation), the frequency of exchanging increased, and the mean circulation time of needles declined. Had these changes not occurred or had there been observed changes in the composition of the study population, the plausibility of the observed effect (i.e., reduction in the rate of infected needles) attributable to the program would have been undercut. Evidence about the program processes strongly suggests that the reduction in the rate of infected needles is plausibly due to the program. Similarly, reduction in the rate of infected needles strongly suggests (but does not directly test) that there should be a reduction in HIV incidence on the order of magnitude projected by Kaplan's models.

In the panel's view, the empirical data clearly indicate that needles used by program participants have a lower probability of being infected and, consequently, program participants are less likely to become infected.

THE TACOMA STUDIES

The first legally authorized needle exchange program in the United States was implemented in Tacoma, Washington, in 1988. There are several reasons for examining the research on the Tacoma needle exchange in some detail. The needle exchange was the dominant HIV prevention effort in the local area, so there is less confounding with other simultaneous HIV prevention efforts than in other geographic areas. Also, several studies have been conducted on the Tacoma needle exchange program, making it possible to assess consistency across different outcome measures and study designs. As a U.S. city with an ethnically diverse population of injection drug users and high rates of both heroin and cocaine injection, Tacoma may be more relevant to the circumstances of other U.S. cities than the European and Australian cities in which other needle exchange programs have been implemented.

The importance of the Tacoma studies on needle exchange programs is the fact that they provide direct evidence of the incidence of a blood-borne viral disease, spread by needles and sexual contact, among individuals who attended and those who did not attend a needle exchange program. In Tacoma, the prevalence of HIV infection among injection drug users was low, indicative that incident HIV infections would be expected to be rare. However, the rates of two other blood-borne infections, hepatitis B (HBV) and hepatitis C (HCV), were higher and therefore considered as surrogates for HIV infection.

The Program

The Tacoma needle exchange program began operating "unofficially" in August 1988. After informing city officials that a needle exchange would be opening, a community-based organization set up a folding table on a sidewalk in an area of downtown Tacoma where there was a visible concentration of drug users and began exchanging syringes. The unofficial program was officially sanctioned and funded by the local health department beginning in January 1989. A few months later, the health department filed a lawsuit to settle the issue of the legality of the program in view of existing drug paraphernalia laws. In early 1990, a Pierce County Superior Court judge declared that needle exchange was legal in the county. During the past 6 years, the needle exchange has developed into a broad public health program of prevention and education for injection drug users.

At present, the Tacoma needle exchange program consists of two fixed outdoor exchange sites, one located two blocks from the original location and another in a Tacoma neighborhood. Both fixed sites are located near shelters or food kitchens that provide services to homeless persons and operate in areas of the city where there are many injecting drug users. The fixed outdoor sites are open 5 hours per day, 5 days per week. In addition, a community-based organization also operates a mobile needle exchange that can be accessed by phoning exchange workers and arranging to meet and exchange syringes at a mutually agreed-on location within the county. The mobile exchange can be reached during business hours weekdays and Saturdays; exchanges are arranged before or after the fixed sites' hours of operation. A van is used to transport supplies and staff to each of these exchange sites. Syringe exchange is also available within the local public health department clinic pharmacy for 8 hours each weekday.

There are few regulations governing the Tacoma needle exchanges. Participants do not need to register or show identification or proof of drug injection to participate in any exchange program. However, all programs operate on a strict one-for-one basis, and participants must return a syringe for each new syringe they receive. At the pharmacy exchange, a maximum of 20 syringes may be exchanged at any time. At the fixed outdoor and mobile exchanges, there is no maximum number of syringes that may be exchanged at any time, and single exchanges of more than 1,000 syringes have been recorded. The purpose of imposing no limit on the number of syringes is to encourage injection drug users to build up a large reserve of clean syringes to perhaps enable them to better avoid high-risk situations when they have exhausted their supply. It is estimated that 900,000 syringes were exchanged in Tacoma needle exchange programs in 1994 (90,000 from the pharmacy, the remainder from the fixed outdoor and mobile programs).[6]

Assistance from injection drug users willing to act as "secondary exchangers" is encouraged, and several have been identified via the mobile exchange program. They have included representatives from groups of gay and bisexual injection drug users and other injection drug user groups who report they are fearful of being exposed as drug injectors if they come to the fixed sites. With each of the secondary exchanges, there is an explicitly stated expectation that syringes will not be sold. Although for a few months in 1993 the pharmacy exchange asked needle exchange participants for donations, at present there is no cost for syringes or any services provided directly by any exchange.

The Tacoma needle exchange program has been the primary source of AIDS education for injection drug users in the county. Exchange workers spend time each day talking with individuals about their own and other injection drug users' behavior in relation to risk of exposure to HIV and other pathogens and about specific prevention strategies. When it was apparent that the exchange was a better setting for one-to-one education than were ad hoc encounters on street corners, the local health department's small-scale "bleach and teach" outreach campaign moved to the needle exchange site. Eventually, needle exchange staff assumed responsibility for providing one-to-one education and counseling to local injection drug users, primarily because regular and frequent visits to the exchange by their clientele offered an opportunity for follow-up contact and counseling. From January to November 1994, a monthly average of 511 one-to-one contacts were made (range 411-724), which consisted of individualized education, counseling, and referral to other services.

Condoms and sexual risk reduction education have been included among the basic services since the program began. The fixed outdoor exchange sites are both within police-defined areas of prostitution in the city, and there are many female and male sex workers among needle exchange participants. In the first 11 months of 1994, approximately 2,900 condoms (range from 2,100 to 3,900) were distributed each month at the exchange sites.

The fixed needle exchange sites have become the primary locations in the county for bringing health and social services to local injection drug users. Since 1990, a public health nurse has been stationed at the fixed outdoor sites to administer tuberculosis screening tests (the PPD skin test). Those who are given the screening test return to the exchange to have their results read, and further medical workup is arranged for those with positive skin tests. Patients who require antituberculosis medications are scheduled to receive directly observed therapy at the needle exchange. Tuberculosis prevention education is provided to all needle exchange participants through one-to-one counseling and a small-media approach. An average of 175 tuberculosis screening tests are administered to exchange participants each year (Hagan et al., 1992b:8).

HIV testing has also been provided to exchange participants to a limited extent; full implementation has been hindered by the physical setting of the exchange. Both asymptomatic HIV-positive participants and those who have progressed to AIDS are eligible to receive AIDS case management services. The support services given to case management clients provide stability in housing and health care access.

The needle exchange has also become an important source of referral to drug treatment programs in the community. In the first 11 months of 1994, an average of 65 persons were referred to treatment each month. Methadone drug treatment programs, in particular, noted that recruitment at the exchange resulted in enrolling a higher proportion of injection drug users with no previous history of treatment. Furthermore, in 1991 and 1992, the needle exchange was the largest single source of recruitment to methadone treatment programs in the county (Hagan et al., 1993:1694-1695). Since that period, referrals to methadone treatment from the exchange have increased, but program capacity has not kept up with the demand as the number of low-cost, publicly funded treatment slots has plateaued.

In the Tacoma community, the exchange's function of safe disposal of contaminated injection equipment has been considered important. In fact, the local police chief cited public safety and protection of his officers from accidental needlestick injury as the basis for his support of the exchange program (affidavit of Raymond Fjetland, in Tacoma Pierce County Health Department v. City of Tacoma). In addition, a maintenance supervisor responsible for keeping public areas in the vicinity of one of the fixed outdoor sites free of trash and litter noted a dramatic decline in the number of discarded syringes picked up by his crews (affidavit of James Burgess, in Tacoma Pierce County Health Department v. City of Tacoma). In 1990, a sample of returned syringes was collected from the exchange and tested for HIV (Hagan et al., 1991). The virus was detected in 1 percent of 1,200 syringes tested; 2 percent of syringes with visible blood or dirt were HIV-positive. That year, approximately 120,000 used syringes were collected and safely disposed of by the needle exchange.

In Table 7.6 appears a list of five studies that examine various aspects

TABLE 7.6 Tacoma Studies

Study	Design	Results	Alternative Explanation
HIV seroprevalence[a]	• CDC non-link 5-year survey protocol • Injection drug user entering methadone treatment • $N = 1,109$ • To 1992	2 to 4 percent over 5 years' time	• Low HIV prevalence and incidence imply no presence of transmission risk; needle exchange program does not matter • Other HIV interventions

Hepatitis surveillance case reporting[a]	• CDC sentinel pre-post needle exchange program
	• To 1990
		1985—HBV
		  injection drug user = 40
		  Sex = 9
		  Unknown = 13
		1990—HBV
		  injection drug user = 7
		  Sex = 12
		  Unknown = 6
			• Due to normal fluctuation in incidence; saturation in injection drug user community (exhaustion of susceptibles)
			• Local health department implemented other prevention interventions

Hepatitis B and C case control[b]	Case from injection drug user CDC sentinel surveillance 28 injection drug user—HBV 20 injection drug user—HCV Control from injection drug user from • HIV testing and counseling • Treatment 38 injection drug user no serologic markers HBV 26 injection drug user no serologic markers HCV	HBV • Case—75 percent never used needle exchange program • Control—26 percent never used needle exchange program • OR = 8.4 HCV • Case = 75 percent never used needle exchange program • Control = 26 percent never used needle exchange program • OR = 8.1	• Case control not equivalent groups • Controls are a bias sample • Self-selection bias in use of needle exchange program

Interview study 1[b]
- To 1989
- Retrospective pre-post
- $N = 204$ random selection of needle exchange program participants

Overall unsafe injection
Pre = 58 percent
Post = 33 percent
Past used
Pre = 100 per month
Post = 62 per month
Rent
Pre = 56 per month
Post = 30 per month
Bleach
Pre = 69 per month
Post = 105 per month

- Decline in self-report data due to response bias (social desirability)
- Self-selection

Interview study 2[b]
- To 1991
- Cross-sectional
- Exchange users $N = 265$
- Non-exchange $N = 93$
- Random selection of needle exchange participants

Frequency injection no change
Unsafe injection
Needle exchange program users = 21 percent
Non-needle exchange program = 45 percent
HIV
Needle exchange program users = 2 percent
Non-needle exchange program = 7 percent
HIV rates remained stable at follow-up

- Decline in self-report data due to response bias (social desirability)
- Self-selection

NOTE: OR = odds ratio.
[a]Community-level data.
[b]Individual drug user-level data.

of the Tacoma needle exchange program experience. We consider these studies in the order shown there.

HIV Seroprevalence Studies

Beginning in June 1988, individuals entering the health department's methadone drug treatment program were enrolled in an HIV seroprevalence study conducted as part of the CDC Family of HIV Seroprevalence Surveys. A *nonlinked design* was used in accordance with the CDC unlinked survey protocols, with all eligible clients being enrolled so that an unbiased estimate of seroprevalence is obtained. Eligible clients included those who were not coming to the methadone clinic solely for HIV testing and who had not been previously admitted during the survey period, which corresponded to the calendar year. Demographic and risk behavior information was abstracted from data routinely collected for client records. All persons entering drug treatment were required to have a Venereal Disease Research Laboratory test, and any remaining serum was tested for HIV (Hagan and Hale, 1993).

From June 1988 through December 1992, 1,109 drug treatment clients were enrolled in the seroprevalence survey. HIV seroprevalence remained between 2 and 4 percent during each year of the 5-year period. There was no variation in seroprevalence in relation to gender, age, or race/ethnicity (Hagan and Hale, 1993:10).

The continued maintenance of such a low HIV seroprevalence in a population of injection drug users cannot be unequivocally attributed to the needle exchange program and its many program components. However, this stands in sharp contrast with experience in many places, where no systematic prevention programs were in place and seroprevalence among injection drug users was observed to rise rapidly from low to high levels.

Hepatitis Surveillance and Case Reporting

Pierce County has been one of four U.S. counties participating in the CDC's sentinel hepatitis surveillance system since the late 1970s (Alter et al., 1990a, 1990b).[7] The stimulated reporting system includes laboratory-based reporting of serologic findings suggestive of hepatitis and contact with physicians, hospitals, and other health care providers in the community. All confirmed and suspected cases are reported to the local health department's hepatitis surveillance clinic. Public health nurses at the clinic conduct the case investigations and, using a standardized questionnaire, they interview cases and collect demographic and risk-factor information in accordance with the sentinel county study protocol. Hepatitis serologies are performed to specify type of infection.

The surveillance case definition for hepatitis B has included the presence in serum of hepatitis B surface antigen (HBsAg), elevated liver enzymes (SGOT or SGPT) greater than 2.5 times the upper limits of normal, and no other possible causes of liver injury. For hepatitis C, the case definition included absence in sera of both HBsAg and hepatitis A virus immunoglobulin (HAV-IgM), in conjunction with elevated liver enzymes greater than 2.5 times the upper limits of normal and all other possible causes of liver injury ruled out. Hepatitis C cases were presumptively classified as non-A non-B hepatitis until hepatitis C virus antibody (anti-HCV) assays were introduced to diagnose acute illness. The majority of both hepatitis B and hepatitis C cases were symptomatic at the time they were reported.

An outbreak of hepatitis B was observed among injection drug users in Pierce County beginning in 1985: 43 incident cases as of December 1985 (Figure 7.1). The incident cases of hepatitis B among injection drug users persisted until several months after the needle exchange opened (i.e., Au-

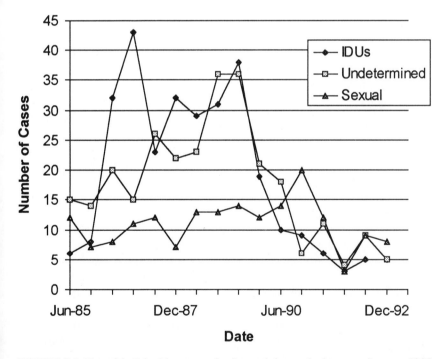

FIGURE 7.1 Hepatitis B incident cases by 6-month intervals, between January 1985 and December 1992. NOTE: IDU = injection drug user. SOURCE: Adapted from Hagan et al. (1991c:1647).

gust 1988) and then declined rapidly (Hagan et al., 1991c). That is, incident cases peaked in December 1986: 43 incident cases among injection drug users were reported, declining to 39 incident cases in December 1989, and further declining to 9 cases as of December 1990. A similar pattern was observed among cases whose source of infection was not identified, whereas the incidence of those cases for which sexual exposure was identified as the primary mode of exposure remained relatively stable over that time period (ranging between 12 and 20 incident cases per 6-month interval between June 1985 and December 1990).

The fact that the reduction of new HBV cases coincided with the introduction of the needle exchange program suggests a plausible positive impact of the exchange. These ecological data alone are subject to alternative explanations. However, when combined with other data from Tacoma, the data support the pattern of evidence suggesting that the abrupt (rather than gradual) reduction in new hepatitis B infections among injection drug users following the opening of the needle exchange program could be in part due to the exchange.

Hepatitis B and C Case-Control Study

Injection drug users who reported to the sentinel hepatitis surveillance system in Pierce County from January 1991 to December 1993 and who met the hepatitis B or hepatitis C case definition (see the previous section) were included in the case series (Hagan et al., in press). Male cases who reported sexual contact with another male were excluded from the study because they may have acquired hepatitis as a result of sexual rather than parenteral exposure to the virus. Cases reporting other risk factors for hepatitis B or C (blood transfusion, health care employment with frequent blood contact, hemodialysis, or sexual or household contact with a confirmed case of hepatitis B or C) were also excluded. In addition to items included in the surveillance questionnaire, a supplemental question was asked about previous use of the needle exchange (Hagan et al., 1994a:5-8).

Control subjects were injection drug users from either of two other health department services, including those attending the HIV-testing center or enrolling in a methadone drug treatment program. Controls were enrolled during the time the cases were being reported. As with the cases, potential controls who were males reporting sexual contact with another male were excluded, and those referred to either health department service by the needle exchange program were also excluded. In addition, hepatitis B controls had to have an absence of any serologic evidence of previous exposure to hepatitis B (negative for HBsAg, antibody to hepatitis B core antigen (anti-HBc), and IgM anti-HBc). Similarly, hepatitis C controls had to have an absence of any serologic evidence of exposure to hepatitis C (anti-HCV negative). Demographic and behavioral data and serum specimens were collected for routine purposes and recorded on client records. Data were abstracted from client records by study personnel. Residual sera were tested for hepatitis B and C markers at the CDC Hepatitis Reference Laboratory in Atlanta, Georgia.

A total of 28 injection drug users with acute hepatitis B and 20 with acute hepatitis C who met study eligibility criteria were reported to the sentinel surveillance system in Pierce County during the time period 1991 to 1993 (Hagan et al., 1994a:8-9). Controls were 38 injection drug users with no serologic markers of exposure to hepatitis B and 26 with no markers for hepatitis C who were attending health department services during the same calendar period and met all study criteria. Of the hepatitis B cases, 75 percent had never used the needle exchange program, compared with 26 percent of hepatitis B seronegative controls (unadjusted odds ratio = 8.4, with a 95 percent confidence interval [CI] 2.4-30.2). Similarly, the risk of hepatitis C was higher among those who never used the exchange (unadjusted odds ratio = 8.1, with a 95 percent CI 1.8-38.7). For both hepatitis B and C infections, there were no differences between cases and controls in the distributions of gender or race. Injection drug users with hepatitis B were somewhat younger and had injected for fewer years than hepatitis B controls. For hepatitis C, there were no differences between cases and controls in relation to age or duration of injection. Adjusted for gender, race, age, and duration of injection, the odds ratio for the association between nonuse of the exchange and hepatitis B was 5.5, with a 95 percent CI 1.5-20.4. For hepatitis C, the adjusted odds ratio was 7.3, with a 95 percent CI 1.6-32.8 (Hagan et al., 1994a:9-10). These case-control studies indicate a powerful retardant effect of needle exchange program attendance on infection with two blood-borne viral infections, offering support to the wholly independent indications from the New Haven study.

Interview Studies with Injection Drug Users

The first interview study with injection drug users in the county was carried out between November 1988 and December 1989. A systematic random sample of 204 injection drug users attending the needle exchange was drawn and asked to participate in a brief interview (Hagan et al., 1993:1692-1693). Subjects were asked about their behavior during the month prior to their enrollment into the needle exchange program and their behavior during the most recent month following their enrollment. Pre- versus postexchange behavior was compared for individual study subjects.

In the pre- versus postexchange comparison of behavior among exchange users, there were no changes in the rate of injection. However, there were statistically significant declines in the frequency of unsafe injections. Study subjects reported a mean of 155 injections per month before first use of the exchange compared with 152 injections per month while participating. The number of injections with rented or borrowed syringes declined from 56 per month pre-exchange to 30 per month while participating. The number of occasions when a used syringe was given to another injector also declined from a mean of 100 times to 62 times per month (Hagan et al., 1993:1693-1695). The number of times when bleach was used to disinfect syringes also increased from 69 to 105 times per month. The proportion of exchange users reporting any unsafe injections also decreased, pre- versus postparticipation, from 58 percent to 33 percent (Hagan et al., 1994b:26 and 32).

From 1990 to 1991, a referent group of Pierce County injection drug users not participating in the exchange (nonexchangers) was enrolled in a cross-sectional study (Hagan et al., 1991b). The systematic sampling scheme used in the pre- versus postexchange study was used to select exchange users for the referent group study. Nonexchangers were recruited from health care and social service agencies and street locations in areas where the exchange did not operate. In addition, chain-referral sampling was used to increase the sample size of nonexchangers. Data were collected from both exchange users and nonexchangers through interview and HIV testing. Analysis compared recent behavior reported by exchange users (while participating in the program) with recent behavior reported by nonexchangers during the same calendar period.

In their second interview study, 265 exchange users were compared with 93 nonexchangers. Significantly fewer exchange users (21 percent) reported any unsafe injections than nonexchangers (45 percent) (Hagan et al., 1991b:3 and 5). And 2 percent of exchange users versus 7 percent of nonexchangers were HIV positive. A larger proportion of exchange users were living on the street or in shelters (20 percent) than nonexchangers (8 percent) (Hagan et al., 1991b:3 and 4). There have been no HIV seroconversions detected in either exchange users or nonexchangers in follow-up HIV testing (67 person years follow-up for nonexchangers, 223 person years for exchange users) (Hagan et al., 1994b:27).

Potential Alternative Explanations

We now discuss one or more alternative explanations for the results in each of the separate studies (Table 7.6). First, it should be noted that the magnitude of the observed effects in each of the studies is relatively large, and that the findings are consistent across different potential outcome measures and methodological approaches. HIV seroprevalence has remained low and stable in the area, implying low community seroincidence. HIV seroincidence in a cohort of injection drug users enrolled in the needle exchange program is low, less than 0.5 per 100 person years at risk. Incidence of acute hepatitis B among injection drug users in the county abruptly declined by 75 percent shortly following the opening of the needle exchange program, whereas incident cases attributable to sexual exposure remained relatively constant.

The case-control studies of incident hepatitis B and C among injection drug users show use of the exchange to be a strong protective factor, and this finding persists after controlling for other potential confounding variables.

The comparison of self-reported risk behavior before and after beginning to use the exchange shows a reduction of almost half. Injection drug users attending the exchange report substantially fewer unsafe injections than those not using it. Those using the exchange also have a substantially lower prevalence of HIV infection.

Although there is at least one alternative explanation for each of the findings from the Tacoma studies, there is no single alternative explanation that could consistently explain the findings across the different studies. Indeed, the possible alternative explanation for one study is often contradicted by findings from another study. For example, low community HIV prevalence and the low incidence of HIV infection in the needle exchange cohort study might have been found simply because the conditions for rapid HIV transmission did not exist in Tacoma even before the needle exchange was implemented. This alternative explanation would not explain, however, why the community rate of hepatitis B virus infections among injection drug users fell dramatically after the implementation of the needle exchange or why the exchange users reported large reductions in risk behavior.

Other potential contributing factors may have been legal sales of syringes by pharmacies or saturation of hepatitis infections in the population of injection drug users. However, by taking into account the results of the two interview studies (i.e., reduction in risk behaviors) and the case-control study (protective effect of the needle exchange program), the credibility of the program having a beneficial effect on hepatitis incidence in the county is strengthened. An outbreak of HBV that *abruptly* subsides several months after the start of the needle exchange program (while sexual cases remain stable) is consistent with a program effect. In outbreaks, an abrupt downward slope in the epidemic curve suggests the impact of an intervention, whereas exhaustion of susceptible or other epidemic features is usually associated with a more gradual decline. This is a generalization, but it piques interest in the data.

An important alternative explanation is that the health department geared up and achieved momentum in case finding and contact tracing and delivered hepatitis B hyperimmune globulin and HBV vaccine. However, this potential rival explanation still would not explain why no such abrupt decline was observed with the sexually transmitted cases. Moreover, as stated earlier, Pierce County has been part of CDC's hepatitis surveillance system since the late 1970s, and no changes in protocol have been implemented since then. Furthermore, no hepatitis vaccine campaign was ever undertaken in the county (H. Hagan, personal communication, January 1995).

Social desirability effects (telling the interviewer what you believe he or she wants to hear) might explain why needle exchange users report large reductions in their risk behavior and lower frequencies of injection risk behavior than injection drug users not using the exchange (even though the interviews were conducted by research staff separate from the exchange staff). The alternative explanation of social desirability for self-reported risk behavior does not match the findings from the hepatitis case-control studies (Hagan et al., in press), in which injection drug users who used the exchange were much less likely to have been recently infected with hepatitis B and hepatitis C viruses.

Self-selection or volunteer bias might explain why the injection drug users who use the exchange report low levels of current risk behavior and have low incidence of HIV, hepatitis B, and hepatitis C virus infections. The exchange might simply have attracted injection drug users who were concerned about health and were practicing safer injection prior to the implementation of the needle exchange. However, this alternative explanation is not consistent with the exchange users' report of their frequent risk behavior prior to beginning use of the exchange and the community-wide reduction in hepatitis B incidence and the low community prevalence rate of HIV infection.

Case-control studies are always open to the objection that cases and controls may differ in important respects. If cases and controls in the Tacoma study (Hagan et al., in press) were not arising from the same source population, it would result in biased estimates of the associations between needle exchange participation and incident cases of hepatitis B and C. Nonequivalence between controls and cases was not detected on measured demographic characteristics for hepatitis C (sex, race, age, and duration of injection). Hepatitis B cases and controls differed regarding age and duration of injection. Nonetheless, after statistically controlling for such disparities, the association between needle exchange participation and hepatitis B was still found to be significant.

Another concern that may arise is that hepatitis B cases may not be representative of nonselected cases in the community because they were symptomatic. It is true that immunocompromised individuals (e.g., from renal dialysis, steroid use, HIV, and age extremes) are less likely to be symptomatic. However, given the low HIV prevalence, the age range of study cases, and other factors, these seem unlikely to be a major factor operating in the Tacoma study.

The case-control study report (Hagan et al., in press) can be viewed as having design issues that affect confidence in the inferences that can be drawn. One is the selection of controls.

Controls for this study were injection drug users who were ascertained through entry into drug treatment or enrollment in the county's HIV testing program. Although cases in this study can be argued to be representative of all cases for hepatitis B (Pierce County is a CDC sentinel surveillance site), the selection of controls through the two stated mechanisms raises questions. The underlying issue is the extent to which new drug treatment admissions or enrollees for HIV testing are "representative" of the overall uninfected population (including those not in treatment or uninterested in HIV testing). The descriptive epidemiologic literature on the characteristics of persons with a *history* of treatment versus *no history* of treatment suggests demographic differences; this literature hints at the possibility for bias when limiting ascertainment to treatment or testing programs (Alcabes, 1993). However, analyses of drug-use risk factors for infection for those in treatment compared with those out of treatment indicate that, despite differences in distribution of certain characteristics, patterns of drug-use risk behaviors and infection are similar for both groups. This argues that treatment samples are not biased as far as susceptibility to infections is concerned (Alcabes et al., 1993). Also, prospective studies of factors associated with entry into treatment note similar injection risk behaviors, but increased complications of drug abuse in those entering treatment (Schütz et al., 1994); this suggests that the effect of sampling treatment entrants for the purpose of studying viral infection is likely to be minor.

Nevertheless, the issue of potential of bias for controls selected among treatment entrants and injection drug users who arrive for HIV testing could be real if the needle exchange program makes active referrals into treatment and HIV testing. In the case of the Tacoma study, this apparently occurred, *but* the researchers made explicit the point that direct referrals were identified and excluded from analysis.

The issue remains whether the probability that controls who were picked from treatment and testing were somehow more likely to have used needle exchange than HBV-seronegative drug users not going into treatment or testing. If the proportion of drug users in a community that used needle exchange was small (e.g., 5 percent) and the proportion in this sample was high, then the discrepancy might be attributed to sampling. However, as Hagan and colleagues note, the proportion of the entire Tacoma community of injection drug users that has been estimated to be enrolled or covered by needle exchange is high (i.e., 50 to 70 percent; see Hagan et al., 1994a:10-

11) and not inconsistent with the proportion estimated in the controls in this study. This suggests that the effect of selection bias is probably minor.

In sum, the choice of controls for the study of hepatitis B and C virus infections and needle exchange in Tacoma is intuitively open to criticism. A broader cross section of approaches to sample injection drug users might add confidence in the inferences drawn. However, on closer inspection, there is evidence from other studies to suggest that (1) the sampling approach is not obviously biased; (2) the investigators excluded those who might have biased the sample (referrals); (3) the sample estimates and population estimates for use of needle exchange are not dissimilar; and (4) no mechanism for differential bias could be identified. Taken together, these suggest that, whereas it is prudent to be cautious about the results of any case-control study, the effect of selection bias in this situation is likely to be minimal.

The lack of any consistent alternative explanation for the Tacoma findings leads the panel to accept the primary hypothesis that implementation of the needle exchange program led to substantial risk reduction among local injection drug users, which then led to reduced transmission of blood-borne viruses (both HIV and hepatitis). Although different study designs were used, there was consistency among the results; under these circumstances, it is less likely that the findings are due to bias (Rothman, 1986). Thus, the panel concludes that the Tacoma studies show that a needle exchange program can lead to behavior change and reduced transmission of blood-borne viruses.

Program Effects on New Initiates to Drug Use or Abuse

The Tacoma and New Haven studies and previous reviews had few, if any, empirical data on the impact of needle exchange programs on drug initiation or drug abuse among noninjection drug users. This leaves any conclusion regarding the impact of such programs on nondrug users to be theoretical at best. Although few empirical data are available on how these programs may impact overall drug use in communities that choose to implement such programs, a sizable literature does exit on the etiology of drug use. In this section we first briefly summarize what factors have been found to influence drug-use initiation and progression to drug abuse. Based on that knowledge base we attempt to foresee how needle exchange programs may potentially impact drug-use initiation and/or progression to drug abuse.

Some research suggests that the reasons people begin using drugs are different from the reasons they continue or escalate their use, which is to say, the factors that influence initiation are different from those that influence progression to more serious use (e.g., injection drug use). Several researchers have found that initiation is often strongly tied to social and peer influences, whereas biological and psychological processes appear to be associated with abuse (Carman, 1979; Kandel et al., 1978; Newcomb and Bentler, 1990; Paton et al., 1977). Even though data may as yet be too sparse to establish firmly that the causes of use are different from the causes of abuse, the evidence consistent with this hypothesis is accumulating (Glantz and Pickens, 1992).

Moreover, the more risk factors to which someone is exposed that encourage use, the more likely he or she is to use or abuse drugs. Exposure to a greater number of risk factors is not only a reliable correlate of use, but it also influences the increase in drug use over time, implying a true causal role for those variables that together make for increased risk (Schreier and Newcomb, 1991). It appears that the presence of particular factors that can encourage drug use are not as important as the accumulation and interaction of such factors in a person's life.

The existing knowledge about risk and protective factors suggests that certain social influences to use drugs have the *potential* to be impacted by needle exchange programs (Hawkins et al., in press; Clayton and Leukefeld, 1994). Impacting such factors can theoretically either increase or decrease the risk of nondrug users moving from nonuse to use and abuse. Known risk factors include peers who use drugs, current involvement of parents and siblings in drug use, favorable societal and community norms regarding drug use, and favorable personal attitudes toward drug use, which include perceived risk of harm. The effect of needle exchange programs on other risk and protective factors is not likely.

On the positive side, needle exchange and bleach distribution programs may decrease the number of new initiates to drug use or abuse. As described earlier in this chapter, treatment referral and entrance has been a documented result of such programs. Since parental and peer drug use are risk factors for drug initiation and abuse, needle exchange and bleach distribution program participants who are referred to treatment and become abstinent are likely to reduce the likelihood that their children and their close family and friends make the transition from nondrug to drug user.

On the negative side, the presence of needle exchange programs may affect risk factors for drug use and abuse. This includes an increase in favorable community or personal norms and attitudes toward drug use. An increase in clean needles and syringes may lead to a reduction in the perceived risk of AIDS and other blood-borne diseases associated with injection drug use. Furthermore, changes in federal regulations banning the use of federal funds for needle exchange programs may result in the perception that societal resolve against drug use is weakened. However, there is no evidence of an impact of needle exchange programs on these community attitudes and, in general, little evidence of an increase in the number of nondrug users that move to drug use as a result of such programs in their community. If the effect of needle exchange programs on nondrug users is evident only over the long term because of an extended temporal causal chain—including weakened societal antidrug abuse resolve first affecting community norms and personal attitudes, which, in turn, affect the transition from nonuse to use—then the effect on nondrug users may not be evident in the short term. Although this long-term effect may be possible and should be investigated, there is also reason to believe that the existing evidence of no effect will hold in more controlled and long-term investigations. The relationship between drug-use norms and perceived risk of drug use indicates that the effect of these norms and attitudes is *drug specific* (Bachman et al., 1990). Since needle exchange programs are likely to affect only risk due to injection, and because nondrug users are extremely unlikely to begin their drug-using careers by using injectable drugs (Kandel et al., 1978, 1992), it is not likely that changes in community or personal norms and attitudes as a result of having needle exchange and bleach distribution programs will increase the risk of the transition of nondrug users into drug use.

Alternatively, it may be possible to curtail the emergence of these theoretical potential negative effects of needle exchange programs on norms and attitudes. There is evidence that drug-use norms and attitudes are manipulable by intervention (Hansen et al., 1988; Hansen and Graham, 1991), and it may be possible, through active norm change strategies, to avoid the potential negative effects of needle exchange programs on norms and attitudes. By stressing to the public the fact that these programs are health approaches taken to curb the spread of contagious diseases (e.g., AIDS, HBV, HCV), rather than remaining neutral or leaving interpretation solely to community and personal impressions, it may be possible to avoid potentially adverse community norm changes.

All of these issues need to be properly addressed in future research to clarify whether possible long-term harms associated with the implementation of needle exchange programs are tenable.

SUMMARY

The following conclusions and recommendations are necessarily built on the progressive presentation of information and research data found in this and earlier chapters. This presentation reflects the cumulative development of the panel's understanding about issues inherent in the establishment of needle exchange and bleach distribution programs and, ultimately, their anticipated effects, based on the *pattern of evidence* discerned by the panel from its collective activities, primarily its reviews of pertinent studies.

Conclusions

The panel found sufficient evidence among the studies reviewed to reach the following conclusions:

• Needle exchange programs increase the availability of sterile injection equipment.

• For the participants in a needle exchange program, the fraction of needles in circulation that are contaminated is lowered by this increased availability. This amounts to a reduction in an important risk factor for HIV transmission.

• The lower the fraction of needles in circulation that are contaminated, the lower the risk of new HIV infections.

The first two conclusions are amply supported by empirical evidence. The third is a logical consequence: if a needle has a lower probability of being contaminated, then it necessarily has a smaller chance of infecting the user. Direct empirical evidence (from a case-control study) confirms this proposition when hepatitis B virus and hepatitis C virus (more virulent than HIV) are the infections in question. HBV and HCV are spread by contaminated needles in the same population, and needle exchange was shown to reduce the incidence of new cases of these (less rare) blood-borne viral infections.

The panel further concludes that:

• Additional possible positive outcomes are reported by the users of needle exchange programs, including:

— increased cleaning of used needles;
— decreased sharing of needles; and
— uncertain and probably small improvements in risky sexual behaviors (fewer partners, more condom use).

• Needle exchange programs report increased referrals to drug abuse treatment and, in the few studies that examined this issue, no increase in the number of dirty needles discarded in public places (e.g., parks, streets, alleys).

Unfavorable aspects of needle exchange and bleach distribution programs also demand consideration. The act of giving a needle—however clean—to an injection drug user has a powerful symbolism that has sparked fears about the potential negative effects of needle exchange programs. Similar fears sometimes appear in response to proposals to distribute bleach to injection drug users. However, the record shows little evidence in support of these concerns.

• There is no credible evidence to date that drug use is increased among participants as a result of programs that provide legal access to sterile equipment. (Long-term effects are necessarily not yet known, providing a reason for continued monitoring for potential negative effects.)

• The available scientific literature provides evidence based on self-reports that needle exchange programs:

— do not increase the frequency of injection among program participants and
— do not increase the number of new initiates to injection drug use.

• The available scientific literature provides evidence that needle exchange programs:

— have public support, depending on locality, and
— have public support that tends to increase over time (where trend data are available).

The high level of concern about potential negative effects of needle exchange and bleach distribution programs cannot be ignored, despite the paucity of supporting evidence. Communities wracked with drug abuse and addiction, AIDS, crime, and poverty may well resent the institution of needle exchange and bleach distribution programs, seeing the programs as a wholly inadequate response to the key problems. Attention to comprehensive responses to the drug epidemic is clearly important, especially the expansion of drug treatment to make it more available. Needle exchange programs should be regarded as a public health promotion and disease prevention strategy that fits within the broader harm reduction approach to public health.

It is essential that prevention programs (including initiation of needle exchange programs) must vary regionally and locally to reflect those infected or at risk in any area. Thus, although the panel supports the use of needle exchange and bleach distribution programs as part of a nationwide HIV prevention strategy, it is absolutely critical that their use should be driven by the nature of the epidemic in different locales.

Recommendations

The specific charge to this panel was to examine the effectiveness of syringe exchange and bleach distribution as methods of reducing HIV transmission. This necessarily led to some consideration of other methods of reducing HIV transmission.

Reducing drug use would serve to reduce HIV transmission as well as to achieve other important social and public health goals. Comprehensive drug treatment is one important way to reduce drug use. However, (1) treatment, especially comprehensive treatment, is inadequately available; (2) treatment does not work for all individuals who enter it; and (3) not all drug abusers currently are willing ("wish") to enter treatment.

For all of these reasons, researchers have explored the efficacy of more limited programs, such as needle exchange and bleach distribution, as a means of reducing the risk of HIV infection by providing users not able to undertake drug treatment access to uncontaminated injection equipment.

Based on a comprehensive review of the research literature, the panel concludes that well-implemented needle exchange programs can be effective in preventing the spread of HIV and do not increase the use of illegal drugs. Hence, we recommend that:

• **The Surgeon General make the determination called for in P.L. 102-394, section 514, 1993, necessary to rescind the present prohibition against applying any federal funds to support needle exchange programs.**

Observe that the panel does not recommend a mandated national program of needle exchange and bleach distribution. As documented in this report, regional variation in prevalence of HIV infection, the extent and kind of drug use, the presence of other AIDS programs, operational characteristics of existing needle exchange programs, and the attitudes and needs of local communities all influence the potential effects of needle exchange programs and militate against such a mandate. The recommendation is to *allow communities that desire such programs to institute them,* using resources at their disposal and unencumbered by the specific funding handicap that is now in place.

If needle exchange programs become available tools of public health and disease prevention, certain implementation measures become desirable. In particular, the panel recommends that:

• Local community members (e.g., police, church, treatment providers, pharmacists, local public health authorities) should be involved in determining whether such programs should be implemented locally and how they should be institutionalized.

• Attention must be given to the development of site-specific programs that are community based, culturally sensitive, and capable of demonstrating respect for the concerns of the communities in which they are to be based. The importance of flexibility and community control is strongly emphasized.

• Appropriate health agencies should make available technical assistance and relevant epidemiologic data to local organizations and groups within the communities to assist them in making informed decisions about needle exchange and bleach distribution programs.

• Needle exchange programs should promote HIV prevention not only by providing sterile equipment, but also by means of education, drug treatment referral, and materials, including bleach, alcohol pads, and condoms.

• Needle exchange programs should make special efforts to reach and retain hard-to reach subgroups of injection drug users, such as young injection drug users and women.

• The National Institutes of Health, the Centers for Disease Control and Prevention, and the Agency for Health Care Policy and Research should support evaluation research examining the programs and the key outcomes, including HIV risk behavior and reduced HIV transmission.

The panel further recommends that in meeting the need for increasing the treatment capacity, as described above,

• Incremental funds for needle exchange programs and other AIDS prevention strategies should be appropriated but should not be taken from resources now supporting drug treatment programs.

In addition, such a diversion of funds would be unwise because drug treatment programs have been shown to be effective in treating the underlying disorder of drug abuse and can be effective in curtailing HIV risk behaviors. Moreover, for many program participants, needle exchange and bleach distribution programs have been found to serve as a bridge to drug treatment for many needle exchange program clients. Indeed, the panel further recommends that:

• The appropriate legislative bodies should enact legislation (and should appropriate monies) to increase drug treatment capacity and establish better links between treatment and AIDS prevention programs that target injection drug users.

Finally, the panel recommends that:

• The National Institutes of Health (e.g., National Institute on Drug Abuse) and the Centers for Disease Control and Prevention should support research that evaluates the effect of needle exchange and bleach distribution programs on the severity of abuse and addiction among needle exchange and bleach distribution program participants.

• A better monitoring system should be established for assessing long-term societal changes in drug use at the community level due to needle exchange programs.

NOTES

1. Specifically the GAO was requested to: (1) review the results of studies addressing the effectiveness of needle exchange programs in the United States and abroad; (2) assess the credibility of a forecasting model developed at Yale University that estimates the impact of a needle exchange program on the rate of new HIV infections; and (3) determine whether federal funds can be used in support of studies and demonstrations of needle exchange programs.

2. The U.S. project sites were Berkeley, California; Boston, Massachusetts; Boulder, Colorado; New Haven, Connecticut; New York City, New York; Portland, Oregon; San Francisco, California; Santa Cruz, California; Seattle, Washington; and Tacoma, Washington. Sites abroad included: Montréal, Toronto, and Vancouver (Canada); Amsterdam, the Netherlands; and London, England.

3. To derive the estimate of the relative impact, Kaplan and his colleagues developed a model based on a circulation theory. The basic idea is that each time an infected needle is removed from circulation among a population of injection drug users and replaced with a sterile needle, the risk of infecting some member of that population is decreased. This model was based on a two-state continuous time Markov process and assumed that uncontaminated needles become infected at a rate that does not change over time, and infected needles become uncontaminated at another rate that also does not change over time. Under these assumptions, a formula was developed for the expected proportion of circulating needles that were infected. This formula involved these rates and the mean circulation time. Data from the Syringe Tracking System developed for the New Haven project were used to estimate these rates as well as the mean circulation times of needles before and after the initiation of the needle exchange program. These estimates and formulas were used to determine that the relative reduction in the expected proportion of circulating needles that were infected was 33 percent.

4. In order to compute absolute reduction in incidence, estimates of the baseline HIV incidence rate before the initiation of the needle exchange program were required. This was determined by introducing some additional modeling assumptions concerning the dynamics of the epidemic. These calculations, together with additional assumptions about the proportion of infections among injection drug users resulting from needle sharing as opposed to sexual transmission, estimated that between 1 and 4 HIV infections were prevented per 100 injection drug users per year. This range of the estimated number of infections averted was derived by two methods: (1) the equilibrium method and (2) the backcalculation method (involving 7 years of AIDS incidence data for New Haven). The equilibrium method estimates 1.2 to 2.8 averted infections; the backcalculation method estimates 1.07 to 3.73

(assumes 30 percent of infections are sexually transmitted) or 0.92 to 3.2 (assumes 40 percent derived from sexual exposure) averted infections.

5. In a footnote, Heimer et al. (1993) explain that, for demographics to account for these results, assuming that needle exchange programs have no effect, the contribution to the overall prevalence rates for earlier and late time periods should be proportionate to the fractional size of each group at each time point. Solving these two equations reveals the impossible value for white participants. Therefore, they reject the plausibility of this explanation.

6. The community-based organization submits monthly reports to the health department detailing syringe exchange activities; somewhat less detailed reports are provided by the health department pharmacy. These were used to estimate numbers of syringes, client contacts, referrals, and prevention materials distributed January to November 1994.

7. A program of stimulated case reporting of hepatitis in the county has resulted in approximately 50 percent of all hepatitis being reported in Pierce County, compared with about 17 percent nationwide (Alter et al., 1987).

REFERENCES

Alcabes, P., E.E. Schoenbaum, and R.S. Klein
  1993   Correlates of rate of decline of CD4+ lymphocytes among intravenous drug users infected with human immunodeficiency virus. *American Journal of Epidemiology* 137:989-1000.
Alter, M.J., A. Mares, S.C. Hadler, and J.E. Maynard
  1987   The effect of underreporting on the apparent incidence and epidemiology of acute viral hepatitis. *American Journal of Epidemiology* 125:133-139.
Alter, M.J., S.C. Hadler, and H.S. Margolis
  1990a   The changing epidemiology of hepatitis B in the United States. *Journal of the American Medical Association* 263:1218-1222.
Alter, M.J., S.C. Hadler, and F.N. Judson
  1990b   Risk factors for acute non-A, non-B hepatitis in the United States and association with hepatitis C virus infection. *Journal of the American Medical Association* 264:2231-2235.
Bachman, J.G., L.D. Johnston, and P.M. O'Malley
  1990   Explaining the recent decline in cocaine use among young adults: Further evidence that perceived risks and disapproval lead to reduced drug use. *Journal of Health and Social Behavior* 3(June):173-184.
Bruneau, J., F. Lamothe, E. Franco, N. Lachance, J. Vincelette, and J. Stoto
  1995   Needle Exchange Program (NEP) Attendance and HIV-1 Infection in Montreal: Report of a Paradoxical Association. Abstract for International Conference on the Reduction of Drug Related Harm, Palazzo dei Congressi, Florence, Italy, March 26-30.
Carman, R.S.
  1979   Motivations for drug use and problematic outcomes among rural junior high school students. *Addictive Behaviors* 4:91-93.
Clayton, R.R., and C.G. Leukefeld
  1994   Drug Use and Its Progression to Drug Abuse and Drug Dependence: Implications for Needle Exchange and Bleach Distribution Programs. Paper commissioned by

the Panel on Needle Exchange and Bleach Distribution Programs, National Research Council and Institute of Medicine.

Cordray, D.S.
1986   Quasi-experimental analysis: A mixture of methods and judgment. *New Directions for Program Evaluation* 31:9-27.

Davoli, M., C.A. Perucci, D.D. Abeni, M. Arcà, G. Brancato, F. Forastiere, P.M. Montiroli, and F. Zampieri
1995   HIV risk-related behaviors among injection drug users in Rome: Differences between 1990 and 1992. *American Journal of Public Health* 85(6):829-832.

Des Jarlais, D.C.
1994   Current Findings in Syringe Exchange Research: A Report to the Task Force to Review Services for Drug Misusers. United Kingdom: Department of Health.
in press   HIV epidemiology and interventions among injecting drug users. *Journal of the Royal Society of Medicine.*

Des Jarlais, D.C., and H. Maynard
1992   *Evaluation of Needle Exchange Program on HIV Risk Behaviors: Supplemental Final Report.* American Foundation for AIDS Research. September 10.

Des Jarlais, D.C., S.R. Friedman, and W. Hopkins
1985   Risk reduction for the acquired immunodeficiency syndrome among intravenous drug users. *Annals of Internal Medicine* 103:755-759.

Des Jarlais, D.C., S.R. Friedman, J.L. Sotheran, J. Wenston, M. Marmor, S.R. Yancovitz, B. Frank, S. Beatrice, and D. Mildvan
1994a   Continuity and change within an HIV epidemic: Injecting drug users in New York City, 1984 through 1992. *Journal of the American Medical Association* 271(2):121-127.

Des Jarlais, D.C., D. Paone, M. Marmor, S. Titus, J.L. Sotheran, and S.R. Friedman
1994b   New York City Syringe Evaluation: The New York City Syringe Exchange Program: Evaluation of a Public Health Intervention. Paper presented at a Conference of the American Public Health Association, Washington, DC, November.

Des Jarlais, D.D., D. Paone, M. Marmor, S. Titus, Q. Shi, T. Perlis, J.L. Sotheran, and S.R. Friedman
1995   New York City Syringe Evaluation: HIV Risk Behavior and Seroincidence Among Injecting Drug Users in the New York City Syringe Exchange Programs. Paper submitted for publication.

Doherty, M.C., R.S. Garfein, B. Junge, P. Beilenson, and D. Vlahov
1995   Discarded Needles Do Not Increase With a Needle Exchange Program. Paper presented at The Second National Conference on Human Retroviruses and Related Infections, American Society for Microbiology, Washington, DC.

Dolan, K., M. Donoghoe, S. Jones, and Stimson, G.
1991   *A Cohort Study of Syringe Exchange Clients and Other Drug Injectors in England, 1989 to 1990.* The Centre for Research on Drugs and Health Behaviour. April.

Donoghoe, M.C. G.V. Stimson, K. Dolan, and L. Alldritt
1989   Changes in HIV risk behavior in clients of syringe-exchange schemes in England and Scotland. *AIDS* 3:267-272.

Donoghoe, M., K. Dolan, and G. Stimson
1991   Changes in Injectors' HIV Risk Behavior and Syringe Supply in UK 1987-90. Abstract ThC 45 in *Final Program and Abstracts of the VII International Conference on AIDS*, Florence.

Feldman, H. P. Biernacki, T. Knapp, and E. Margolis
1989   Modification of Needle Use in Out-of-Treatment Intravenous Drug Users. Ab-

stract ThDP 62 in *Final Program and Abstracts of the V International Conference on AIDS*, Montréal.

Glantz, M.D., and R.W. Pickens
1992   Vulnerability to drug abuse: Introduction and overview. Pp. 1-14 in M. Glantz and R. Pickens, eds., *Vulnerability to Drug Abuse*. Washington, DC: American Psychological Association.

Guydish, J. A. Abramowitz, W. Woods, J. Newmeyer, G. Clark, and J. Sorensen
1989   Sharing Needles: Risk Reduction Among Intravenous Drug Users in San Francisco. Abstract ThDP 34 in *Final Program and Abstracts of the V International Conference on AIDS*, Montréal.

Guydish, J. J. Bucardo, M. Young, W. Woods, O. Grinstead, and W. Clark
1993   Evaluating needle exchange: Are there negative effects? *AIDS* 7:871-876.

Hagan, H., and C.B. Hale
1993   HIV-1 Seroprevalence Surveys in Pierce County. Report available from Tacoma-Pierce County Health Department.

Hagan, H., D.C. Des Jarlais, D. Purchase, S.R. Friedman, T. Damrow, R. Ip, N. Mellor, T.R. Reid, and D. Villareal
1991a   Syringe seroprevalence in relation to seroprevalence among syringe exchange users and accidental HIV transmission. Proceedings of the 119th Meeting of the American Public Health Association, November 10-14, Atlanta, GA.

Hagan, H., D.C. Des Jarlais, D. Purchase, T.R. Reid, and S.R. Friedman
1991b   Lower HIV Seroprevalence, Declining HBV and Safer Injection in Relation to the Tacoma Syringe Exchange. Abstract WC 3291 in *Final Program and Abstracts of the VII International Conference on AIDS*, Florence.

Hagan, H., D.C. Des Jarlais, D. Purchase, S.R. Friedman, T.R. Reid, and T.A. Bell
1991c   The incidence of HBV infection and syringe exchange programs [letter]. *Journal of the American Medical Association* 266:1646-1647.

Hagan, H., D.C. Des Jarlais, S.R. Friedman, D. Purchase, and T. Bell
1992a   Oral presentation at Kaiser Foundation Conference, Menlo Park, CA.

Hagan, H., D.C. Des Jarlais, S.R. Friedman, D. Purchase, and T.R. Reid
1992b   Potential for multiple public health functions of a syringe exchange. Proceedings of the 120th Annual Meeting of the American Public Health Association, November, Washington DC.

Hagan, H., D.C. Des Jarlais, D. Purchase, S.R. Friedman, T.R. Reid, and T.A. Bell
1993   An interview study of participants in the Tacoma, Washington, syringe exchange. *Addiction* 88:1691-1697.

Hagan, H., D.C. Des Jarlais, S.R. Friedman, D. Purchase, and M.J. Alter
1994a   Reduced risk of hepatitis B and hepatitis C among injecting drug users participating in the Tacoma syringe exchange program. Manuscript submitted for review.

Hagan, H., D.C. Des Jarlais, S.R. Friedman, and D. Purchase
1994b   Risk for human immunodeficiency virus and hepatitis B virus in users of the Tacoma syringe exchange program. Pp. 24-34 in *Proceedings, Workshop on Needle Exchange and Bleach Distribution Programs*. National Research Council and Institute of Medicine. Washington, DC: National Academy Press.

Hagan, H. D.C. Des Jarlais, S.R. Friedman, D. Purchase, and M.J. Alter
in press Reduced risk of hepatitis B and hepatitis C among injecting drug users participating in the Tacoma syringe exchange program. *American Journal of Public Health*.

Hankins, C., S. Gendron, J. Bruneau, and E. Roy
1994   Evaluating Montréal's needle exchange CACTUS-Montréal. Pp. 83-90 in *Proceedings, Workshop on Needle Exchange and Bleach Distribution Programs*. National Research Council and Institute of Medicine. Washington, DC: National Academy Press.

Hansen, W.B., and J.W. Graham
1991   Preventing alcohol, marijuana, and cigarette use among adolescents: Peer pressure resistance training versus establishing conservative norms. *Preventive Medicine* 20(3):414-430.
Hansen, W.B., J.W. Graham, B.H. Wolkenstein, B.Z. Lundy, J. Pearson, B.R. Flay, and C.A. Johnson
1988   Differential impact of three alcohol prevention curricula on hypothesized mediating variables. *Journal of Drug Education* 18(2):143-153.
Hartgers, C., E.C. Buning, G.W. van Santen, A.D. Verster, and R.A. Coutinho
1989   The impact of the needle and syringe-exchange programme in Amsterdam on injecting risk behaviour. *AIDS* 3:571-576.
Hartgers, C., E. van Ameijden, J. van den Hoek, and R. Coutinho
1992   Needle sharing and participation in the Amsterdam syringe exchange among HIV-seronegative injecting drug users. *Public Health Reports* 107:675-681.
Hawkins, D., M.W. Arthur, and R.F. Catalano
in press Preventing substance abuse. In D. Farrington and M. Tonry, eds., *Crime and Justice: A Review of Research*, Vol. 18. Crime Prevention. Chicago: University of Chicago Press.
Hawkins, J.D., R.F. Catalano, and J.L. Miller
1992   Risk and protective factors for alcohol and other drug problems in adolescence and early adulthood: Implications for substance abuse prevention. *Psychological Bulletin* 112(1):65-105.
Heimer, R.
1994   Presentation at Focus Group on HIV and Substance Abuse, July 28, Washington, DC.
Heimer, R., E.H. Kaplan, K. Khoshnood, B. Jariwala, and E.C. Cadman
1993   Needle exchange decreases the prevalence of HIV-1 proviral DNA in returned syringes in New Haven, Connecticut. *American Journal of Medicine* 95(2):214-220.
Hill, A.B.
1965   The environment and disease: Association or causation? President's address at January 14 meeting. *Proceedings of the Royal Society of Medicine* 163(seriesB):295-300.
Hunter, G.M., M.C. Donoghoe, G.V. Stimson, T. Rhodes, and C.P. Chalmers
1995   Changes in the injecting risk behaviour of injecting drug users in London, 1990-1993. *AIDS* 9:493-501.
Kandel, D.B., R.C. Kessler, and R.S. Margulies
1978   Antecedents of adolescent initiation into stages of drug use: A developmental analysis. *Journal of Youth and Adolescence* 7:13-40.
Kandel, D.B., K. Yamaguchi, and K. Chen
1992   Stages of progression in drug involvement from adolescence to adulthood. *Journal of Studies on Alcohol* 53(5):447-457.
Kaplan, E.H.
1994a   A method for evaluating needle exchange programmes. *Statistics in Medicine* 13:2179-2187.
1994b   Operational modeling of needle exchange programs. Pp. 202-249 in *Proceedings, Workshop on Needle Exchange and Bleach Distribution Programs*. National Research Council and Institute of Medicine. Washington, DC: National Academy Press.
in press Probability Models of Needle Exchange Programs. Operations Research.

Kaplan, E.H., and R. Heimer
1992   HIV prevalence among intravenous drug users: Model-based estimates from New
         Haven's legal needle exchange. *Journal of Acquired Immune Deficiency Syn-
         dromes* 5:163-169.
Kaplan, E.H. and R. Heimer
1994a   A circulation theory of needle exchange. *AIDS* 8(5):567-574.
1994b   HIV incidence among needle exchange participants: Estimated from syringe tracking
         and testing data. *Journal of Acquired Immune Deficiency Syndromes* 7(2):182-
         189.
in press HIV incidence among New Haven needle exchange participants: Updated esti-
         mates from syringe tracking and testing data. *Journal of Acquired Immune Defi-
         ciency Syndromes*.
Kaplan, E.H., and E. O'Keefe
1993   Let the needles do the talking! Evaluating the New Haven needle exchange.
         Interfaces 23:7-26.
Kaplan, E.H., and D. Soloshatz
1993   How many drug injectors are there in New Haven? Answers from AIDS data.
         Mathematical and Computer Modelling 17:109-115.
Klee, H., and J. Morris
1994   Needle Exchange Schemes: Increasing the Potential for Harm Reduction Among
         Injecting Drug Users. In *Tenth International Conference on AIDS*, Yokohama,
         Japan.
Klee, H., J. Faugier, C. Hayes, and J. Morris
1991   The sharing of injecting equipment among drug users attending prescribing clinics
         and those using needle-exchanges. *British Journal of Addiction* 86:217-223.
Lamothe, F., J. Bruneau, R. Coates, J.G. Rankin, J. Soto, R. Arshinoff, M. Brabant, J. Vincelette,
and M. Fauvel
1993   Seroprevalence of and risk factors for HIV-1 infection in injection drug users in
         Montréal and Toronto: A collaborative study. *Canadian Medical Association
         Journal* 149(7):945-951.
Lange, W.R., F.R. Snyder, D. Lozovsky, V. Kaistha, M.A. Kaczaniuk, and J.H. Jaffe
1988   Geographic distribution of human immunodeficiency virus markers in parenteral
         drug abusers. *American Journal of Public Health* 78(4):443-446.
Lewis, D.K., and J. K. Watters
1994   Sexual behavior and sexual identity in male injection drug users. *Journal of
         Acquired Immune Deficiency Syndromes* 7:190-198.
Lurie, P., A.L. Reingold, B. Bowser, D. Chen, J. Foley, J. Guydish, J.G. Kahn, S. Lane, and J.
Sorensen
1993   *The Public Health Impact of Needle Exchange Programs in the United States and
         Abroad, Volume 1*. San Francisco, CA: University of California.
National Research Council and Institute of Medicine
1994   *Proceedings, Workshop on Needle Exchange and Bleach Distribution Programs*.
         Washington, DC: National Academy Press.
Newcomb, M.D., and P.M. Bentler
1990   Antecedents and consequences of cocaine use: An eight-year study from early
         adolescence to young adulthood. Pp. 158-181 in L. Robins, ed., *Straight and
         Devious Pathways from Childhood to Adulthood*. Cambridge, Mass.: Cambridge
         Press.
O'Brien, M.U., J. Murray, F. Cannarozzi, A. Jimenez, W. Johnson, L. Ouellet, and W. Wiebel
1995   Needle Exchange in Chicago: The Demand for Free Needles and Their Effect on
         Injecting Frequency and Needle Use. Draft manuscript.

O'Keefe, E., E. Kaplan, and K. Khoshnood
1991   Preliminary Report: City of New Haven Needle Exchange Program. City of New Haven, July 31.

Oliver, K. S.R. Friedman, H. Maynard, and D.C. Des Jarlais
1991   Behavioral Impact of the Portland Syringe Exchange Program: Some Preliminary Results. Presentation at Third National AIDS Demonstration Research Conference.

Oliver, K., S. Friedman, H. Maynard, D. Des Jarlais, and D. Fleming
1992   Comparison of Behavioral Impacts of Syringe Exchange, and Community Impacts of an Exchange. Abstract PoC 4284 in *Final Program and Abstracts of the VII International Conference on AIDS*, Amsterdam.

Oliver, K., H. Maynard, S.R. Friedman, and D.C. Des Jarlais
1994   Behavioral and community impact of the Portland syringe exchange program. Pp. 35-46 in *Proceedings, Workshop on Needle Exchange and Bleach Distribution Programs*. National Research Council and Institute of Medicine. Washington, DC: National Academy Press.

Paone, D., D.C. Des Jarlais, S. Caloir, and P. Friedmann
1993   AIDS Risk Reduction Behaviors Among Participants of Syringe Exchange Programs in New York City, USA. Abstract PO-C24-3188 in *Final Program and Abstracts of the IX International Conference on AIDS*, Berlin.

Paone, D., D.C. Des Jarlais, S. Caloir, P. Friedmann, I. Ness, and S.R. Friedman
1994a   New York City syringe exchange: An overview. Pp. 47-63 in *Proceedings, Workshop on Needle Exchange and Bleach Distribution Programs*. National Research Council and Institute of Medicine. Washington, DC: National Academy Press.

Paone, D., D.C. Des Jarlais, S. Caloir, B. Jose, and S.R. Friedman
1994b   New York City Syringe Exchange: Expansion, Risk Reduction, and Seroincidence. Abstract for Tenth International Conference on AIDS and STD, Yokohama, Japan, August 7-12.

Paton, S., R.C. Kessler, and D.B. Kandel
1977   Depressive mood and illegal drug use: A longitudinal analysis. *Journal of Genetic Psychology* 131:267-289.

Rothman, K.
1986   *Modern Epidemiology*. Boston, MA: Little, Brown and Company.

Schreier, L.M., and M.D. Newcomb
1991   Psychological predictors of drug use initiation and escalation: An expansion of the multiple risk factors hypothesis using longitudinal data. *Contemporary Drug Problems* 18:31-37.

Schutz, C.G., D. Vlahov, J.C. Anthony, and N.M. Graham
1994   Comparison of self-reported injection frequencies for past 30 days and 6 months among intravenous drug users. *Journal of Clinical Epidemiology* 47(2):191-195.

Schwartzkoff, J.
1989   *Evaluation of the New South Wales Needle and Syringe Exchange Program*. Department of Health. November.

Stimson, G.V., L.J. Aldritt, K.A. Dolan, M.C. Donoghoe, and R.A. Lart
1988   *Injecting Equipment Exchange Schemes: Final Report*. The Centre for Research on Drugs and Health Behaviours.

Stimson, G., M. Donoghoe, and K. Dolan
1989   Changes in HIV Risk Behavior in Drug Injectors Attending Syringe-Exchange Projects in England and Scotland. Abstract WAP 108 in *Final Program and Abstracts of the V International Conference on AIDS*, Montréal.

Stimson, G.V., J. Keene, N. Parry-Langdon, and S. Jones
    1991   Evaluation of the Syringe Exchange Programme in Wales, 1990-91: Final Report
            to Welsh Office. Centre for Research on Drugs and Health Behaviour. December.
U.S. General Accounting Office
    1993   Needle Exchange Programs: Research Suggests Promise as an AIDS Prevention
            Strategy. (GAO/HRD-93-60). Washington, DC: U.S. Government Printing Of-
            fice.
van Ameijden, E.J.C., J.A.R. van den Hoek, and R.A. Coutinho
    1993   A Major Decline in Risk Behavior Over 6 Years Among IDUs. Abstract WS-C21-
            2 in Final Program and Abstracts of the IX International Conference on AIDS,
            Berlin.
van Ameijden, E.J.C., J.A.R. van den Hoek, C. Hartgers, and R.A. Coutinho
    1994   Risk factors for the transition from noninjection to injection drug use and accom-
            panying AIDS risk behavior in a cohort of drug users. American Journal of
            Epidemiology 139:1153-1163.
Watters, J.K.
    1994   Trends in risk behavior and HIV seroprevalence in heterosexual injection drug
            users in San Francisco, 1986-1992. Journal of Acquired Immune Deficiency Syn-
            dromes 7:1276-1281.
Watters, J., and Y. Cheng
    1991   Syringe Exchange in San Francisco: Preliminary Findings. Abstract ThC 99 in
            Final Program and Abstracts of the VII International Conference on AIDS, Flo-
            rence.
Watters, J.K., M.J. Estilo, G.L. Clark, and J. Lorvick
    1994   Syringe and needle exchange as HIV/AIDS prevention for injection drug users.
            Journal of the American Medical Association 271(2):115-120.

8

Directions for Future Research

As this report demonstrates, needle exchange programs have been shown to have the ability to retard the spread of HIV infection among the injection drug users who participate in them. It is also true that bleach distribution programs offer promise of being useful in a similar way. Improving the effectiveness of HIV and AIDS prevention programs such as needle exchange and bleach distribution programs is an important and valid public health goal. Such improvement would be much easier to accomplish if the knowledge base were broader and more secure.

On the basis of our review of the epidemiologic data, program characteristics, community views, legal constraints, and the impact of the programs on an array of outcomes (both positive and negative), the panel notes that there is substantial room to expand and improve the current state of knowledge. Several areas must be explored further to enhance understanding of the dynamic process of managing the myriad aspects of the HIV epidemic in the United States and limiting the imminent danger it poses for the public health. In this chapter we briefly discuss some of the most salient areas in which further study has the potential to more effectively limit the spread of this deadly infectious viral agent. We note, however, that our intent is not to set priorities for the funding of needed research, but rather to point out research issues that need to be addressed to enhance the current knowledge base.

RESEARCH ON PROGRAM EFFECTIVENESS

Needle Exchange Evaluation

As illustrated by the literature reviewed in Chapter 7, previous evaluation studies have provided valuable insights into issues to be considered for future research endeavors. Such issues include (but are not limited to): categorization of exposure to the intervention condition (ever/never, secondary exchangers); measurement of alternative sources of sterile syringes other than needle exchange programs (e.g., pharmacies, diabetics); opportunistic comparison groups; eligibility requirements; temporal associations of participation program and HIV seroconversion; accounting for alternative modes of HIV transmission; and consolidation and coordination of program effects. A discussion of these issues follows.

Categorization of Exposure to Intervention Condition

Many studies have simply compared "ever" versus "never used" a needle exchange, with no provisions to allow the researcher to distinguish between different intensity (or frequency) of program exposure across participants. This creates a problem because most needle exchange reports to date identify a substantial proportion of needle exchange participants who have used the program only once. To consider the single-time users similar to frequent users, but different from never users, dilutes any potential effect due to program participation. At a minimum, analyses of the effects of needle exchange program use should stratify by the frequency with which the program is used, to allow for an assessment of a dose response.

At the other extreme, a small proportion (e.g., <25 percent) of program participants have been known to exchange extraordinarily large numbers of needles (e.g., in Tacoma, Chicago, and San Francisco), unlike the single-time users who are not interested in continuing participation for undetermined reasons. Regular low or moderate users who are engaged in personal risk reduction are unlike the high-frequency users who exchange large numbers and are likely to be *secondary exchangers*. This phenomenon raises serious concerns about the common practice of using *means* as a summary statistic in the analyses of program effect. Employing this method equates all exchangers and may lead to masking trends in subgroups. Therefore, it is important to delineate subgroups and define risks accordingly.

The role of secondary exchangers is controversial because a small portion of exchange users obtains a large portion of syringes distributed by the programs. The number of syringes exchanged by these participants typically exceeds the number of syringes that would be used by a single individual. Although this could lead to individuals making money to support their drug habit, it also could facilitate the much wider dissemination of sterile syringes, particularly in areas in which limited program hours allow only a small number of injection drug users to be served directly by the program. More research on secondary exchange is warranted.

Measurement of Alternative Sources of Sterile Syringes

To properly measure sources of sterile syringes, asking injection drug users only if they use or do not use the needle exchange program is insufficient. Other extant sources of sterile syringes can impact enrollment and measurement of outcomes from the program.

Prior studies in Baltimore (Gleghorn, in press) show that about half of injection drug users had sterile sources of needles *prior* to the opening of the needle exchange program, which were primarily from diabetics and pharmacies in a city with a paraphernalia—but *no prescription*—law. If needle exchange programs differentially attract people with nonsterile street sources but not those who already have sources of sterile needles, then, when comparing participants and nonparticipants, an evaluation study might show no relative reduction in HIV incidence resulting from program participation. This may partially explain the lack of significant findings in the Amsterdam case-control study (in which nonparticipants had access to unrestricted pharmacy sales) and appears to contribute, in part, to the findings of the Montréal needle exchange program (see Appendix A). Evaluations of needle exchange programs should collect and analyze information about sources of needles and syringes for all study participants, regardless of their program participation status.

Community-Based Studies

Some studies to date have collected data from programs on needle exchange participants and then sought data on a group of nonparticipants to generate comparisons. However, the different settings in which data are collected are likely to raise concerns about differential bias of interviewers and recall among participants.

The panel recommends the use of *prospective* community-based studies of injection drug users—independent of the operation of needle exchange programs—while gathering information on program use. Comparison groups of nonparticipants might nevertheless have contact with program users and even obtain needles from the program, although they are not directly enrolled. Therefore, information on contacts with persons who use needle exchange programs and are the recipients of secondary exchange should be collected and incorporated into the analysis.

Appropriate Selection of Respondents

Studies that follow injection drug users over time should not restrict themselves to only the highest-risk users. Although this strategy would seem to efficiently select persons at highest risk of seroconversion and thereby make evaluations statistically efficient, a drawback of this strategy is that such selection may be subject to effects of *regression to the mean* (i.e., the highest-risk persons have nowhere to go except down in terms of behavioral and HIV risk). Analyses of offsetting trends using person-time analysis, which uses time intervals rather than individuals as units of analysis, can mask these offsetting trends; they should be maintained in analysis to consider these possible effects.

Temporal Association of Participation in Programs and HIV Seroconversion

The incubation period for HIV seroconversion is generally within 2 weeks to 3 months. Within prospective epidemiologic studies, the date of seroconversion is generally calculated as the midpoint between the last seronegative and the first seropositive serological test visit. This estimation procedure creates a window of uncertainty that needs to be carefully considered in evaluation studies (see Appendix A). Specifically, if an injection drug user is a recent enrollee in a needle exchange program and seroconverts within the next several months, it will be difficult to determine whether the seroconversion can be ascribed to activities engaged in prior or subsequent to use of the exchange program. Particular care needs to be exercised in establishment of inferences related to individuals who seroconvert soon after enrollment in a needle exchange program.

Accounting for Alternative Risk Behaviors

Needle exchange and bleach distribution programs are intended to reduce the risk of HIV and other blood-borne infections due to sharing of contaminated syringes. However, the use of sterile needles and bleach disinfection alone does not have an impact on risks from indirect sharing (e.g., sharing cookers) or sexual risk behaviors. As noted in Chapter 1, *sexual transmission is not uncommon among injection drug users*. Unless significant efforts to determine the risk associated with indirect sharing and more efficient sexual risk reduction strategies are developed within the context of such programs, the effect of needle exchange programs on HIV incidence is likely to be somewhat limited.

The needle exchange research community should bear in mind that there are multiple routes of transmission, each with multiple transmission mechanisms, and that direct needle sharing constitutes only one of many potential sources of transmission. Unless needle exchange programs consistently provide a full range of sterile equipment and adequate education regarding these risky behaviors, it is likely that some transmission stemming from these other practices will continue. To date, no studies to quantify the risk associated with these other behaviors in relation to direct needle sharing are available.

In short, the effect of needle exchange on HIV incidence is likely to be confounded with other sources and modes of transmission. At best, these considerations point to the need for needle exchange programs to institute multidimensional approaches to prevention and not simply rely on distribution and exchange of needles. Providing sterile needles and syringes is necessary but insufficient to adequately address the problem of HIV transmission. Therefore, the relative effects of different components of needle exchange programs that target different risk behaviors associated with the different transmission routes (sexual risk versus sharing of contaminated injection equipment) need to be studied.

Consolidation and Coordination of Program Effects

What is learned about program effectiveness at one site may be of value at another; sharing and consolidating information increases its value. It is also essential to develop standard terms and a common format for record-keeping, as a way to ensure consistency in the collection of data from different programs at different sites. Consistency in data collection makes it possible to supply program operators and evaluators with more valid feedback about program effectiveness: what works in Denver may not work in Miami, but, without consistent information, it may not be possible to analyze the results of program evaluations across sites.

In funding considerations, coordination is also essential. The efficiency of needle exchange and bleach distribution programs would benefit from some centrally supplied funding and some central coordination of what could be a primarily collaborative enterprise. This could make provision for more reliable and swift learning from the experiences of programs already in operation.

Program Characteristics

Most evaluation research to date has focused on program effectiveness in isolation. Needle exchange and bleach distribution programs vary considerably in their characteristics (as noted in Chapter 3) and their effectiveness. Their success depends in part on the choices they make in setting their hours of operation, their location(s), their eligibility rules, and their exchange policies. Some programs insist on one-for-one exchange, and others do not. Some programs limit the number of needles that may be exchanged at one time, and others do not. Each of these policies has pros and cons, but we know too little about them, in terms of what balance is optimal in maximizing gains, minimizing harm, and contributing to the ultimate goal of the program—prevention of HIV transmission.

Also, as Chapter 2 describes in detail, the aims of needle exchange and bleach distribution programs are broader than simply providing sterile needles to injection drug users. Other goals include linking users to needed health care and social services, providing drug abuse counseling, and facilitating entry into drug treatment. Research on how to improve these ancillary services is virtually nonexistent and should be pursued. The most effective ways to pursue these goals presumably depends in part on the characteristics of the participants, such as age, ethnicity, education, drug-using career, and socioeconomic status.

Identification of program characteristics that enhance or inhibit effectiveness is needed. The limited available research on the organizational characteristics of needle exchange programs and case studies presented in Chapter 3 hints at specific operational characteristics that may facilitate program effectiveness—for example, user-friendliness (see Stimson et al., 1988).

Evaluation research in this area of study would also benefit from adopting programmatic research strategies that acknowledge the need for feeding back information to program administrators to allow rational modification of procedures and operational characteristics. This type of iterative research process attempts to identify optimal procedures for maximizing the overall effectiveness of programs or identifying problematic components resistant to effectiveness modification. Quality assurance programs are witness to the value of systematic internal research with feedback as a method for improving the operations of almost any kind of organization.

In addition to examining the relative effects of different operational characteristics of programs (such as staffing, location, hours of operation, program policies) and various combinations of ancillary services on traditional outcomes (e.g., risk behaviors, infection rates)—more attention must be given to understanding how these characteristics may also impact the recruitment and retention of program participants.

The relationships between program characteristics and success at both the individual and the community levels should be examined. For example, it may be possible for a needle exchange program to be effective when limited to a small number of injection drug users, yet it may show no noticeable effect on either risk behaviors or HIV infection rates among the broader local population of injection drug users. By the same token, programs that reach larger populations may show a more modest effect among participants, but also show that the effect extends into the broader community. Studies are needed to determine the relative effectiveness of programs that concentrate on intensively serving a limited client base versus those serving a broad population and providing fewer services.

An issue related to the policy of setting limits on the number of syringes provided to individual participants per visit was raised earlier in this report. The potential effects of such program policies need to be further researched. Enforcing limits may discourage unintended consequences (e.g., individuals selling the needles they obtain); however, it could discourage participation because it may be inconvenient from the viewpoint of program participants (especially if participants have to travel a distance to reach the exchange). Specifically, research in this area should address questions such as: What are the relative benefits and risks associated with program policies related to the number of needles distributed? What are the potential benefits (e.g., broader diffusion of sterile equipment, reduced sharing) and harms (e.g., source of income for participants that may impact severity of drug addiction) that are related to other environmental and personal characteristics of program participants?

Differential effectiveness of these programs across racial/ethnic, age, and gender populations must be further explored. Little is currently known about the relative effectiveness of these programs across population subgroups. In addition to research on the demographic characteristics, more research needs to be done to better understand how programs can have the most impact while taking into account the risk behaviors of program participants (i.e., drug use, sexual risks), both across and within programs. For example, the severity of drug addiction may be more pronounced in certain programs or within subsets of program participants, reflecting different risks that should be considered by program operations. Such research (e.g., development of needs assessment methods) could assist program operators in establishing the most effective combination of ancillary services particular to specific situations.

The panel's review revealed that little is known about the effects of these programs on the level of illicit drug use in the community at large. Research indicates that the programs do not affect the level of drug use of their participants and do not appear to recruit new drug abusers to injection drug use. But results in this country necessarily relate to a relatively short time horizon. In principle, findings on a time scale of, say, a decade might be different. Here, then, are questions calling for research.

Another unexplored area of research concerns the potential adverse effects these programs may have on certain risk behaviors of program participants (e.g., severity of drug use and sexually transmitted diseases). Do they inadvertently generate new social networks of drug users, which then may serve as a mechanism to facilitate viral spread, depending on the risk characteristics—drug and sexual—of the new social network and the seroprevalence background level of infection of new groups? Similar concerns were raised when methadone maintenance treatment programs were first introduced. Understanding these interactions across social networks is crucial to developing a better perspective on the changing patterns of risks and the progression of the HIV epidemic.

RESEARCH ON BLEACH EFFICACY IN DISINFECTION

In addition to the issues listed above regarding needle exchange programs that are also relevant to evaluation studies of bleach distribution programs, there are others specific to bleach distribution programs.

Although limited in some ways (see Chapter 6), laboratory studies have shown that bleach is an effective disinfection agent for HIV-contaminated materials. Yet current epidemiologic studies have revealed that bleach disinfection, as currently practiced by injection drug users, does not appear to have a protective effect. It is therefore crucial that educational methods be developed to improve the level of compliance by injection drug users with the recommended disinfection protocol.

Laboratory studies are needed that carefully characterize the efficacy of bleach disinfection of needles and syringes under conditions that mimic field or actual use situations, accounting for bioburden and minimum effective contact times. These efforts should identify the optimal procedure while incorporating bioburden/consistency of use/contact time characteristics. Although some data are available, the panel noted limitations in current methods to assess efficacy (see Chapter 6).

In terms of recommended field procedures, studies are needed to determine if injection drug users can perform, and under what circumstances are willing/or not to perform, the multistep procedures that are recommended (e.g., ethnographic research). If current procedures are too complex or unacceptable to injection drug users, then research is needed to identify safe and effective procedures that can be performed by them. Moreover, effective educational strategies are urgently needed. Information on the diffusion of education intervention effects over time and the possible benefit of booster sessions to ensure sustained beneficial effects needs to be further studied. In addition, effective modes of disseminating bleach information to injection drug users need to be further explored (e.g., relative effectiveness of media, outreach).

EPIDEMIOLOGIC RESEARCH

The HIV and AIDS epidemiologic data clearly document the critical role of injection drug use in the current and future course of the HIV epidemic in this country. Our review of HIV infection rates among population subgroups of injection drug users (Chapter 1) indicates wide variation in geographic distribution of HIV infection. Likewise, there is considerable geographic diversity in patterns of injection drug use (e.g., drug used, frequency of injection) (see Chapter 2). The risk of transmission in a population depends on the reservoir of infection (as measured by HIV and other blood-borne pathogen seroprevalence) and the levels of risk behaviors that transmit infection. As these two parameters evolve, so does the epidemic. In order to minimize the occurrence of new infections, ongoing monitoring systems of HIV seroprevalence, seroincidence, and levels of risk behaviors can help guide interventions aimed at curbing new infections. The documented connection between injection drug use and AIDS points to the need to better understand the underlying dynamics of sexual/drug-use behaviors of high-risk groups, and how these networks are linked to other social networks within the intravenous drug user populations. Such an understanding could benefit from the development of theoretical research and alternative methodologies for studying such sensitive topic areas as drug-use and sexual behavior. To better achieve this goal, future research should include the following:

• Ongoing coordinated studies are needed of the seroprevalence and seroincidence of HIV, HBV (hepatitis B virus), and HCV (hepatitis C virus) among local populations of injection drug users, using standardized methodologies across locations.

• Extensive and repeated surveys of seropositivity rates are needed to determine the incidence and prevalence of infection by age, race/ethnicity, geographic area, and sex. Such studies should be performed locally with standardized protocols developed to ensure comparability of the collected data.

• Improved estimation procedures (including enhanced surveillance systems, modeling techniques, and ethnographic methods) should be developed for obtaining more accurate and time-relevant estimates of the number of drug users by city/county rather than attempting to obtain accurate national estimates. Detailed surveys that allow better characterization of specific drug-use behaviors and dynamics of drug-use patterns are needed. This will enable better-targeted prevention efforts.

• Developing a typology/demography of HIV infection that identifies high-risk groups in terms of prevalence and incidence and of risk behaviors is necessary to prevent the creation of potential epicenters. Attention should also be given to identifying subgroups or clusters within the broader defined risk groups—e.g., whether there are identifiable groups at relatively different levels of risk within the population of local injection drug users. Delineating the characteristics of these subgroups of injection drug users along such characteristics as the disparities in risk behaviors and/or patterns of risk behaviors would greatly assist targeting and tailoring prevention interventions.

• Regular, geographically detailed information about the prevalence of HIV (and, as useful surrogates, hepatitis B and C) could help guide priorities in mounting public health initiatives.

• Improved measurements of injection drug use and sexual risk behaviors are needed. Such measures should include information on: (1) patterns of drug use (e.g., drug type, route of administration, frequency of use, source of needles, patterns of reuse of needles); (2) direct and indirect sharing behavior; (3) patterns of sexual contacts (e.g., heterosexual, homosexual, frequency, number of patterns) and activities (e.g., receptive anal sex); (4) sexually transmitted diseases; and (5) drug and sexual social networks.

• Better understanding of certain biological and social parameters is needed, including the relative efficiency of different transmission routes, the kinetics, and the relative efficiency of known transmission routes (i.e., direct and indirect sharing).

• There is an urgent need to identify the key determinants of illicit drug injection at both the individual and the community levels. In particular, it is important to conduct etiologic studies of the transition from noninjection to injection drug use.

• Most individuals who inject illicit drugs begin this behavior in late adolescence or early adulthood (Gerstein and Green, 1993; Newcomb and Bentler, 1988; Chen and Kandel, 1995). Moreover, as mentioned in Chapter 2, a substantial number of those who reported having injected a drug in the past year were between the ages of 12 and 25. Chapter 3 also shows that needle exchange programs do not recruit a sizable number of young injectors. This highlights the need for recruiting study cohorts of younger individuals as part of ongoing efforts to further our understanding of injection drug use and improve AIDS prevention strategies. This is especially urgent because some studies have shown that seroconversion typically occurs during the early stages of injection drug use after initiation has occurred (Nicolosi et al., 1992; Moss et al., 1994; Nelson et al., in press).

RESEARCH ON COMMUNITY ISSUES

Chapter 4 of this report highlighted the severity of the drug abuse problem in our society. Injection drug use ruins the lives of users and of those close to them. HIV and AIDS have only worsened the situation. Coping with these public health problems is *much* more likely to succeed if we fully understand them. Moreover, critical to the effective implementation of HIV and AIDS preventive interventions is a better understanding of local community concerns.

• More systematic research is needed on other ethnic groups who are known to be at high risk of infection (e.g., Puerto Ricans in New York City). This panel recognized its own limitations in attempting to address the issues and concerns of the multitude of communities that are summarized simply as Hispanic/Latino. More detailed investigation and response are needed.

• Although some pharmacists, law enforcement officers, and treatment service providers have been supportive of needle exchange programs, others have expressed concerns and reservations about their potential role in making sterile injection equipment more readily available to injection drug users. A better understanding of the beliefs, attitudes, values, and motivational factors that influence these reservations needs to be developed through both qualitative and quantitative research efforts.

OTHER FUTURE RESEARCH ISSUES

Deregulation of Syringe Sale and Possession

Within the context of deregulation of pharmacy sales and possession of needles, important issues warrant further research. For example, the practice of sharing needles and syringes continues in industrialized countries other than the United States. Some of these countries have needle exchange programs and no paraphernalia or prescription laws limiting the availability of sterile injection equipment. These circumstances lead the panel to suggest that:

• Researchers need to identify the causal agents involved in sharing after legal constraints are removed. Ethnographic research should identify why needles and syringes continue to be shared when community availability is no longer a constraint (see Chapter 5, time of injection versus community availability issues).

• In terms of the deregulation of syringe sale and possession (allowing injection drug users to purchase syringes in pharmacies), one important concern that requires immediate attention is that of developing efficient disposal methods for used needles and syringes. Pharmacies, with numerous locations and hours of operation, are convenient and accessible for obtaining syringes. However, the issue of appropriate needle and syringe disposal needs further consideration and planning.

Incarcerated Populations

Members of highly vulnerable populations, such as injection drug users, are known to frequently come in contact with various social institutions. These include public medical facilities, such as drug treatment facilities, clinics for treating sexually transmitted diseases, emergency rooms, and correction facilities. For example, more injection drug users can be found in prisons than in drug treatment programs, hospitals, and social services (Brewer and Derrickson, 1992). It is plausible that preimprisonment drug-use behavior among incarcerated injection drug users will be more heterogeneous than that of users in treatment facilities or needle exchange programs (Vlahov and Polk, 1988). Moreover, Siegal et al. (1994), in a study that examined the relationship between level of HIV risk behavior and history of exposure to jail or prison, report that active injection drug users with the highest HIV risk behaviors were those most likely to spend time in jail. These findings, combined with the fact that more than 4 million people are incarcerated annually in the United States, argue for devoting more prevention research efforts to this subpopulation of injection drug users.

Randomized Trial of Needle Exchange Programs

The emphasis of this chapter has been on identifying research issues that need to be vigorously pursued in order to improve the current knowledge base. In addition, we feel that the issue of randomized trials of needle exchange programs should be addressed, because some researchers have argued for their implementation to adequately answer issues concerning the effectiveness of such programs.

As was stressed in a previous National Research Council evaluation report on AIDS (Coyle et al., 1991), the randomized experiment might be the ideal scheme to adopt when attempting to assess the effect of AIDS prevention strategies. That report acknowledged, however, that because of practical constraints (e.g., complying with true random assignments of individuals or communities, inability to provide "blinding" of behavioral interventions, treatment attrition, cost), one may choose to focus instead on well-conceived observational epidemiologic designs. These practical constraints are severe in the case of needle exchange and bleach distribution programs.

The more important problems associated with randomized trials (i.e., randomized field experiments) are practical. There are currently over 55 cities in the United States that have implemented needle exchange programs. This places serious constraints on finding comparable communities that do not have needle exchange programs and would be willing to be randomized. Moreover, given the sensitive nature of these programs (in contrast with smoking cessation programs, for example), many volunteer communities may not be capable of initiating proper legislative change (of paraphernalia and prescription laws) to legally allow such programs to take place. Furthermore, given the results of the two recent government-sponsored reports that have concluded that these programs have positive effects and do not appear to have negative impacts (U.S. General Accounting Office, 1993; Lurie et al., 1993), it may not be ethical to withhold treatment from communities willing to initiate such programs. Problems may also arise because communities eager to participate may proceed with program implementation after having been informed that they have been assigned to the control condition.

In addition, one major concern with these designs in prevention research is differential attrition rates across conditions. As Booth and Watters (1994) point out in their review of risk reduction interventions, participation in the treatment condition is more demanding than in the control condition, which typically leads to experimental attrition.

Cost is a factor, particularly when treatments are randomized across large units, such as cities or communities, rather than across individuals. Only a small number of units may be assigned to conditions. Yet the strength of randomization depends on the random assignment of a sufficiently large number of units to substantially weaken the possibility that confounding factors would coincidentally vary with the random assignment. When only a small number of units are randomly assigned to conditions, given the low probability that the treatment and control conditions will be equivalent on unmeasured factors, sensitivity is necessarily reduced.

• The panel recommends adopting strong observational epidemiologic designs (i.e., prospective and case-control studies) rather than attempting to conduct large-scale randomized experiments to evaluate needle exchange and bleach distribution programs.

BROADER ISSUES

To better understand the workings of needle exchange and bleach distribution programs and how to render them more effective, we need a deeper understanding of many phenomena that are not specific to needle exchange and bleach distribution programs but are more general in scope. For example, we need to know about the processes of addiction, about the propagation of infectious diseases, about the dynamics of social networks, about the underlying factors in personal failure and success, and about the role of sexual behaviors in the lives of injection drug users.

• Motivation and attitude are central to behaviors that are implicated in the spread of HIV infection: intravenous drug use and unprotected sex. It would be particularly valuable to explore how the underlying attitudes and motivations can be modified.

• Social networks, especially among injection drug users, appear to exert large effects on recruitment to, and attrition from, needle exchange and bleach distribution programs. They are also implicated in needle-sharing behavior. Research in this area would contribute to better understanding of how social networks affect program participation (and nonparticipation).

CONCLUSION

The HIV epidemic in the United States is growing largely because of infection spread by contaminated needles in the population of injection drug users. Needle exchange and bleach distribution programs can help to retard this spread. And, to the extent that these programs can be made to be more effective, their retardant effect will be greater. To improve the effectiveness of needle exchange and bleach distribution programs calls for additional research, including arrangements for collecting findings across sites and coordinating studies at various locations. Good, up-to-date local measures of seroprevalence, not only of HIV but also of HBV and HCV, would help greatly to target program efforts and resources.

Finally, to make a difference, resources must flow to these research tasks. An infusion of funds, personnel, and training would all yield important returns. To live now with this epidemic without knowledgeably combating it would be shortsighted. In the long-term control of HIV and AIDS, the kinds of research we propose would be thoroughly worthwhile.

REFERENCES

Booth, R.E., and J.K. Watters
    1994   How effective are risk-reduction interventions targeting injecting drug users? [edi-
            torial]. *AIDS* 8(11):1515-1524.
Brewer, T.F., and J. Derrickson
    1992   AIDS in prison: A review of epidemiology and preventive policy [editorial].
            AIDS 6(7):623-628.
Chen, K., and D.B. Kandel
    1995   The natural history of drug use from adolescence to the mid-thirties in a general
            population sample [comment]. *American Journal of Public Health* 85(1):41-47.
Coyle, S.L., R.F. Boruch, and C.F. Turner, eds.
    1991   *Evaluating AIDS Prevention Programs: Expanded Edition.* Panel on the Evalua-
            tion of AIDS Interventions. Washington, DC: National Academy Press.
Gerstein, D.R., and L.W. Green, eds.
    1993   *Preventing Drug Abuse: What Do We Know?* Committee on Drug Abuse Preven-

tion Research, National Research Council. Washington, DC: National Academy Press.

Gerstein, D.R., and H.J. Harwood, eds.
1992   *Treating Drug Problems: Volume 1.* Committee for the Substance Abuse Coverage Study. Washington, DC: National Academy Press.

Gleghorn, A., T.S. Jones, M. Doherty, D. Celentano, and D. Vlahov
in press   Acquisition and use of needles and syringes by injecting drug users in Baltimore, Maryland. *Journal of Acquired Immune Deficiency Syndromes.*

Lurie, P., A.L. Reingold, B. Bowser, D. Chen, J. Foley, J. Guydish, J.G. Kahn, S. Land, and J. Sorensen
1993   *The Public Health Impact of Needle Exchange Programs in the United States and Abroad, Vol. 1.* San Francisco, CA: University of California.

Moss, A.R., K. Vranizan, R. Gorter, et al.
1994   HIV seroconversion in intravenous drug users in San Francisco, 1985-1990. *AIDS 1994* 8:223-231.

Nelson, K.E., D. Vlahov, L. Solomon, S. Cohn, and A. Muñoz
in press   Temporal trends of incident HIV infection in a cohort of injection drug users in Baltimore, Maryland. *Annals of Internal Medicine.*

Newcomb, M.D., and P.M. Bentler
1988   Impact of adolescent drug use and social support on problems of young adults: A longitudinal study. *Journal of Abnormal Psychology* 97(1):64-75.

Nicolosi, A., M.L.C. Leite, S. Molinari, et al.
1992   Incidence and prevalence trends of HIV infection in intravenous drug users attending treatment centers in Milan and Northern Italy, 1986-1990. *Journal of Acquired Immune Deficiency Syndromes* 5:365-373.

Siegal, H.A., M.A. Forney, R.G. Carlson, and D.C. McBride
1994   Incarceration and HIV risk behaviors among injection drug users: A Midwestern study. *Journal of Crime and Justice* XVI(1):85-101.

Stimson, G.V., L.J. Aldritt, K.A. Dolan, M.S. Donoghoe, and R.A. Lart
1988   *Injecting Equipment Exchange Schemes. Final Report.* London: Monitoring Research Group, Goldsmith's College.

U.S. General Accounting Office
1993   *Needle Exchange Programs: Research Suggests Promise as an AIDS Prevention Strategy.* Washington, DC: U.S. Government Printing Office.

Vlahov, D., and R.S. Brookmeyer
1994   The evaluation of needle exchange programs [editorial]. *American Journal of Public Health* 84(12):1889-1891.

Vlahov, D., and B.F. Polk
1988   Intravenous drug users and human immunodeficiency virus infection in prison. *AIDS Public Policy Journal* 3:42-46.

Appendixes

A
Description and Review of Research Projects in Three Cities

As the panel was completing its review of available research on needle exchange and bleach distribution programs and related issues, the Assistant Secretary for Health made public statements that a number of unpublished needle exchange evaluation reports had raised doubts in his mind about the effectiveness of these programs. The panel deemed these statements to be significant in the public debate, therefore necessitating appropriate consideration in order for the panel to be fully responsive to its charge. We therefore reviewed the unpublished studies—by investigators in San Francisco, Montréal, and Chicago—that had raised concerns. As unpublished findings, these studies lack the authority provided by the peer review and publication process. They have been considered, however, in the panel's presentation of its approach to the pattern of evidence on the effectiveness of needle exchange programs, which is discussed in Chapter 7. This appendix describes the individual studies and provides the panel's detailed review of the reported findings.

SAN FRANCISCO

The investigators (Hahn et al., 1995) collected data on demographic, sexual, and drug-use risk behaviors, treatment experience, living arrangements, HIV status, needle exchange participation, and number of needles exchanged through a structured interview in order to "examine use of the needle exchange program in San Francisco in the first two years after its commencement" (p. 1). The information on "needle exchange use" reported by study participants allowed these researchers to examine predictors of needle exchange participation and to estimate HIV seroconversion rates among needle exchange users and nonusers. According to these authors, this information allowed them to "assess whether the San Francisco needle exchanges are reaching their intended clientele and whether the exchanges affect risk reduction and HIV incidence" (p. 3).

This study recruited 1,093 injection drug users from nine methadone maintenance and 21-day detoxification programs from 1989 through 1990, following the November 1988 opening of the Prevention Point needle exchange program in San Francisco. Each participant completed structured interviews (questionnaire) and had an HIV test performed at each repeat visit. Of those recruited, repeated questionnaire data and serostatus test results were available from 412 participants (38 percent). Needle exchange participation was determined by examining participants' questionnaire responses (needle exchange participation items) for their most recent treatment visit (methadone maintenance, 21-day detoxification, or both).

Descriptive analyses based on the entire sample of 1,093 study participants showed that males, frequent injectors, homeless people, residents of hotels and shelters, homosexuals and bisexuals, and participants who were aware of their HIV status were more likely to use the needle exchange. No association was detected between needle exchange use and the education level of study participants, the age of first injection, the number of years injecting, bleach use, or prostitution.

During the 1989 through 1990 study period, nine seroconversions were detected among the 412 repeaters who were initially assessed as HIV negative. The time at risk for study participants who remained HIV negative was years from first interview to last interview, whereas the time at risk measure for those who seroconverted was years from first interview to first HIV-positive interview. This resulted in an estimated overall seroconversion rate of 1.1 per 100 person years (95 percent confidence interval [CI]: 0.5 to 2.0 percent per person years) among the 412 repeaters. The estimated seroconversion rates for those who had *never used the needle exchange* was 0.33 percent per person years (95 percent CI: 0.05 to 1.02 percent per person years) compared with an estimated rate of 3.49 percent per person years (95 percent CI: 1.49 to 6.75 percent per person years) for those who had *ever used needle exchange*. More specific estimates of seroconversion rates among needle exchange users were derived for those study participants who had used the needle exchange for fewer than 3 months (6.26 percent per person years) and for those who had used the needle exchange for 3 months or more (2.19 percent per person years).

Results of a proportional hazard model indicated that, among the 412 repeat study participants, the hazards ratio for seroconverting was higher for those who had used the needle exchange (10.60; 95 percent CI: 2.20 to 51.06) compared with those who had not.

Finally, in an attempt to control for potential selection bias due to the self-selection of the 412 repeaters, standardized seroconversion rates accounting for differences in age, sex, race, and participation in methadone maintenance between repeaters and nonrepeaters were derived. The estimated standardized rates were found to be 1.12 percent per person years for the entire group, 0.51 percent per person years for those who had never used needle exchange, and 2.97 percent per person years for those who had ever used the needle exchange.

These findings were interpreted by the authors as indicating that needle exchange programs attract a high-risk, chaotic, and indigent population of injection drug users. The authors conclude that needle exchange programs are well suited for implementing HIV preventive interventions, in view of their findings that such programs provide direct access to high-risk injectors. Moreover, the authors state that it is unlikely that the extremely high HIV seroconversion rate among study participants who had ever used the needle exchange compared with participants who had never used the needle exchange, or that the large hazards ratio for seroconversion associated with needle exchange participation, is the result of needle exchange use itself. Several possible explanations are offered by the investigators: (1) most participants had a very brief exposure period to the needle exchange; (2) the highest seroconversion rates were observed in the subgroup with the lowest amount of time exposed to the needle exchange, which is less than 3 months, less than the typical detection window for the HIV antibody; and (3) seroconversion rates were not based on a fixed schedule (i.e., voluntary re-enrollment).

Review

The panel's main concern about this research is the potential misinterpretation of the reported findings. Although the authors do not attribute the observed disparities in seroconversion rates between needle exchange program participants and nonparticipants to exposure to these programs, their readers may misinterpret these study findings as reflecting the causal effect of needle exchange programs on seroconversion. As indicated by one of the investigators, the study design and analytical methods used by the researchers preclude such an assessment (Moss, 1995).

Indeed, for a number of reasons, the existing data are inadequate to assess a needle exchange effect by comparing the seroconversion rates of needle exchange users and nonusers. One possible strategy for attempting to make such an assessment would have been to estimate the seroconversion rate per injection drug user per unit of time at risk while exposed to the needle exchange with the seroconversion rate per injection drug user per unit of time at risk while not exposed to the needle exchange. This would have allowed a direct inferential test of the null hypothesis that the seroconversion rate per unit of time exposed to the needle exchange equals the seroconversion rate per unit of time not exposed to the program. However, the data needed to test such a hypothesis were not available.

Another reason the data are inadequate to draw inferences about needle exchange effects is because needle exchange exposure was measured as weekly, monthly, infrequent, or never, so it is impossible to derive an accurate estimate of time at risk while exposed to the needle exchange. It is likewise difficult or impossible to draw sound inferences from this study about the effects of needle exchange on seroincidence rates because of uncertainties about the times of infection and the times of entry into the needle exchange program. The dates on which several seroconverters were first detected as HIV positive (note that we do not know when they actually seroconverted) were very close to the reported dates of entry into the needle exchange program; therefore, it is uncertain whether these individuals entered the program prior to exposure to the virus or after. This creates serious concerns regarding the quality and accuracy of the reported seroconversion rate estimates. Different methods of imputing these times could lead to substantially different results (Brookmeyer and Gail, 1994).

Another reason for the inadequacy of the data is that the "time at risk" measure for computing the seroconversion rates in this study was operationalized as being the years from first interview to last interview for study participants who remained HIV negative, whereas the time at risk measure for those who seroconverted was equal to the number of years from the first interview to the first HIV-positive interview. Another, more commonly used method for computing time at risk for seroconverters is to use midpoint imputation; that is, to compute the time estimate of infection by averaging the times of the last negative and first positive test results. Estimating in this way would substantially impact the reported seroconversion rates for needle exchange users and nonusers by changing their estimated time of becoming infected. A drastic change in the number of seroconversions occurring among needle exchange user and nonuser subgroups would result: five of the seven seroconversions among needle exchange users would be classified as having occurred prior to their participation in the needle exchange program. This example, taken in consideration with the small number of seroconverters, illustrates why it is impossible to reach any conclusion about seroincidence from this study.

Even if detailed information on needle exchange exposure times and times of infection were available, the tenability of the inferences that could be drawn from such an analysis would be subject to substantial challenges on the basis of sampling biases: bias in the HIV seroconversion rate estimates are bound to be present. First, the sample was decidedly not extracted from the needle exchange user and nonuser populations: the sample was drawn from a treatment population and as a consequence represents, at best, a very select subpopulation group of injection drug users. Second, the sampling strategy adopted appears to have been dependent on client exposure time to treatment, meaning that treatment clients who spent extended periods in methadone treatment or made frequent visits to detoxification programs were more likely to be sampled, again creating a bias.

The panel concurs with the conclusions made by the authors that the observed differences in seroincidence rates across groups cannot be attributed to program participation, given the uncertainty regarding the time of infection and the lack of information concerning the needle exchange participants' intensity (dose) of exposure to the program. Moreover, although there are serious selection bias concerns associated with the reported HIV incidence estimates among program participants and nonparticipants, the San Francisco program does appear to attract individuals who are at high risk of infection, at least among injection drug users who have recently been in contact with treatment services.

MONTRÉAL

The Montréal CACTUS (Centre d'Action Communautaire Auprès des Toxicomanes Utilisateurs de Seringues) needle exchange program opened on July 9, 1989. It is a fixed-site program that operates 7 days a week from 9 p.m. to 4 a.m. In addition to exchanging needles, staff disseminate information on AIDS and the prevention of HIV transmission and distribute condoms, alcohol swabs, lubricants, bottles of bleach, and distilled water. CACTUS practices a policy of one-for-one exchange to a maximum of 15 needles with 1 extra needle per visit. The number of visits to the program stabilized at approximately 1,200 visits per week after 1 year of operation (Hankins et al., 1994).

Two research projects have provided needle exchange participation data on the Montréal program. The first is a formal attempt to evaluate the effect of the needle exchange program on risk behaviors, HIV prevalence, and HIV incidence (Hankins et al., 1992, 1994; Hankins et al., 1993). The second is a prospective epidemiologic study of HIV infection among injection drug users in Montréal that was initiated in 1988, one year prior to the opening of the needle exchange program (Bruneau et al., 1995; Lamothe et al., 1995).

Needle Exchange Evaluation Project

The evaluation study (Hankins et al., 1994) recruited volunteer program participants who were leaving the needle exchange site on one randomly chosen evening per week. Study participants were asked to provide a blood specimen for HIV antibody testing. Serology test results were linked by means of a random bar code identifier to individual demographic and risk behaviors (in the previous 7 days) that were collected at each visit on a questionnaire on service delivery and behavior. Overall, 25 percent of the individuals approached agreed to provide a specimen; the 75 percent of program participants who declined indicated they were in a hurry. Yearly HIV prevalence estimates for the period of January 1990 through January 1993 are presented in Table A.1.

Seroincidence

Repeat test results on the same individuals using the random bar code identifiers were used to identify seroconversions and to estimate seroincidence for the same 3-year period (January 1990 through January 1993). The date of seroconversion was estimated as the midpoint between the last negative and first positive result. Hankins et al. (1993, 1994) reported that during that 3-year period a total of 13 of the 136 repeat participants seroconverted, for an overall incidence rate of 12.9 per 100 person years of observation (95 percent CI: 6.9 to 22.0).

Separate incidence estimates per year are provided in Table A.2. Participants who reported having borrowed or loaned needles in the previous 7 days were found to be substantially more at risk of seroconverting. Seroconversion was not found to be associated with age, sex, cocaine use, condom use, or the sexual orientation of males.

Data from Correctional Institutions

In a separate investigation undertaken to assess the degree of needle exchange program participant awareness, use, and satisfaction, Hankins et al. (1992) recruited injection drug users from three medium-security correctional institutions ($n = 319$) and one drop-in detoxification clinic ($n = 173$) for a brief structured interview (5 to 10 minutes). The sample of incarcerated injection drug users was originally recruited as part of an ongoing

TABLE A.1 HIV Prevalence Among Montréal Needle Exchange Participants

Year	Seropositive	Total	Proportion (%)	95% CI
1990	49	442	11.1	8.4 to 14.4
1991	51	345	14.8	11.3 to 19.0
1992	45	270	16.7	12.4 to 21.7

SOURCE: Adapted from Evaluating Montréal's Needle Exchange CACTUS-Montréal (Hankins et al., 1994:86).

TABLE A.2 HIV Incidence Rate Among the 25 Percent of Needle Exchange Participants Followed (Repeaters)

	1990	1991	1992	Total
Seroconversion	6/111	7/85	0/19	13/136
Percent	(5.4)	(8.2)	(0)	(9.6)
Person days	16,510	16,707	3,588	36,805
Incidence[a]	13.3	15.3	0	12.9
95 percent CI	(4.9 to 28.9)	(6.1 to 31.5)	—	(6.9 to 22.0)

[a]Per 100 person years.

SOURCE: Adapted from Evaluating Montréal's Needle Exchange CACTUS-Montréal (Hankins et al., 1994:89).

research project on risk factors for HIV infection among inmates in medium-security correctional institutions and included HIV antibody testing (Hankins et al., 1994). Results indicate that 73 percent of those interviewed had heard of the needle exchange program; 55 percent of this number had participated and 76 percent of them had used the program more than five times. Attenders expressed a very high level of satisfaction with the personnel (88 percent liked the staff), and 98 percent indicated that they had received the services they had requested.

An analysis of the serology test results shows that the overall HIV prevalence rate among incarcerated injection drug users was 10 percent (29/293). When needle exchange attenders were compared with nonattenders, program participants were found to be twice as likely to be HIV positive (14 and 7 percent, respectively). When the data are stratified by sex, this sizable disparity in HIV prevalence rates was not observed for female inmates; however, the rate was substantially higher for men (Table A.3).

Finally, Hankins and colleagues (1993) have reported meaningful reductions in risk behaviors among needle exchange participants. After the program opened, lending needles declined from 31 to 20 percent, and 62 percent of those who injected with used needles were doing so after having cleaned them with bleach compared with 30 percent in the first 2 months of operation.

Review

As with the San Francisco study, one of the panel's primary concerns with this research is the potential for severe bias in the prevalence and incidence estimates among needle exchange program users and nonusers. Given the nature of the samples studied and the shortfalls in the study

TABLE A.3 HIV Seroprevalence Rates (%) Among Incarcerated Injection Drug Users by Needle Exchange Participation

	Attenders	Non-Attenders	Total
Men	8/39 (20.5)	6/124 (4.8)	14/163 (8.6)
Women	8/69 (11.6)	7/61 (11.5)	15/130 (11.5)
Total	16/108 (14.8)	13/185 (7.0)	29/293 (10.0)

SOURCE: Adapted from Evaluating Montréal's Needle Exchange CACTUS-Montréal (Hankins et al., 1994:90).

design, it would be difficult for researchers to disentangle the potential causal effects of needle exchange programs on the outcome measures studied.

The seroprevalence base rates among needle exchange users reported by Hankins et al. (1994) are based on a 25 percent study participation rate. Clearly, this low participation rate raises concerns about the representativeness of the estimates and their accuracy in reflecting the HIV prevalence of the needle exchange user population. Moreover, the authors state that needle exchange participation stabilized at approximately 1,200 visits per week after the first year of operation. By assuming that a standard recruitment strategy was adopted over the 3 years of data collection, the number of recruited study participants—on which prevalence rates are based—dropped steadily over those 3 years and precipitously during the third year following the program opening (Table A.1). This latter observation further jeopardizes the representativeness of the derived prevalence estimates.

The same potential bias issues are relevant for the incidence rates reported in Table A.2. These are based on even smaller subgroups of those initial study participants who agreed to be tested more than once in a given year. Furthermore, the proportion of the initial base rate groups that were followed up in a given year also dropped substantially in the third year. Of the original 442 study participants in 1990, 25 percent were repeaters (111 of 442); this proportion remained stable in 1991 and dropped to 7 percent (19 of 270) in 1992.

To assess the potential effect of needle exchange participation on HIV prevalence, the investigators relied on data collected from a sample of incarcerated injection drug users who were part of an ongoing research project with another objective: identifying risk factors for HIV infection among inmates. The substantially higher prevalence rate observed among needle exchange program users compared with nonusers (especially for men) is disconcerting. Hankins et al. (1994) also report that incarcerated needle exchange program users were engaging in many more high-risk behaviors— e.g., using needles previously used by an HIV-positive person, receiving income from prostitution—than inmates who did not use the needle exchange program. Because this study examines only seroprevalence rates, neither the timing of the infections nor the temporal link needed to establish the viability of a causal effect for the observed relationship between serostatus and needle exchange program participation (i.e., seroconversion before attending needle exchange) can be determined.

The population sampled also precludes generalizing these findings to the needle exchange user population or to the total population of injection drug users in Montréal. Specific idiosyncrasies of the studied samples directly impact the magnitude of the observed relationships (i.e., properties of the distribution of the variables studied). Although the magnitude of the observed associations (as assessed by odds ratios) is not affected by the shapes of the conditional distributions, their shapes (as assessed by the sample studied) are nonetheless assumed to be representative of the population distributions to which the estimated associations are being generalized.

Given the severe selection bias issues associated with the reported HIV seroprevalence and seroincidence rates among program participants and with the seroprevalence rates among the sampled incarcerated population, the panel concludes that this evaluation study cannot provide valid estimates of program effects on HIV prevalence and incidence.

Epidemiologic Study

Researchers at St.-Luc Hospital in Montréal (Lamothe et al., 1995; Bruneau et al., 1995) initiated a prospective epidemiologic study of HIV infection among injection drug users in September 1988. Active injection drug users who had injected drugs in the past 6 months were recruited from the street (with offers of free HIV testing and precounseling) and from drug treatment programs. The proportion of study participants recruited from treatment programs represents approximately 10 to 15 percent of the total cohort (Bruneau, 1995). Study participants were followed at 6-month intervals and were paid $10 at each visit to complete a structured interview including information on sociodemographic, sexual, and drug-related behaviors and to provide a blood sample for HIV antibody testing. Bruneau et al. (1995) reported on the association between needle exchange attendance (as assessed by one questionnaire item) and HIV infection status among injection drug users by conducting three series of analyses to identify: (1) baseline determinants of HIV seroprevalence, (2) entry determinants of HIV seroincidence, and (3) follow-up determinants immediately preceding HIV seroconversion.

Seroprevalence

By September 1994, the open cohort had an enrollment of 1,506 participants. At entry, 11.1 percent (167/1,506) were HIV positive. The odds ratio of HIV positivity at entry for needle exchange program attenders (i.e., those who had attended at least once in the last 6 months) versus nonattenders was 3.4 (95 percent CI: 2.4 to 3.9). The final solution of the logistic regression model revealed that the adjusted odds ratio for HIV positivity at entry and needle exchange program attenders versus nonattenders was 2.7 (95 percent CI: 1.8 to 4.1). Adjustments were made for study entry, gender, language, age, and several other sociodemographic and sexual and drug-use risk behaviors. In addition to needle exchange program participation, variables found to be associated with seropositivity at entry included: education, income level, and the number of sex partners in the last 6 months. Furthermore, several drug-use risk behaviors were found to be associated with HIV positivity at entry, including: drug of choice; number of times injected drugs in the last month; participated in the needle exchange during the last 6 months; injected drugs in shooting galleries during last 6 months; injected drugs while in prison; ever shared injection equipment; acquaintances known to be HIV positive; and ever shared injection equipment with HIV-positive person.

Seroincidence

Of the 1,339 study participants who were not seropositive at entry, 75 had no follow-up data due to their recent enrollment date and 354 (25 percent) were lost to follow-up. Of the remaining 910 participants followed up (median follow-up was 15.3 months), 77 seroconverted, for an overall incidence of 5.0 per 100 person years (95 percent CI: 3.9 to 6.2). An upward trend in incidence rates was found when these rates were examined over three consecutive 18-month periods: for the period of September 1988 through February 1990, an estimated incidence rate of 4.5 percent was observed. This was followed by an incidence rate of 7.5 percent during the second 18-month period and a 9.8 percent rate during the 18 months after September 1991. At entry, the odds ratio of becoming HIV positive based on needle exchange participation (attenders versus nonattenders) was 2.5 (95 percent CI: 1.6 to 4.0).

To further explore the association between needle exchange participation at enrollment and subsequent seroconversion, a proportional hazards model was used with adjustments for the following variables: age; entry period; number of times used drugs in previous month; number of partners sharing injection equipment in previous month; number of acquaintances known to be HIV positive; participation in drug abuse treatment; other sources of injection equipment; and drug of choice. Although noteworthy, the resulting hazards ratio for needle exchange program attendance did not reach statistical significance.

Finally, to try to identify potential determinants immediately preceding

HIV seroconversion, a logistic regression model was fit to a nested case-control design, with the 77 seroconverters as cases and 279 matched controls (matched on gender, language, year of enrollment, and age). This analysis used information on sociodemographic variables, sexual behaviors, and drug-use risk behaviors collected during the last follow-up interview session preceding seroconversion. For the purpose of this analysis, a needle exchange program use variable was derived based on the sources of needles available to the participants, and cases were categorized as the participant: (1) had never used the needle exchange program as a source of needles, (2) had used the needle exchange program as the exclusive source of needles, and (3) had used the needle exchange program as one of several sources for obtaining needles. After controlling for multiple covariates in the logistic model (number of partners sharing equipment in previous month; number of times having used new injection equipment; number of acquaintances known to be HIV positive; booting; practicing disinfection; and drug of choice), the odds ratio (OR) associated with participants having used the needle exchange program as their exclusive source of needles in the last 6 months prior to seroconversion was found to be 5.19 (95 percent CI: 1.9 to 14.5). Those who did not make exclusive use of the needle exchange program as their source of needles were found to be 16.78 times more likely to seroconvert than needle exchange nonusers (i.e., OR = 16.78; 95 percent CI: 2.7 to 06.0).

Review

As with the other research discussed above, biases in parameter estimates due to the use of limited sampling strategies pose serious concerns for the generalizability of these findings either to the population of injection drug users or to the population of needle exchange program users in Montréal. One of the panel's concerns with this study is that the authors use causal language to describe the purpose of their analysis. In their abstract, Bruneau et al. (1995) state that they performed a series of analyses to assess the baseline determinants of HIV prevalence, entry determinants of HIV seroincidence, and follow-up determinants immediately preceding HIV seroconversion. The use of the term *determinants* would seem to indicate that these researchers are attempting to assess the causal effect of needle exchange participation on HIV prevalence and incidence. However, given the limitations of the study design and the analytical methods used, this study is incapable of sorting out the independent causal effects of each predictor on the outcome variables. It should be noted that, during a briefing session with the panel (Bruneau, 1995), the authors clearly communicated to us that they did not attempt to assess the causal effect of needle exchange on seroprevalence or seroincidence. They consider their study to be purely descriptive in nature and not evaluative.

One difficulty associated with trying to assess needle exchange program effects on seroprevalence and seroincidence with these data relates to properly identifying and measuring confounding factors. The choice of variables for control is not well specified. This makes it extremely difficult to know whether the list of controls is relevant or complete enough to address the selectivity processes that might distinguish attenders from nonattenders. The measurement level of most variables is weak, consisting mostly of dichotomized or trichotomized variables, and this can significantly limit the capacity of the statistical adjustment process to adjust fully for the potential influence of those variables. Moreover, no attempt to assess the influence of interactions was discussed.

The key variable used in this study to assesses needle exchange program participation is limited, consisting of a single item asking respondents if they have used the needle exchange program at least once in the last 6 months. The use of a single item to categorize individuals as having participated in the needle exchange program raises concerns about measurement errors—mainly systematic errors in this case—in the variable being measured, which can produce serious biasing effects. *Systematic measurement error* refers to measurement validity. This type of error occurs when the true variable of interest has not been measured (e.g., time at risk while exposed to the needle exchange) and some other variable or proxy is used in its place (e.g., use of program at least once in last 6 months). When more than one covariate is used in the analysis, the effects of random and systematic errors become quite unpredictable and may overestimate or underestimate the regression coefficients.

Another noteworthy consideration is that injection drug users who do not use the needle exchange program in Montréal have access to sterile injection equipment through pharmacies (there is a pharmacy a block away from the exchange program that sells syringes and is open 24 hours a day). Furthermore, although the seroprevalence and seroincidence among needle exchange participants are higher than among nonparticipants, both groups have high rates of infection, although the nonexclusive needle exchange users were found to be at substantially higher risk than the exclusive users of the program.

Having access to sterile needles in Montréal through sources other than needle exchange is not problematic. It is clear that some selectivity processes are at work. Something is attracting high-risk injectors to the exchange program. Without a more detailed understanding of the characteristics that distinguish nonusers from users, we cannot ascribe the differences in the seroprevalence and seroincidence rates to the needle exchange program. Again, we note that the authors themselves do not attribute the observed differences to the program.

CHICAGO

Investigators in Chicago have recently reported in two unpublished manuscripts the results of an investigation of the relationship among access to free needles through needle exchange program participation, drug-use behaviors (injection frequency, needle use, needle exchange use), other HIV risk behaviors, and HIV incidence to disentangle the causal effect of the Chicago needle exchange on these critical variables.

Demand for Free Needles and Their Effect on Injecting Frequency and Needle Use

In their first paper, O'Brien et al. (1995a) attempt to examine the causal effect of needle exchange use on individual needle and drug use. The Chicago needle exchange program was initiated in 1992. Before the program was initiated, these investigators had been monitoring trends in risk behaviors and HIV incidence among out-of-treatment injection drug users in an effort to assess the impact of an extensive outreach HIV intervention program (discussed in detail in Chapter 6). This study's participants are part of three distinct cohorts that were recruited from three different inner-city neighborhoods: the South Side (mostly African American), North Side (ethnically mixed), and Northwest Side (largely Puerto Rican). The three cohorts were recruited from these three neighborhoods by outreach workers in local community settings, such as street corners, copping areas, and shooting galleries.

The first cohort (1988 cohort) was assembled as part of a longitudinal outreach HIV prevention study and consisted of 850 injection drug users, of which 25 percent were found to be HIV positive at baseline. An additional cohort of 244 injection drug users (baseline HIV prevalence was 32 percent) not exposed to the outreach HIV prevention program was recruited in 1992 (1992 cohort) to supplement the original cohort. Finally, a third cohort of 323 injection drug users, also not exposed to the outreach HIV prevention program, was recruited in 1994 (1994 cohort) and found to have a 24 percent baseline HIV prevalence rate. Results of the analyses presented in this manuscript are based on demographic characteristics, drug-use risk behaviors, sexual risk behaviors, and HIV serology test results collected in 1994 as part of the baseline assessment for the 1994 cohort and as part of a 1994 follow-up assessment for the 1988 and 1992 cohorts for members that were still injecting ($n = 728$) at the time. They are also based on interview data (demographic characteristics and risk behaviors) and serologies collected in a 1993 follow-up (n = 405) for the 1988 and 1992 cohorts.

Drug-use behavior measures included the number of injections for which participants had used their last needle, the total number of injections over the past 4 weeks, and the amount of money spent on drugs in the last week. From these, a measure of injection frequency per week was derived (number of injections over past 4 weeks/4) and a measure of needles used per week was constructed as a linear function of the number of injections per week and the number of times the participant's last needle was used (number of injections per week/number of times used last needle). Two measures of needle exchange use were obtained, a dichotomous measure (use/nonuse in past 4 weeks) and an extent of use measure (nonuse in last 6 months; used in the last 6 months but not in last 4 weeks; used at least once in last 6 months but at a current annual rate of less than 25 times a year; and used at a current rate of over 25 times per year). Needle exchange users were asked to report the number of needles they exchanged in the last 4 weeks; from this, a measure of extra needles per week was derived by taking the difference between the number of needles exchanged per week and the number of needles used per week. The street price of needles in the three areas was reported by the 1994 cohort, and the average was used to compute the value of needles used per week. A relative measure of per-injection cost of drugs was derived for each area and treated as an indicator of injecting drug prices. Other structured interview measures included the number of injection drug user associates and coinhabitants, various injecting and sexual HIV-related risk behaviors, the extent of self-reported frequency of worry about becoming infected with HIV via injection drug use, and having enough money.

A two-step approach was used to assess the effect of free needles on needle exchange participants' current drug use (drug expenditure and current injection frequency) and needle use (number of times a needle is used). First, predictors (potential explanatory variables) of needle exchange use, total needles exchanged, and extra needles were examined, while initially accounting for preexisting level of drug use (past injection frequency) by using 1988 and 1992 cohort data (n = 405). Then, 1994 data (n = 728) were used to predict the same three outcome measures, while ignoring the preexisting level of drug use (past injection frequency). The purpose of repeating the analyses without the preexisting level of drug use in the regression models was to examine the stability of the estimated coefficients of those predictors found to be significantly related to the outcome measures in the initial equations when the preexisting level of drug use was included as a covariate in the equations. That approach was needed because information pertaining to the preexisting level of drug use (past injection frequency)

TABLE A.4 Predictive Models of Chicago Needle Exchange Use, Number of Needles Exchanged, and Extra Needles

	EQ1: Exchange Use [OR/(.95% CI)]		EQ2: Total Needles Exchanged [β/(t statistic)]		EQ3: Extra Needles [β/(t statistic)]	
	Panel	All	Panel	All	Panel	All
Intercept	.011	.03	8.2	4.6	3.9	1.4
	(.01–0.9)	(.006–.12)	(0.9)	(0.68)	(0.49)	(0.2)
Weekly needle	1.6	1.7	2.99	4.17	1.96	2.6
expense (log)	(1.4 –1.9)	(1.5–1.9)	(6.17)	(9.1)	(4.1)	(6.4)
Prior level of	1.04	—	0.32	—	0.28	—
injecting	(1.02–1.07)		(3.59)		(3.47)	
HIV status	2.14	1.14	2.85	2.7	1.59	1.79
	(1.26–3.6)	(.79–1.6)	(1.13)	(1.46)	(0.79)	(1.1)
Relative drug	2.2	4.3	11.28	8.2	10.6	7.0
prices	(.24–19.4)	(1.9–9.6)	(1.2)	(2.0)	(1.2)	(1.94)
Needle prices	1.4	.88	–4.0	–1.9	–3.76	–1.54
	(.46–4.4)	(.69–1.1)	(–0.87)	(–1.49)	(–0.87)	(–1.36)
Race: Puerto	1.57	1.37	2.3	–.53	1.28	–0.28
Rican	(.7–3.4)	(.89–2.1)	(0.7)	(–0.25)	(0.42)	(–0.15)
Race: white	1.26	1.44	3.6	1.11	1.5	–0.05
	(.62–2.55)	(.90–2.3)	(1.2)	(0.46)	(0.54)	(–0.02)
Age	1.0	1.21	–0.95	0.39	–0.48	0.71
	(.69–1.4)	(.96–1.5)	(–0.6)	(0.33)	(–0.35)	(0.68)
Worry about	0.94	1.05	–0.6	–0.11	–0.47	–0.12
AIDS	(.85–1.04)	(.98–1.11)	(–1.5)	(–0.35)	(–1.3)	(–0.4)
Worry about	1.0	1.01	–0.46	–0.54	–0.36	–0.39
money	(.9–1.1)	(.94–1.08)	(–1.1)	(–1.56)	(–1.0)	(–1.2)
1992 cohort	0.8	1.22	–3.2	–1.3	–2.45	–
	0.87(.4–1.5)	(.7–2.1)	(1.29)	(–0.48)	(–1.0)	(–0.3)
1994 cohort	—	1.03	—	2.58	—	2.6
		(.65–1.6)		(1.1)		(1.2)
χ²	125 (df = 12)	151 (df = 12)	—	—	—	—
	(p < .001)	(p < .001)				
Hosmer-Lemeshow	6.3	10	—	—	—	—
Goodness-of-fit						
measure	(p = .61)	(p = .26)				
R²	—	—	.13	.16	.10	.076

SOURCE: From Needle Exchange in Chicago: The Demand for Free Needles and Their Effect on Injecting Frequency and Needle Use (O'Brien et al., 1995a:Table 3).

was not available for a substantial portion of the 1994 data. Table A.4 summarizes the results of these analyses.

The results of the logistic regression of needle exchange use on potential explanatory variables show that only the "weekly needle expense" variable was found to be significant in both sets of equations (i.e., using the 1988 and 1992 cohorts while controlling for the preexisting level of drug use and with the entire set of 1994 data). Moreover, the estimated effect for weekly needle expense was the same in both equations, and the relative drug price became significant when complete data from the 1994 cohort were used.

Most variables used to predict *total needles exchanged* and *extra needles* were not found to be significantly related in the multivariate regression equation to these two outcome measures. Both *weekly needle expense* and *relative drug prices* were found to be associated with these two outcome measures.

The second step of the analyses called for using two-stage least-squares regressions to estimate the effects of free needles on drug expenditure, current injection frequency, and number of times a needle is used. If the coefficients for free needles (i.e., extra needles) could be found to be significantly different from zero, free needles were considered to have a causal effect on current level of drug use. Again, the 1988 and 1992 cohorts ($n = 405$) were first used to take into account the preexisting level of drug use to assess the causal effect of prior drug use levels on 1994 data (drug expenditure, current injection frequency, and number of times a needle is used).

Then, as was the case earlier, the two-stage least-squares regression equations were reexamined while making use of the entire 1994 data ($n = 728$) without including preexisting levels of drug use (past injection frequency) in the equations (i.e., once using only 1988 and 1992 follow-up data, and once using all 1994 data). As stated above, these latter sets of equations were carried out to examine the stability of the parameter estimates (coefficients). Furthermore, these equations were reestimated with the 1988 and 1992 cohorts using Maddala's formulation (using both needle exchange users and nonusers) of Heckman's method in an attempt to eliminate selection bias. Using this procedure, the effects of extra needles remained significant in each set of equations (i.e., for drug expenditure and current injection frequency).

Although the authors did not specifically provide their predictive equations, the text can be interpreted as reflecting the following primary elements of the causal models (Figure A.1):

$$D = f(Y, X); \tag{1}$$
$$J = g(Y, P, X, J'); \text{ and} \tag{2}$$
$$N = (J, X); \tag{3}$$

where: D = drug expenditure; Y = current income; X = number of extra needles; P = current price; J' = past injection frequency; J = current injection frequency; and N = number of times a needle is used.

Partial results of the two-stage least-squares regressions are depicted in

Causal Models

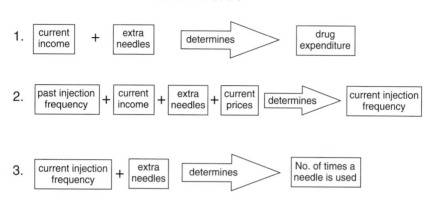

FIGURE A.1 Causal models proposed by O'Brien et al. (1995a).

Table A.5. The solution of the first equation regarding drug expenditure per week indicates that weekly drug expenditure increases as both weekly income and extra needles increase. This is true for the 1988 and 1992 cohorts, regardless of whether past injection frequency is included in the equation. Moreover, the results of the two-stage least-squares regressions, based on the 1994 data, show little variation in the magnitude of the *extra needles* effect in the subsamples of 405 panel members or in the entire sample of 728). The authors interpret this finding as showing that current cash income and current extra needles exchanged determine drug expenditure. They also state that the positive effect of extra needles exchanged on drug expenditures implies that exchangers spend more for drugs than can be expected from only their level of weekly cash income and in proportion to the number of extra needles.

The *current injection frequency* equations indicate that, when *past injection frequency* is incorporated into the model while using the 1988 and 1992 cohorts, the latter does not contribute to explaining variations in the current level of injection frequency. Estimated effects for the extra needles variable were found to be relatively stable when data from the 1988 and 1992 cohorts were used compared with fitting the model to the 1994 data. The investigators state that the positive coefficient of extra needles exchanged in the drug expenditure model and the positive effect of extra needles on current injection frequency indicate that extra free needles are increasing the frequency of drug injecting.

The last set of equations presented in Table A.5 pertains to the *number of times a needle is used*. The effect of the number of needles exchanged was not found to be significant in any of the regression equations, whereas

TABLE A.5 Chicago's Two-Stage Least-Squares Regression Results[a]

	1988-1992 Cohort[b]	1988-1992 Cohort[c]	1994 Cohort[c]
Drug expenditure			
Weekly income	0.45 (6.9)	0.45 (6.0)	0.54 (9.4)
Extra needles	0.95 (4.4)	1.2 (4.1)	0.58 (3.1)
R^2	0.14	0.11	0.27
Current injection frequency			
Past injection frequency	−0.20 (−1.1)	—	—
Extra needles	2.4 (4.0)	2.3 (4.6)	2.15 (4.8)
Current drug price	−0.12 (−0.9)	−0.10 (−0.78)	−0.21 (−1.6)
R^2	0.06	0.06	0.08
Injections per needle			
Current injection frequency	−0.27 (−3.4)	−0.27 (−1.4)	−1.0 (−2.3)
No. of needles exchanged	−0.14 (−0.31)	−0.14 (0.3)	0.8 (0.9)
R^2	0.06	0.07	0.08

[a]Entries are standardized coefficients (asymptotic t statistics).
[b]Past injection frequency (i.e., 1993 data) included.
[c]Past injection frequency not included.

SOURCE: Adapted from Needle Exchange in Chicago: The Demand for Free Needles and Their Effect on Injecting Frequency and Needle Use (O'Brien et al., 1995a:Table 4).

the effect of current injection frequency was found to be negative and significant. As current injection frequency increases, the number of times a needle is used decreases. The authors conclude that the lower number of times a needle is used among exchangers is not due to free needles, but rather to the higher level of current injection frequency among the exchangers.

These authors also compared their data with results of Kaplan's New Haven needle exchange evaluation findings (see Chapter 7 for a review of Kaplan's work). Using data from their 1994 cohort, the investigators regressed information reported by injection drug users regarding *how long they keep a used needle* on use of the exchange program, needles used per week, risky injecting, HIV status, handing off a used needle, and number of times a needle was used for injecting. The only significant predictor of how long a needle was kept was the number of times a needle was used. The authors interpreted this as showing that the use of a needle exchange did not affect the circulation time of needles as measured in their study. Moreover, to explore the potential effect of needle exchange programs in recapturing used needles (removing them from circulation), the authors regressed study participants' (1994 cohort) reported method for disposing of used needles (throwing away needles) on the same variables mentioned above. The only variable found to be associated with throwing a needle away was handing off a used needle; needle exchange use was not found to reduce throwing away needles after use. This latter finding was interpreted by the authors as indicating that the utility of needle exchange in recapturing used needles is limited. Finally, researchers reported that exchange users do not report a significantly higher level of worry about HIV infection than nonusers.

Review

This research (O'Brien et al., 1995a) reported that needle exchange users injected more frequently than nonusers and, on average, obtained three times more than the number of needles that they were estimated to use personally. The estimates of drug expenditures and current injection frequency were positively associated with the number of needles exchanged. These authors infer that access to free needles results in increased drug expenditure and injection frequency among exchange users. Moreover, the effect of free needles (number of needles exchanged) on the number of times a needle is used was reported not to be related, while the current level of drug use (current injection frequency) was reported to be negatively related to the number of times a needle was used. This latter finding is interpreted as indicating that needle exchange participation (or access to free needles) does not impact the number of times a needle is used and that current injection frequency determines the number of times a needle is used.

Several concerns arise in assessing the soundness of the conclusions drawn by these investigators. The attempt to disentangle causal relationships on the basis of observational data has always been problematic and controversial, and the problems are considerably greater when the data are cross-sectional (as is the case here). There are numerous strategies possible (i.e., covariance analysis, structural equation models, and selection models); the strategy adopted by the Chicago research team was to use a two-stage least-squares (2SLS) procedure (i.e., a selection model) to estimate their equations. This procedure allows for estimating effects when one variable is both a dependent (response) variable and an independent (explanatory) variable. In addition, sample selection bias was investigated, using a procedure developed by Heckman (1979).

The panel's primary concerns relate to (1) the absence of any presentation or consideration of plausible alternative or competing models and (2) serious potential for bias in estimates due to measurement error.

With respect to alternative models, the Chicago researchers assert that current injection frequency is a function of prior injection frequency, current income, extra needles, and price. But one alternative model would assert that current income is a function of current injection frequency. That is, the frequency with which a person injects drugs leads to the need for additional money and engaging in money-gathering activities (legal and otherwise). This very plausible alternative model would have major implications for the estimates derived from the model. The lack of consideration of this and other plausible alternative models renders the manuscript's conclusions far from compelling.

The 2SLS method is appropriate under fairly stringent conditions. In particular, in order to achieve identification of the parameters being estimated, there need to be "instrument" variables that are unrelated to the measured causes of the endogenous variables. In this particular application, the method is appropriate only if there are predictor variables presented in the manuscript's Table A.4 that should be excluded (based on a priori consideration) from the regressions in Table A.5. One problem is that there is no discussion in the manuscript about this issue, and another is that there may not be a plausible argument to be made. In this specific case, the manuscript does not present the actual equations estimated, making it difficult to determine which variables have been excluded on an a priori basis. *Weekly needle expense* may be one such variable, but it seems likely that this would have a direct effect on all dependent variables in Table A.5. Thus, in addition to the weakness of lack of consideration of plausible alternative models, the manuscript fails to provide adequate consideration of the assumptions underlying the particular model that was estimated.

O'Brien et al. (1995a) did attempt to eliminate selection bias in their estimation of coefficients. Nonetheless, it should be noted that "the potential uses of selection modeling in evaluation have generated considerable controversy. . . . At present there are divergent and strongly held opinions about the potential uses and misuses of these procedures" (Coyle et al., 1991:175). The Chicago researchers used the Heckman method, as described in Maddala (1983:Chapter 9). However, this procedure has some major difficulties. Indeed, in certain situations, Heckman-type selection models may not improve estimates in observational data (Little, 1985; Stolzenberg, and Relles, 1990; Winship and Mare, 1992). Moreover, the method requires that there exist measured variables in the data set that can predict—in this specific case—the use (versus nonuse) of a needle exchange program. To the extent that needle exchange use is not well predicted, then the selection model may have little effect on parameter estimates.

Additional concerns are related to problems with measurement properties of some key variables. Although the reliability of the measures is not discussed, it may have important implications. For example, the effect of prior injecting is not significant in the panel sample predicting current injecting frequency in the 2SLS. But the 2SLS method assumes that these variables are measured without error (as does the ordinary least squares method—OLS). In fact, there is likely to be considerable measurement error in these variables, and thus the "true" correlation or covariation between them may be substantially attenuated. The lack of fully controlling for the effect of prior injecting may lead to an overestimate of the effect of extra needles. These sorts of issues are always present in regression models. Modern structural equation models involving latent variables usually attempt to address them, though not necessarily successfully. But particularly when one method (OLS) shows a nonsignificant effect of extra needles on current injecting frequency, and another method (2SLS) shows a significant effect, caution in drawing causal conclusions should be stressed.

Another measurement issue is that no detailed information on the properties of the distribution of variables (e.g., variance, skewness) is provided. The authors report mean measures, some of which have large standard errors, which seem to indicate the possible presence of outliers; these, in turn, may have substantial impact on the reported results. For example, data reported in the manuscript are inconsistent with records maintained by the Chicago needle exchange program. That is, the exchange records show a mean of 15 needles obtained per week by exchangers compared with a mean of 30 per week (with a standard error of 37) reported by these authors. When comparing actual records with self-report data (as used by these investigators), it is to be expected that some disparity will be observed, but the magnitude of these disparities is of concern. The Chicago needle exchange records also show that the distribution of needles obtained per week is highly skewed, and that the median of 8 needles per week would be a better measure of central tendency than the mean. Another measurement concern relates to their *extra needles measure*. It does not allow for passing needles to other injectors who are not cohabitants and/or sharing partners.

With regard to systematic error, several of the measures used appear to be problematic. For example, the measure of *worry about HIV* was assessed after study participants had joined the needle exchange program (i.e., they may no longer worry as a result of having joined the program). Therefore, it is not surprising to find that such a measure was not related to needle exchange use.

Another source of concern is the representativeness of the sample of study participants of the population of needle exchange users and nonusers. The authors state that needle exchange users in their cohorts represent 20 percent of the total population of needle exchange users. But the critical issue that must be addressed is where these 20 percent fall on the distribution of the critical variables used in the model: if they are extreme cases, it may bias the reported estimates. Again, data from the Chicago needle exchange records show a median of one visit per month, with 75 percent visiting two or fewer times per month—compared with the 50 percent visiting weekly or more frequently in the self-report data used by the authors. It appears that these investigators are attempting to test the tenability of an aggregate model to explain the behaviors of needle exchange users and nonusers without giving appropriate attention to the potentially biasing effect of outliers in their data set.

Another design concern relates to the investigators' assumption that needle exchange nonusers are not gaining access to needle exchange needles. If a large number of nonusers is obtaining sterile needles that have originated from the exchange programs, it could be argued that they are indirectly participating in the needle exchange program or at least benefiting from it.

The method used to verify the stability of coefficients also poses some difficulties. The paper indicates that the final equations that use the data from all cohorts ($n = 728$) also incorporate the 1988 and 1992 cohorts ($n = 405$) on which the original coefficients were derived. This nonindependence of samples raises questions about the ability of this approach to reliably assess the stability of coefficient estimates across samples (especially because more than half of the final sample were members of the original sample).

It is inappropriate for the investigators to apply the circulation theory concept used in the New Haven evaluation study. The Chicago program is not a one-for-one program, and the protocol it follows allows for the number of distributed needles to exceed the number of returned needles by 5 on a per-visit basis. Kaplan's circulation theory requires that needles be exchanged on a one-for-one basis; as derived in Kaplan's work, it is this law of conservation of needles that provides the link between needle exchange rates and the level of infection in needles. In the absence of a one-for-one exchange, there is no physical guarantee that needle circulation times will decline as the numbers of needles distributed increases, because there is a net increase in the total number of needles in circulation.

In sum, based on the panel's interpretation, we cannot say that the data justify the conclusions the researchers have reached.

Effects of Exchange Use on HIV Risk Behavior and Incidence

In a second paper, the same investigators (O'Brien et al., 1995b) explore the potential effect of needle exchange programs on HIV risk behaviors and incidence. Data from the 1994 interview and HIV serology test results of current injection drug users from all three cohorts ($n = 728$; 1988, 1992, and 1994 data), as well as data from the 1993 follow-up of the 1988 and 1992 cohorts ($n = 405$) described above, form the basis of the reported analyses.

Four measures of injection risk behaviors were derived. A dichotomous variable indicating overall risky injecting behavior based on injection drug users' reported *use of others' used needles, consistent use of bleach, sharing cotton, cookers, or water,* and *backloading* (see Wiebel, 1990, for a description of the measure). Two additional dichotomous drug-related variables were constructed, one based exclusively on whether the injection drug user used other injection drug users' needles without using bleach and the other based on whether drug users passed their own used needles to other injectors. A final syringe-sharing variable consistent with Watters et al. (1994)—injecting risk behavior—was derived. This latter variable is based on information concerning an injector's use of someone else's needle and ignores possible cleaning practice with bleach. The sexual risk behavior variable assessed whether a respondent had multiple sex partners in the past 6 months or an injection drug user sex partner and did not always use a condom.

Three measures of needle exchange were derived: dichotomous use/ nonuse in the past 4 weeks; use over two interview waves; and a four-category measure of frequency of use similar to the Watters et al. (1994) measure. Other information collected during the follow-up and baseline interviews included: number of injection drug users' associates and cohabitants; frequency of worry about becoming infected with HIV via injection drug use; and having enough money.

Of the overall 1994 data ($n = 728$), 8 percent used the needle exchange once in the previous 4 weeks; 12 percent used it 2 to 3 times; and 19 percent used it once a week or more. This represents 40 percent ($n = 285$) of the total sample having used the exchange in the past 4 weeks, which also represents approximately 21 percent of all injection drug users who had used the program at least once since February 1, 1994.

With respect to HIV risk behaviors assessed in 1994, a comparison of needle exchange users and nonusers revealed no statistically significant difference in the proportion of study participants reporting having engaged in injection drug use risk behaviors, whereas nonusers were found to be more likely to report multiple sex risk (43 compared with 40 percent). The investigators used logistic regressions to examine the effect of exchange use on each risk behavior when prior level of risk was accounted for (using 1993 follow-up data on the 1988 and 1992 cohorts; $n = 405$). The results showed that the measure of prior risk behavior was the only significant predictor of current risk level; the main effect of needle exchange use, as well as its interaction with age, was nonsignificant for all risk variables. Moreover, these logistic regressions were reexamined using the 1994 data as a cross section, ignoring prior risk behavior, and the results showed that each risk variable was unaffected by frequency of exchange use.

There were 258 current injection drug users from the 1988 and 1992 cohorts known to be at risk of seroconverting at the 1994 follow-up. An equal proportion of these HIV-negative study participants were needle exchange users and nonusers. Three seroconverted over an average 9-month observation period. Of the 177 who did not use the needle exchange, 1 person seroconverted in the same period (0.56 percent or 0.75 per 100 person years); of the 81 who had used the needle exchange, 2 seroconverted (2.50 percent or 3.0 per 100 person years). This difference in incidence is not statistically significant.

Review

The reported findings from this second paper by O'Brien and colleagues suggest that the needle exchange program has no protective effect on the risk behaviors and HIV infection rates among program participants. This research suffers from the same selectivity problems associated with the Chicago paper reviewed above. That is, there are problems with measurement error, and underadjustments originating from the unreliability of the measures used may explain, at least in part, the lack of effects. The control conditions (i.e., nonusers of the program) are sufficiently different as to render them unusable as a counterfactual condition.

Moreover, no observed reduction in risk behavior may be explained by the fact that a substantial proportion of the studied sample (i.e., the 1988 cohort) was exposed to an extensive HIV prevention program. Findings from that original study have shown significant declines in injection drug use risk behaviors (see Chapter 6).

The reported null results for program effect on HIV incidence are not surprising given the small number of years at risk chosen and the low power associated with the inferential test used. These findings do not prove that the needle exchange program has no protective effect on the rate of new HIV infections among needle exchange participants. That is, not being able to reject the null hypothesis (i.e., rates of HIV incidence in exchange users and nonusers are equal) does not establish that the null hypothesis is true (i.e., incidence rates are the same in both groups).

CONCLUSION

The study designs and analytical methods employed in the San Francisco, Montréal, and Chicago studies preclude making causal inferences about the effect of needle exchange programs on risk behaviors and HIV prevalence or incidence. In addition, none of these studies has used adequate sampling strategies to ensure that risk behavior and HIV prevalence and incidence estimates are representative of the injection drug-using populations who use and do not use the respective exchange programs. Nonetheless, the studies have reported measures of associations—although there is some question about the populations to which they apply—that are sizable and should be further studied with proper study designs, measurement, and analytical methods to properly investigate the tenability of such causal relationships.

REFERENCES

Brookmeyer, R., and M.H. Gail
1994   *AIDS Epidemiology: A Quantitative Approach.* New York, NY: Oxford University Press.
Bruneau, J.
1995   Presentation at a meeting of the Panel on Needle Exchange and Bleach Distribution Programs, Washington, DC, April 5.
Bruneau, J., F. Lamothe, E. Franco, N. Lachance, J. Vincelette, and J. Soto
1995   Needle Exchange Program (NEP) Attendance and HIV-1 Infection in Montréal: Report of a Paradoxical Association. Abstract for International Conference on the Reduction of Drug Related Harm, Palazzo dei Congressi, Florence, Italy, March 26-30.
Coyle, S.L., R.F. Boruch, and C.F. Turner, eds.
1991   *Evaluating AIDS Prevention Programs: Expanded Edition.* Panel on the Evaluation of AIDS Interventions, National Research Council. Washington, DC: National Academy Press.
Hahn, J.A., K. Vranizan, and A.R. Moss
1995   Needle Exchange Among Injection Drug Users in San Francisco. Draft manuscript.
Hankins, C.
1994   Appendix E in *The Proceedings of the Meeting on HIV Infection Among Injection Drug Users in Canada*, Montréal, Québec, December 12-13.
Hankins, C., S. Gendron, J. Bruneau, F. Rouah, N. Paquette, M. Jalbert, F. Prévost, and B. Gomez
1992   Consumer Awareness, Utilization, and Satisfaction with CACTUS-Montréal's Needle Exchange. Eighth International Conference on AIDS, Amsterdam, July 19-24.
Hankins, C., S. Gendron, F. Rouah, C. Godbout, I. Mayr, and D. Lepine
1993   Rising Prevalence? Declining Incidence? Montréal's Needle Exchange: A Successful Verdict or Is the Jury Still Out? IXth International Conference on AIDS, Berlin, June 6-11.
Hankins, C., S. Gendron, J. Bruneau, and E. Roy
1994   Evaluating Montréal's needle exchange CACTUS-Montréal. Pp. 83-90 in *Proceedings, Workshop on Needle Exchange and Bleach Distribution Programs.* National Research Council and Institute of Medicine. Washington, DC: National Academy Press.
Heckman, J.J.
1979   Sample selection bias as a specification error. *Econometrica* 47:153-161.
Lamothe, F., J. Bruneau, J. Soto, N. Lachance, E. Franco, J. Vincelette, and M. Fauvel
1995   Risk Factors for HIV Seroconversion Among Injecting Drug Users in Montréal: The Saint-Luc Cohort Experience. Abstract number 074C. Tenth Annual International Conference on AIDS, Yokohama, Japan.
Little, R.J.A.
1985   A note about models for selectivity bias. *Econometrica* 53:1469-1474.
Moss, A.
1995   Presentation at a meeting of the Panel on Needle Exchange and Bleach Distribution Programs, Washington, DC, April 5.

O'Brien, M.U., J. Murray, F. Cannarozzi, A. Jimenez, W. Johnson, L. Ouellet, and W. Wiebel
  1995a   Needle Exchange in Chicago: The Demand for Free Needles and Their Effect on Injecting Frequency and Needle Use. Draft manuscript.
  1995b   Needle Exchange in Chicago: The Effects of Exchange Use on HIV Risk Behavior and Incidence. Draft manuscript.
Stolzenberg, R.M., and D.A. Relles
  1990   Theory testing in a world of constrained research design: The significance of Heckman's censored sampling bias correction for nonexperimental research. *Sociological Methods and Research* 18:395-415.
Watters, J.K., M.J. Estilo, G.L. Clark, and J. Lorvick
  1994   Syringe and needle exchange as HIV/AIDS prevention for injecting drug users. *Journal of the American Medical Association* 271(2):115-120.
Wiebel, W.W.
  1990   Identifying and gaining access to hidden populations. Pp. 4-11 in E.Y. Lambert and W.W. Wiebel, eds., *Collection and Interpretation of Data in Hidden Populations.* Rockville, MD: National Institute on Drug Abuse.
Winship, C., and R.D. Mare
  1992   Models for sample selection bias. *Annual Review of Sociology* 18:327-350.

B
Professional Association Positions on Needle Exchange and Bleach Distribution Programs

Chapter 4 summarized the panel's efforts to obtain views on needle exchange and bleach distribution programs from professional and trade associations that represent service providers. The panel contacted 25 such organizations; 13 responded, and 8 provided statements of their formal or informal positions. This appendix summarizes the responses by the panel to this request for information.

Alcohol and Drug Problems Association of North America (ADPANA)

No response was received.

American Academy of Health Care Providers in the Addictive Disorders (AAHCPAD)

No response was received.

The American Academy of Psychiatrists in Alcoholism & Addictions (aaPaa)

We are very pleased that the American Academy of Psychiatrists in Alcoholism & Addictions has been asked for their position on the issue of needle exchange programs. We believe that the expertise represented by our membership must be seriously considered in any study of drug use behaviors, research and treatment.

Although aaPaa has no formal policy on needle exchange, we are currently reviewing the American Psychiatric Association's [APA's] policy [see below] which has been approved by the APA board. Our Public Policy Committee has not formally endorsed the APA policy but is very likely to recommend endorsement at our next board meeting.

We feel that further study of needle programs is useful and may be an adjunct to other psychosocial approaches in addition to methadone in the treatment of injecting drug users. If you have questions or require additional information, please contact us.

We would welcome the opportunity to meet with you to more fully inform you regarding the philosophy, goals and priorities of aaPaa. Thank you for the opportunity to express our views on this important issue.

American Association of Public Health Physicians (AAPHP)

No response was received.

American College of Addiction Treatment Administrators (ACATA)

ACATA deals almost exclusively in professional development and credentialing of administrators in the field. Consequently, it has not dealt with needle exchange and bleach distribution programs and does not have a position on this issue.

American Medical Association (AMA)

Whereas, AMA policy 20.977 recognizes the urgent need to decrease transmission of human immunodeficiency virus (HIV) and calls for "pinpoint(ing) effective strategies (including needle exchange programs)" to reduce the spread of HIV infection among intravenous drug abusers; and

Whereas, Negative consequences of needle exchange programs have not been detected, i.e., no increase in injection drug use or changing of drug use behavior from non-injection to injection; and

Whereas, Syringe and needle exchange (SANE) programs reduce the rising incidence of HIV infection among intravenous drug users; and

Whereas, Difficulty in obtaining sterile needles and syringes is significantly and independently associated with needle sharing; therefore be it

RESOLVED, That the American Medical Association encourage needle exchange programs.

American Medical Association House of Delegates Resolution 231 (I-94)

American Psychiatric Association (APA)

APA Policy on Clean Needle and Syringe Exchange: Addiction treatment on demand may be the most effective means of reducing HIV transmission among injecting drug users (IDUs). Treatment on demand, however, does not exist in most areas where injecting drug use is prevalent. In addition, a significant number of IDUs do not seek treatment. The APA recommends that clean needle and syringe exchange programs be developed and independently evaluated in terms of their efficacy in reducing HIV transmission and their impact on the prevalence of injecting drug use. The APA believes that those areas where treatment on demand is available are the most appropriate sites for evaluating this promising but unproven intervention. Further, the APA supports all efforts to increase addiction treatments to meet the need.

American Psychological Association (APA)

No response was received.

American Public Health Association (APHA)

Policy: In 1989, APHA passed a policy resolution, "Illicit Drug Use and HIV Infection," that addresses the issue. Our policy process requires that resolutions be based on scientific fact. Because of the lack of research findings on needle exchange at that time, the policy only goes so far as to call for the research and evaluation of needle exchange programs. The AIDS Working Group of APHA's Special Initiative on AIDS is drafting a new policy on needle exchange which will take into account current research and will be submitted for the 1994 policy resolution process.

Commentary: Public health strategies such as needle exchange and bleach distribution are critical components necessary to fight the twin epidemics of substance abuse and HIV infection. In January 1990, APHA's Special Initiative on AIDS published a report on "Illicit Drug Use and HIV Infection." The reports in the AIDS series are sold to our members and the general public for a low price and are a good source of basic information on topics such as needle exchange. This particular report examines needle exchange and bleach distribution programs, and contains an appendix that describes programs that existed at that time.

American Society of Addiction Medicine (ASAM)

Background: Needle Exchange Programs are a crucial component of a spectrum of HIV prevention services to drug injectors which effectively reduce the transmission of the Human Immunodeficiency Virus. The preferred options within the spectrum are abstaining from the injection of drugs and engagement within the drug treatment system. Other public health interventions which will reduce the transmission of blood borne pathogens include: teaching injection equipment sterilization techniques, teaching safer injecting practices, safer sex education and counseling, the provision of HIV literature and the distribution of risk-reducing materials including condoms, dental dams, and bleach kits.

International and U.S. evaluation studies of needle exchange, as an additional method of risk reduction, have not shown an increase in drug use, an increase in injection as a route of drug administration, nor have they shown an increase in contaminated injection equipment in the community. These studies consistently show decrease in equipment sharing, strongly suggesting a decrease in incidence of new infections of blood borne pathogens such as HIV or Hepatitis B. The programs also serve as a point of contact between heretofore alienated drug dependent persons and service providers who can help them improve their health. In fact, the most requested service by needle exchange clients throughout the world is placement in drug treatment programs.

ASAM Position: For these reasons, ASAM recommends that:

1. Needle/distribution exchange programs be instituted in all communities with injection drug users.

2. Drug paraphernalia laws be amended to eliminate those statutes outlawing the possession of syringes or needles.

3. Proper federal agencies be encouraged to sponsor needle exchange programs on a Federal level. (*Adopted by ASAM Board of Directors, October 2, 1994.*)

Association of Black Psychologists (ABP)

No response was received.

Association of Medical Education and Research in Substance Abuse (AMERSA)

The panel received a call on March 16, 1994, to indicate that its query would be an item for the association's board to discuss at its meeting at the end of April 1994. It was indicated that a statement, if any, would be forwarded for our information in May 1994. No statement was received.

Black Psychiatrists of America (BPA)

No response was received.

Chemical Dependency Treatment Programs Association (CDTPA)

The panel was informed that this association no longer exists.

Drug and Alcohol Nursing Association (DANA)

No response was received.

National Association of Addiction Treatment Providers (NAATP)

NAATP does not have positions on either of these matters.

National Association of Alcoholism and Drug Abuse Counselors (NAADAC)

No response was received.

National Association of Psychiatric Health Systems (NAPHS)

Informal Position: Although NAPHS does not have a formal position on these issues, its view is that the clear nexus between HIV-infected needles and transmission of the virus is so powerful that we can ill afford to ignore any opportunity to intervene in the prevention of the infection.

National Association of Social Workers (NASW)

AIDS/HIV Statement—Recommendation: HIV and AIDS prevention and treatment efforts must incorporate substance abuse issues into their models. By impairing judgment, alcohol and other drug use leads to increased participation in high-risk activities and contributes to the increase in HIV infection. The sharing of any kind of injection equipment will contribute to the spread of the virus. Additionally, although the percentage of cases resulting from men having sex with men is decreasing, the rate of infection resulting from substance use is increasing, that is, the person with AIDS was an injection drug user or had sex with an injection drug user. HIV/AIDS prevention and education must therefore include needle exchange programs as well as substance abuse prevention efforts that are explicit, relevant, and culturally sensitive. There also needs to be an increase in drug treatment slots, particularly for parents.

All human services and educational institutions, including correctional facilities, have the responsibility to carry out maximum HIV prevention activities, including education and needle exchange and condom accessibility programs, as appropriate.

Agencies should be encouraged to . . . Provide information on prevention and other issues. All agencies have a responsibility to educate clients about risk reduction behaviors, including safer sexual practices, not sharing needles or other injection equipment, proper needle-cleaning techniques, needle exchange programs, tuberculosis prevention, and life skills such as sexual negotiation and assertive communication.

National Association of State Alcohol and Drug Abuse Directors (NASADAD)

The NASADAD Board of Directors formally passed the following resolution on September 18, 1991:

The NASADAD Board of Directors supports the recommendations of the National Commission on AIDS regarding the Twin Epidemics of Substance Use and HIV. Additional alcohol and other drug abuse prevention and treatment services, increased HIV prevention activities, and expanded research and epidemiologic studies are urgently needed to prevent further HIV transmission among highly vulnerable and at-risk populations.

NASADAD recommends support for bleach and/or needle distribution programs in areas and geographic regions where appropriate. However, the decision to conduct bleach and/or needle distribution programs should remain at the discretion of States and Territories and/or local communities (where legally permissible).

National Association of Substance Abuse Trainers and Educators (NASATE)

No response was received.

National Consortium of Chemical Dependency Nurses, Inc. (NCCDN)

The NCCDN has no official position on the issues of needle exchange and bleach distribution. This type of program is quite controversial among treatment professionals and the Board of Directors has chosen to not officially speak to these techniques.

National Nurses Society on Addiction (NNSA)

No response was received.

Social Work Administrators in Health Care (SWAHC)

No response was received.

Therapeutic Communities of America (TCA)

No response was received.

APPENDIX
C

Biographical Sketches

LINCOLN E. MOSES (Chair) is professor emeritus (active) in the Department of Health Research and Policy, Division of Biostatistics, at Stanford University. He has had joint appointments in the Statistics Department and the Medical School since 1952. He is a member of the Institute of Medicine and the American Academy of Arts and Sciences and a fellow of the Institute of Mathematical Statistics and the American Statistical Association. His research interests lie principally in social and biological applications of statistics. Major recent application areas include AIDS policy and meta-analysis of diagnostic tests for HIV infection and for other diseases. From 1987 to 1980 he served at the assistant secretary level leading the statistics arm of the U.S. Department of Energy. He has an A.B. and a Ph.D. in statistics from Stanford University.

RONALD S. BROOKMEYER is professor in the Department of Biostatistics at The Johns Hopkins University School of Hygiene and Public Health, with a joint appointment in the Department of Epidemiology. He has a Ph.D. in statistics from the University of Wisconsin. He has authored over 70 scientific articles and books in biostatistics, epidemiologic methods, and AIDS and is the coauthor of the book entitled *AIDS Epidemiology: A Quantitative Approach.* His research has included statistical methods in epidemiologic studies of AIDS. He was one of the developers of the back-calculation method that is widely used for estimating and projecting the size of the epidemic. In 1992, he was awarded the Spiegelman gold medal by the

American Public Health Association for contributions to health statistics. His committee service includes the Committee on National Statistics and a committee on statistical issues in AIDS research of the National Research Council, as well as the clinical research subcommittee of the AIDS Research Advisory Committee of the National Institute of Allergy and Infectious Diseases. He was on the editorial board of *Statistics in Medicine* from 1985 to 1994 and has served on the regional advisory board of the Biometrics Society and is currently chair of the biometrics section of the American Statistical Association.

LAWRENCE S. BROWN, JR., is an attending physician in the Division of Endocrinology of the Department of Medicine at Harlem Hospital and assistant clinical professor of medicine in the College of Physicians and Surgeons at Columbia University. He is also senior vice president for medical services, evaluation, and research of the Addiction Research and Treatment Corporation in Brooklyn, New York. He has an M.D. from New York University and an M.P.H. from Columbia University. He serves as a consultant to many federal, state, and city agencies, as well as private foundations and organizations, including the National Football League. He has participated in public policy development in health manpower and drug-abuse-related transmission of AIDS through projects, media presentations, and involvement in varied public and private task forces and fora. He is the author of several publications and is a member of the National Medical Association, the American Public Health Association, the New York Academy of Sciences, the Association for the Advancement of the Sciences, the professional section of the American Diabetes Association, the American Society for Internal Medicine, the American College of Physicians, and the Black Leadership Commission on AIDS.

RICHARD F. CATALANO, JR., is professor and associate director of the Social Development Research Group at the University of Washington's School of Social Work in Seattle. He has a B.S. from the University of Wisconsin and a Ph.D. in sociology from the University of Washington. He has been involved in research and program development in the areas of drug abuse and delinquency for over 17 years. His work has focused on discovering risk and protective factors for adolescent problem behavior and designing and evaluating programs to address these factors. He is the principal investigator and coinvestigator on a number of federal grants, which involve family, school, and community-based prevention approaches to reduce risk while enhancing the protective factors of bonding and the promotion of healthy beliefs and clear standards. He has published over 50 articles and book chapters and has served on the Epidemiology and Prevention Review Committee of the National Institute on Drug Abuse and on the Washington

State Advisory Committee for Alcohol and Substance Abuse. He is the codeveloper of the Social Development Model, a parenting program called Preparing for the Drug-Free Years, and the community prevention approach called Communities That Care.

DAVID S. CORDRAY is professor of public policy and psychology and director of the Center for the Study of At-Risk Populations and Public Assistance Policy at the Vanderbilt Institute for Public Policy Studies. Prior to joining the faculty at Vanderbilt, he was an associate professor in the Division of Methodology and Evaluation Research at Northwestern University and the assistant director of federal welfare and statistical policy in the Program and Evaluation Methodology Division of the U.S. General Accounting Office. He has served as president of the American Evaluation Association, a member of the National Academy of Public Administration's Panel on Performance Indicators in Government, and a member of the evaluation review panel for the U.S. Department of Education. He has published dozens of journal articles and books, including *Secondary Analysis of Program Evaluations* (as coeditor); Volume 11 of the *Evaluation Studies Review Annual* (as coeditor); *Explanatory Meta-Analysis: A Casebook* (with Tom Cook et al.); articles on meta-analytic strategies and the quality of research; and articles on methodological issues associated with counting the homeless population. His current research areas include alcohol and other drug abuse among homeless people, the effects of job training on welfare and work, and methods for improving the quality of intervention research. Cordray has a B.A. in psychology and an M.A. in social psychology from California State University and a Ph.D. in social-environmental psychology and applied research methodology from Claremont Graduate School, with postdoctoral training in the Division of Methodology and Evaluation Research of Northwestern University.

DON C. DES JARLAIS is director of research for the Chemical Dependency Institute at Beth Israel Medical Center; deputy director for AIDS Research with National Development and Research Institutes, Inc.; visiting professor of psychology at Columbia University; and professor of epidemiology at the Albert Einstein College of Medicine. A leader in the fields of AIDS and intravenous drug use over the last 15 years, he has published widely on these topics. He has served as consultant to various institutions, including the Centers for Disease Control and Prevention, the National Institute on Drug Abuse, and the World Health Organization. He has been a member of a number of committees of the National Research Council and the Institute of Medicine, including the Committee on AIDS Research and the Behavioral, Social and Statistical Sciences and the Panel on AIDS and IV-Drug Use. He was a member of the President's National Commission on

Acquired Immune Deficiency Syndrome. He has a B.A. in behavioral sciences from Rice University and a Ph.D. in social psychology from the University of Michigan; he also attended the University of the Philippines and the Université de Paris (La Sorbonne).

CASWELL A. EVANS, JR., is director of public health programs and services for Los Angeles County, California. He is responsible for the administration of disease prevention, health promotion, and health protection services for more than 9 million area residents. He serves as adjunct professor in the School of Public Health and the School of Dentistry at the University of California at Los Angeles; he is also associate professor for the Charles R. Drew Postgraduate Medical School. Prior to his associations with the Los Angeles County government, he was director of the County Health Services Division of the Seattle-King County Department of Public Health in Washington. He has an M.P.H. from the University of Michigan School of Public Health and a D.D.S. from the Columbia University School of Dental and Oral Surgery. Evans is a diplomate of the American Board of Dental Public Health and also serves on the board of directors of the U.S. Conference of Local Health Officers. He is a member of the Institute of Medicine. In 1994, he became president of the American Public Health Association.

MARK B. FEINBERG is assistant professor of medicine and microbiology and immunology at the University of California, San Francisco, and assistant investigator at the Gladstone Institute of Virology and Immunology. He directs the Virology Research Laboratory at San Francisco General Hospital and is the associate director of the University of California, San Francisco's Center for AIDS Research. He also serves as an attending physician with the Medicine and AIDS/Oncology Services at San Francisco General Hospital. His basic research activities focus on the regulation of HIV gene expression and the application of contemporary methods in molecular biology to the study of the pathogens of HIV disease. He received a B.A. in biology and anthropology from the University of Pennsylvania and an M.D. and Ph.D. in cancer biology from Stanford University School of Medicine.

HERBERT D. KLEBER is professor of psychiatry and director of the Division on Substance Abuse at the College of Physicians and Surgeons of Columbia University and the New York State Psychiatric Institute. He is also executive vice-president of the Center on Addiction and Substance Abuse. Prior to 1991, he served as the deputy director for demand reduction at the Office of National Drug Control Policy in the White House. Previously he was a professor of psychiatry at Yale University School of Medicine; director of the Substance Abuse Treatment Unit at the Connecticut

Mental Health Center; and chief executive officer of the APT Foundation, the major treatment site for drug abusers in the New Haven area. At Yale he was the director of two centers funded by the National Institute on Drug Abuse: a clinical research center to develop new treatments for opiate and cocaine abuse, and a research training center to train physicians or psychologists for research careers in substance abuse. He has been a pioneer in the research and treatment of narcotic and cocaine abuse for over 25 years. He has a B.A. (cum laude with high distinction) in psychology from Dartmouth College and an M.D. from Thomas Jefferson Medical School. He is the author or coauthor of more than 190 papers, chapters, and books dealing with all aspects of substance abuse, and the editor of the recently published *American Psychiatric Association Textbook of Substance Abuse Treatment*. He is a fellow of the American Psychiatric Association, the American College of Neuropsychopharmacology, the American College of Psychiatrists, the New York Academy of Medicine, the College of Problems of Drug Dependence, and the American Academy of Psychiatrists in Alcoholism and Addictions. He has served on three National Research Council and Institute of Medicine committees and chairs a number of scientific advisory boards as well as government panels.

JACQUES NORMAND is a study director at the National Research Council of the National Academy of Sciences in Washington, D.C. Prior to his work with the Panel on Needle Exchange and Bleach Distribution Programs, he directed a National Research Council/Institute of Medicine panel study on drug use in the workplace and coedited its 1994 report entitled *Under the Influence? Drugs and the American Work Force*. Prior to joining the National Research Council in 1991, he held research psychologist positions in both the private and the public sectors. In that capacity, he was responsible for the development, validation, and implementation of various organizational intervention programs. He has published in various professional research journals and has spoken at numerous professional meetings on evaluation issues. He has also served as a consultant to the National Institute on Drug Abuse and acts as an ad hoc reviewer of applied drug-use research manuscripts for various professional journals. He has served as a technical adviser on the National Institute on Drug Abuse's Technical Review Meeting on Research Methods in Workplace Settings and recently completed a four-year term as a full member of the Drug Abuse Epidemiology and Prevention Research Grant Review Committee at the National Institutes of Health. He has a B.A. from McGill University and M.S. and Ph.D. degrees in psychology from the Illinois Institute of Technology.

PATRICK M. O'MALLEY is research scientist and program director in the Institute for Social Research at the University of Michigan. He has a B.S.

from the University of Massachusetts at Amherst and a Ph.D. in psychology from the University of Michigan. Since 1975, he has been a codirector of the Monitoring the Future project, an ongoing study of the lifestyles and values of American youth. This study, which involves annual national surveys of secondary school students in grades 8, 10, and 12 and young adults through age 35, provides the nation with annual reports on trends in the use of psychoactive drugs, including alcohol, tobacco, and illicit drugs. Since 1987, he has been a member of the Drug Abuse Epidemiology and Prevention Research Review Committee for the National Institute on Drug Abuse. He has published extensively on the use and abuse of psychoactive drugs and is senior author of a major report on the role of minimum drinking age laws in alcohol use by young Americans entitled *Minimum Drinking Age: Effects on American Youth: 1976-1987.*

NANCY S. PADIAN is associate adjunct professor and assistant chief of research in the Department of Obstetrics, Gynecology and Reproductive Sciences at the University of California, San Francisco, where she heads a program in reproductive epidemiology. For the past 10 years, she has conducted a study of the heterosexual transmission of HIV in which she has examined the efficiency of and risk factors for transmission. She also conducts research on other sexually transmitted diseases and on contraceptive behaviors. She has a B.A. in child development and education from Colgate University, an M.S. in reading education from Syracuse University, and an M.P.H. and Ph.D. degrees in epidemiology from the University of California at Berkeley.

MARIAN GRAY SECUNDY is professor and director of the Program in Medical Ethics at the Howard University College of Medicine. She has been a visiting scholar at the University of San Francisco Health Policy Institute, the University of Chicago's Pritzker School of Medicine, the National Leadership Training Program in Clinical Medical Ethics, Michigan State University, and Hiram College. A practicing psychotherapist, she is also editor of *Trials, Tribulations, and Celebrations: African-American Perspectives on Health, Illness, Aging, and Loss.* In 1993 she served as cochair of the Ethics Working Group of Hillary Rodham Clinton's Health Care Task Force. She has an A.B. in political science and sociology from Vassar College, an M.S.S. in community organization from Bryn Mawr College, and a Ph.D. in medical humanities/bioethics from Union Graduate School.

DAVID VLAHOV is associate professor of epidemiology in the School of Hygiene and Public Health at The Johns Hopkins University, with a joint appointment in medicine at the School of Medicine. He has coordinated several large clinical epidemiologic studies of HIV infection among drug users (the ALIVE study) and is the principal evaluator of the Washington, D.C., and Baltimore needle exchange programs. He is also a registered nurse with a certificate in infection control and has worked in this capacity at the Baltimore Veterans Administration Medical Center, the University of Maryland Hospital, and Sinai Hospital of Baltimore, Inc. The author of numerous articles, chapters, and monographs, he has served as a peer reviewer for a number of journals and been a member of editorial boards. He has participated on a number of advisory panels for the National Institutes of Health and served as a consultant for the Health Department in Washington, D.C.; the Municipal Institute of Health in Barcelona, Spain; and the Istituto Superiore d'Sanità in Italy. He is a member of the Society for Epidemiologic Research, the American Public Health Association, and the Infectious Disease Society of America, among others. He has a B.A. in history from Earlham College, a B.S.N. and an M.S. in nursing from the University of Maryland at Baltimore, and a Ph.D. in epidemiology from the Johns Hopkins University.

W. WAYNE WIEBEL is associate professor of epidemiology in the School of Public Health at the University of Illinois at Chicago. He also serves as director of Community Outreach Intervention Projects at the university. Originally trained as an ethnographer, his research interests include the combined use of qualitative and quantitative research methods. He has been active in the field of substance abuse research over the past 20 years and in AIDS intervention research for the past 10 years. He has a B.A. in sociology from Northeastern University and an M.A. and Ph.D. degrees in sociology from Northwestern University.

DAVID R. WILLIAMS is associate professor of sociology and associate research scientist in the Institute for Social Research at the University of Michigan. His previous academic appointment was at Yale University. His research has focused on differences in socioeconomic status in health in general, and the health of the African American population in particular. He has served as a consultant to numerous federal health agencies and private organizations. Currently he is a member of the National Committee on Vital and Health Statistics and chairs its subcommittee on Minority and Other Special Populations. He is also a member of the National Science Foundation's Board of Overseers for the General Social Survey. He has an M.P.H. from Loma Linda University, a M.Div. from Andrews University, and a Ph.D. in sociology from the University of Michigan.

Index

A

Academic research, 69
Activist groups, 75, 77, 80
ACT-UP, 86
Addiction treatment services, 63, 64,
    130-132, 253, 274
  and African American communities,
    117-119
  competition for funding, 8, 117, 126-
    127, 130, 254
  concerns about exchange programs,
    104, 126-133, 135, 136, 273
  and federal regulations, 126, 132,
    144
  history of enrollment in, 65, 66, 96,
    149, 247
  professional association positions,
    127-130, 307-312
  referrals from exchange programs, 8,
    81, 82, 89, 90, 131, 199, 208, 211,
    216, 232, 237, 249, 268, 309, 310
Administration of programs, 77, 80, 94,
    268
Adolescents, *see* Youth and adolescents

African Americans
  AIDS and HIV seroprevalence, 10,
    35-36, 38, 182
  bleach distribution participants, 96,
    182
  church leadership, 117, 118-120
  community concerns, 107, 110, 111,
    114-115, 116-120, 134, 136
  exchange program participation, 83,
    84
  injection drug use, 62, 65, 67
  perinatal transmission, 36
  women with AIDS, 31, 35-36
Age
  bleach distribution participants,
    96
  exchange program participation, 81,
    84, 215, 226, 231-232, 268
  injection drug use estimates, 61, 62
  and needle sharing, 149
  seroprevalence studies, 271
Agency for Health Care Policy and
    Research, 254
AIDS cases, 9-10, 23, 31-32, 33, 34
AIDS Outreach Program (AOP), 177

AIDS, Sexual Behavior, and Intravenous Drug Use, 57, 58
Alaska, laws, 75, 147
Alcohol and alcohol wipes, 8, 82, 170, 174, 176, 219, 254
American Academy of Psychiatrists in Alcoholism & Additions (aaPaa), 128, 307-308
American College of Addiction Treatment Administrators (ACATA), 128, 308
American Medical Association (AMA), 127, 128, 308
American Pharmaceutical Association, 124, 125
American Psychiatric Association (APA), 127, 128, 309
American Public Health Association (APHA), 127, 128, 130, 309
American Society of Addiction Medicine (ASAM), 127, 128, 309-310
Ammonium compounds, 170-171
Amphetamine, 67
Amsterdam, Netherlands, exchange programs, 215, 226, 265
Anal intercourse, 28, 42, 218
Ann Arbor, Michigan, 69n
Anslinger, Harry Jacob, 144
Anti-Drug Paraphernalia Act, 145
Arizona, public opinion, 115
Arrest, 67, 122-123, 216
   perceived risk of, 149, 150, 151
Asbury Park, New Jersey, HIV prevalence, 38
Asian Americans, exchange program participation, 83, 84
Assertiveness training, 82
Assistant Secretary for Health, 7, 45-46, 69, 158, 224
Association for Drug Abuse Prevention and Treatment, 120
Association of Medical Education and Research in Substance Abuse (AMERSA), 310
Atlanta, Georgia, injection drug use estimates, 59

Attitudes, 276
Attrition, 201, 233, 275
Australia
   exchange program, 2
   needle disposal, 6, 157-158

B

Backloading, 26, 27, 187
Bacteria and bacterial infections, 27, 149, 170, 171, 172, 190
Baltimore, Maryland, 151
   disinfection habits, 178, 187-188
   exchange programs, 74, 226, 265
   injection drug use studies, 59, 66, 187
   laws, 265
   prostitution study, 41
   public opinion, 107, 116, 136
Bangkok, Thailand, HIV prevalence, 10, 39
Behavior change models, 86, 87
Berkeley, California, exchange programs, 86
Binge episodes, 57-58
Bisexual men, 32, 40, 218
   sexual partners of, 28, 40-41
Black Election Study, 119-120
Black population, *see* African Americans
Bleach and bleaching methods, 168, 169-172, 190, 220, 302, 303
   CDC recommendations, 5, 13-14, 174-175, 188-189, 190, 191
   effectiveness, 2, 82, 172-175, 186-189, 190-191, 270
Bleach distribution programs, 2, 4-5, 8, 74, 75, 82, 95-99, 175-189, 263, 267, 276
   Chicago, 177-178, 180-186, 192n
   education and outreach services, 5, 13, 97-99, 176, 177-181, 185-186, 192, 270
   evaluation of, 4-5, 218, 270
   limitations on effectiveness, 5, 65, 186-187
   participant characteristics, 96, 179

research needs and funding, 5, 191, 192

Bleachman, 97

Blood-borne pathogens, 27-28, 45, 149, 168, 190
  workplace standard, 125

Booting, 25

Boston, Massachusetts
  exchange programs, 74, 86
  injection drug use estimates, 59

Boulder, Colorado, exchange programs, 82, 84, 86

Breastfeeding, 30

Bureau of Narcotics, 144

Bush administration, 144

C

CACTUS needle exchange program, 285-293

California
  Bureau of Narcotic Enforcement, 121
  condom use, 42
  laws, 77, 147, 175

Canada
  exchange program, 2, 95
  needle sharing, 157

Case-control studies, 214
  Amsterdam, 265
  New York City, 188
  Tacoma hepatitis surveillance, 242-243, 245, 246-248

Case law, 148-149

Case management, 75, 81, 82

Center for Substance Abuse Treatment (CSAT), 5, 13, 188, 190, 191

Centers for Disease Control and Prevention (CDC)
  AIDS case reporting system, 23, 31, 67
  bleaching recommendation, 5, 13-14, 174-175, 188-189, 190, 191
  Connecticut study, 123, 152, 154, 155, 156
  evaluation research, 254-255

HIV infection estimates, 32, 34, 37, 38, 39
  injection drug use estimates, 58-59, 63

Central Intelligence Agency, 117

Chancroid, 29

Chicago, Illinois
  bisexual transmission, 40-41
  bleach distribution programs, 177-178, 180-186, 192n
  exchange programs, 84, 224-225, 293-304
  HIV prevalence, 38
  injection drug use, 59, 67, 224-225
  intranasal heroin use, 68
  public opinion, 114

Chlorine demand, 171

Churches, 117, 118-120

Circulation models, 86, 87, 228-229, 230-231, 255n, 302

Cleaning, 170, 177

Cocaine, 25, 26-27, 40, 43, 57-58, 65, 66, 67, 117. *See also* Crack

Community availability, 149, 157

Community-based studies, 64, 66-68, 69, 265

Community concerns and responses, 5-6, 103-104, 133-137, 252, 253-254, 272-273
  African Americans, 107, 110, 111, 114-115, 116-120, 134, 136
  Latino/Hispanic population, 117, 120-121, 134, 273
  law enforcement officers, 104, 121-123, 133, 134, 136, 156, 273
  moral and ethical arguments, 105-106
  pharmacists, 104, 123-126, 135, 136, 156, 273
  public opinion polls, 4, 104, 106-107, 108-115, 133, 136
  treatment service providers, 104, 126-133, 135, 136, 273

Community Epidemiology Work Group (CEWG), 66-68, 69

Comparison and cross-sectional studies, 93, 95, 201, 202

Connecticut needle deregulation, 154-155
New York City, 89-90
see also General Accounting Office review; University of California (Lurie) report
Condoms, 8, 13, 42, 44, 75, 82, 176, 177, 179, 181, 199, 211, 213, 218, 219, 254
Confounding factors, 188, 201, 266-267, 275
Connecticut
laws, 123, 147, 152-155
public opinion, 112, 113
Consolidation of programs, 151, 267
Constitutionality of drug laws, 147-148
Contact time, 170, 172, 173, 186
Contextual factors, 149
Cookers, 26, 27, 65, 82, 169, 186
Cooperation and coordination among programs, 267
Costs and cost effectiveness, 86-88, 99
Cotton, 26, 27, 82, 181
Counseling services, 75, 81, 82, 97, 179-180
Crack, 43, 179
and women, 34, 41-42

D

Dallas, Texas, exchange programs, 74
D.C., *see* Washington, D.C.
DC*MADS, *see* Washington DC Metropolitan Area Drug Study
Deaths, 67, 68, 182
Decontamination, 170
Delaware, laws, 147
de Ligorio, Alphonsi Mariae, 105
Deliveries, 77, 79
Demographic characteristics, 64-66, 82-84, 99, 143, 149, 268, 269
AIDS and HIV seroprevalence, 10, 31, 40, 45, 271
see also Age; Gender; Race and ethnicity; Socioeconomic status

Demonstration and research projects, 11, 64-66, 95-99, 179-180, 181, 220
Denver, Colorado
bleach distribution program, 97
public opinion, 115
Deontologist approach, 106
Department of Health and Human Services, 11. *See also* Assistant Secretary for Health; Center for Substance Abuse; Centers for Disease Control and Prevention; National Institute on Drug Abuse; Public Health Service; Surgeon General
Departments of Labor, Health and Human Services, and Education, and Related Agencies Appropriation Act (P.L. 102-394), 7, 11, 12, 253
Detroit, Michigan, injection drug use estimates, 59
Diabetics, 151, 153
Dialysis machines, 175
Differential bias, 265
Discarded needles, 8, 80, 99, 136, 157, 200, 216, 217, 226, 237, 251
Disinfection, 168-169, 170, 171, 172-174, 190
Disposal, *see* Discarded needles
Drug abuse, *see* Injection drug use
Drug abuse treatment, *see* Addiction treatment services

E

Education and outreach, 8, 13, 27, 75, 81-82, 199, 236, 267
bleach distribution programs, 5, 13, 97-99, 176, 177-181, 185-186, 192, 270
Eligibility for services, 80, 81, 90, 156, 267
Emergency rooms, 67, 216, 274
Endocarditis, 27
Epidemiologic data, 9-10, 23-24
AIDS cases, 9-10, 23, 31-32, 33, 34

HIV infection rates, 10, 32
injection drug transmission, 1, 9-10, 32, 34, 36, 37-44
injection drug use, 10, 57-69
Montréal study, 289-293
perinatal transmission, 43-44
research needs, 270-272
sexual transmission, 1, 9-10, 32, 34-36, 40-43
Ethanol, *see* Alcohol and alcohol wipes
Ethics, *see* Morality and ethics
Ethnicity, *see* Latino/Hispanic population; Race and ethnicity
Ethnographic research, 67, 223, 271
disinfection strategies, 175-176, 270
needle sharing, 27, 150
Evaluation research, 91, 254-255, 264-270

F

Federal regulation, 125, 143-145
constitutionality, 147-148
exchange program funding, 2, 7, 11-12, 253
reflecting moral arguments, 105
treatment services, 126, 132, 144
Feedback processes, 268
Females, *see* Women
Fixed sites, 77, 79, 80, 235
Focus group studies, 215
Forecasting of drug use, 68, 69
Fort Worth, Texas, injection drug use estimates, 59
France
exchange program, 2
needle sharing, 157
Fraternal Order of Police, 121
Frequency of injection drug use, 4, 57-58, 65, 149, 207, 213, 224-225, 252
in Chicago study, 293-302
Frontloading, 26, 27, 187
Funding
disinfection research, 5, 191, 192
of exchange programs, 2, 7, 8, 11-12, 82, 88, 94, 99, 253

for research programs, 276
of treatment services, 8, 117, 126-127, 130, 254

G

Gays, *see* Homosexuality
Gender
exchange program participation, 83, 84, 232, 233
injection drug use estimates, 62, 65
and needle sharing, 149
seroprevalence studies, 37-38, 271
see also Men; Women
General Accounting Office review, 11, 92, 118, 201, 205-208, 255*n*, 275
Genocidal theories, 107, 116, 117, 118, 134
Geographic variation
HIV infection rates, 10, 37-39, 40, 45, 64, 271, 272
injection drug use, 59-60, 64, 66, 271
Germicides, 170, 172
Great Britain, exchange program, 2

H

Harrison Narcotic Act, 143-144
Head shops, 144
Health care services, 75, 81, 82, 236-237, 268
disinfection recommendations, 174-175
facilities as exchange sites, 77, 79
workers' needlestick injuries, 24-25
Heckman method, 300
Hemodialysis machines, 175
Hemophiliacs, sexual partners of, 28
Hepatitis (HBV, HCV), 27, 45, 149, 168, 172, 190, 238, 251, 310
surveillance and seroprevalence studies, 235, 240-243, 245, 246-248, 271, 272, 276
Heroin, 25, 40, 57-58, 60, 65, 66, 67, 68
Heterosexual cases and transmission, 10, 28, 31, 32, 34-35, 218

High school students, 63
Hispanic population, *see* Latino/
    Hispanic population
HIV infection rates and seroprevalence
    among infants, 29
    geographic variation, 10, 37-39, 40,
        45, 64, 271, 272
    impacts of needle exchange
        programs, 86-88, 199, 211, 214,
        216, 220-224, 229, 234, 240, 266
    surveillance and monitoring, 10, 23,
        32, 38-39, 45-46, 271-272, 276
HIV seroconversion, 45, 272
    Chicago studies, 180, 181-186, 303-
        304
    incubation period, 169, 266
    Montréal study, 221-223, 286-293
    New Haven study, 227-228, 229,
        234
    San Francisco study, 282-285
    Tacoma studies, 237, 240, 244-245
    timing relative to program
        participation, 266, 284
HIV testing and counseling, 75, 81, 82,
    179-180, 237
HIV transmission mechanisms, *see*
    Injection drug use; Perinatal
    transmission; Sexual transmission
Homeless population, 60, 61
Homosexuality, 1, 9, 28, 32, 34, 36, 40,
    218. *See also* Men, who have
    sex with men
Hours of operation, 81, 86, 265, 267
Houston, Texas, injection drug use
    estimates, 59
Human T-lymphotrophic viruses
    (HTLV), 27, 168, 190
Hydrogen peroxide, 170, 174, 176

I

Illegal exchange operations, 75, 77, 81,
    82, 92, 99, 148
Illinois, laws, 77, 147
Income, *see* Socioeconomic status
Incubation period, 169, 266

Indirect needle sharing, 26-28, 44, 65,
    169, 179, 186-187, 266, 267, 272
Infants, *see* Perinatal transmission
Initiation of drug use, 4, 83, 99, 133,
    200, 208, 215, 225-226, 231-232,
    248-250, 252, 269
Injection drug use
    behaviors and use patterns, 7, 25-28,
        39-40, 57-58, 65, 67, 68, 69, 149,
        271
    and Connecticut needle legalization,
        154-155
    duration of, 83, 84, 96, 149, 215,
        226, 232
    frequency of, 4, 57-58, 65, 149, 207,
        213, 224-225, 252
    geographic variation, 59-60, 64, 66,
        271
    HIV infection rates, 1, 9-10, 32, 34,
        36, 37-44
    HIV transmission mechanisms, 2,
        24-28, 149, 167-169, 172-173,
        186-187
    lifetime prevalence, 61
    low-seroprevalence areas, 39
    and perinatal transmission, 2, 10, 29,
        31, 43-44
    and sexual transmission, 2, 28, 36,
        40-43, 44, 96, 218, 266-267
    social networks, 65-66, 149, 269-
        270, 271, 272
    subgroups, 66, 271-272
    surveillance and monitoring, 7, 10,
        57-69
    type of drug, 40, 60, 65, 66, 69, 149
    see also Addiction treatment
        services; Bleach and bleaching
        methods; Bleach distribution
        programs; Demographic
        characteristics; Needle exchange
        programs; Needle sharing
Institutionalized population, 60, 61. *See
    also* Prisons and prisoners
International Conference on AIDS, 221
Interviewer bias, 265
Intranasal heroin use (snorting), 60, 68

Iodine, 170
Iowa, laws, 147
Items distributed, 82, 94, 99
Iterative research processes, 268

J

Jail, *see* Prisons and prisoners
Judicial rulings, 147-149, 156

K

Kaplan model, 86, 87, 228-229, 230-231, 255n, 302

L

Laboratory studies
  disinfection methods, 173-174, 190, 270
  field procedures, 270
Latino/Hispanic population
  AIDS and HIV seroprevalence, 36, 38
  bleach distribution participants, 96
  community concerns, 117, 120-121, 134, 273
  exchange program participation, 83, 84
  injection drug transmission, 10
  injection drug use estimates, 62, 65
  women with AIDS, 36
Law enforcement officers
  concerns about exchange programs, 104, 121-123, 133, 134, 136, 156, 273
  education of, 155-156
  harassment of drug users, 121, 155
  needlestick risk, 121, 122, 155, 237
Legal issues, *see* Federal regulation; Judicial rulings; Paraphernalia laws; Prescription laws; State and local laws
Limits on exchanges, 80-81, 90, 99, 156, 235-236, 268, 269
Longitudinal studies, 131, 180

Los Angeles, California
  HIV prevalence, 38, 39
  injection drug use estimates, 59
Louisiana, prescription laws, 124
Lurie study, *see* University of California report

M

Mail Order Drug Paraphernalia Act, 145, 148
Maine, laws, 147
Malaria, 27
Males, *see* Men
Manchester, U.K., exchange programs, 91-92
Maricopa County, Arizona, public opinion, 114
Martinez, Robert, 144
Maryland, public opinion, 107, 112, 116, 136
Massachusetts
  laws, 77, 147
  public opinion, 114
Maternity, *see* Perinatal transmission
Mathematical models, 38-39, 86, 87, 88
  circulation, 86, 87, 228-229, 230-231, 255n, 302
Men
  AIDS and HIV cases, 31, 37-38, 182
  bleach distribution participants, 96, 182
  exchange program participation, 83, 99
  heterosexual transmission, 10, 34, 35
  homosexual, 1, 9, 28, 32, 34, 36, 40, 218
  injection drug use estimates, 62
  who have sex with men, 32-36
Methadone maintenance, 37, 38, 41, 130-131, 132, 151, 178, 226, 237, 270
Methodological problems and limitations, 3-4, 15, 200-204, 304-305
  Chicago study, 224-225, 299-302, 304

confounding factors, 188, 201, 266-
267, 275
cost effectiveness, 87-88
injection drug use estimates, 58, 60-
61, 272
Montréal study, 287-289, 291-293
randomized trials, 201, 202, 274-
275
respondent characterization, 58, 64-
66, 83, 96, 264-265
San Francisco study, 283-285
selection and sampling, 39, 64, 221,
246, 247-248, 266, 283, 284-285,
288, 291
seroprevalence studies, 23, 32, 38-
39, 182-185, 271-272
temporal relationships, 266, 284
Methylphenidate, 67
Metropolitan areas, 59, 66-67
Miami, Florida
disinfection habits, 178-179
HIV infection, 32
injection drug use rates, 10
shooting gallery studies, 25-26
Mid-City Consortium to Combat AIDS,
175, 177
Midwest/Central region
AIDS and HIV cases, 34, 37
injection drug use, 10, 59-60,
67
Milan, Italy, HIV prevalence, 10, 39
Milwaukee, Wisconsin, exchange
programs, 74
Minnesota, exchange programs,
74
Minority groups, see African
Americans; Latino/Hispanic
population; Race and ethnicity
Mobile sites, 77, 79, 80, 235
Model Drug Paraphernalia Act, 145
Monitoring, see Surveillance and
monitoring
Monitoring the Future Survey, 63
Montréal, Canada, exchange programs,
221-223, 265, 285-293
Morality and ethics, 105-106
of randomized trials, 201, 202, 275

N

Narcotic Drug Import and Export Act,
144
Nashua, New Hampshire, 69n
National AIDS Demonstration Research
(NADR) studies, 64-66, 95-99,
179-180, 181, 220
National Association of Chain Drug
Stores, 124-125
National Association of Psychiatric
Health Systems (NAPHS), 129,
311
National Association of Social Workers
(NASW), 127, 129, 311-312
National Association of State Alcohol
and Drug Abuse Directors
(NASADAD), 129, 312
National Consortium of Chemical
Dependency Nurses, Inc.
(NCCDN), 312
National Household Survey on Drug
Abuse (NHSDA), 60, 62, 63
National Institute on Drug Abuse
(NIDA)
bleach distribution studies, 74, 95, 179
bleaching recommendation, 5, 13,
188, 190, 191
HIV infection estimates, 38
injection drug use estimates, 58, 61,
66, 69, 183
risk behavior surveys, 178
National Institutes of Health, 254-255
Necessity defense, 148
NEED exchange, 86
Needle exchange programs, 2, 4, 11,
74, 75-95, 99, 263, 264-270, 276
administration, 77, 80, 94, 268
ancillary on-site services, 7, 13, 75,
81-82, 94, 99, 254, 268
costs and cost effectiveness, 86-88, 99
and discarded needles, 8, 80, 99,
136, 157, 200, 216, 217, 226,
237, 251
education and information services,
8, 13, 75, 81-82, 199, 236, 267
eligibility rules, 80, 81, 90, 156, 267

in foreign countries, 2, 11, 205, 206, 210
funding, 2, 7, 8, 11-12, 82, 88, 94, 99, 253
hours of operation, 81, 86, 265, 267
illegal operations, 75, 77, 81, 82, 92, 99, 148
impact on HIV transmission and infection rates, 86-88, 199, 211, 214, 216, 220-224, 229, 234, 240, 266
and initiation of drug use, 4, 83, 99, 133, 200, 208, 215, 225-226, 231-232, 248-250, 252, 269
items distributed, 82, 94, 99
legal issues, 6, 75-77, 92-93, 94, 148-149
limits on syringes exchanged, 80-81, 90, 99, 156, 235-236, 268, 269
needle sharing impacts, 199, 206, 207, 211, 212, 218, 219, 220, 251, 302-304
organizational and operational characteristics, 75, 77-82, 89-95, 267-270
participation, 75, 82-84, 268, 269
policies, 80-81, 267-268
as promoting and increasing drug use, 4, 105, 122, 126, 127, 132-133, 200, 214-216, 217, 224-226, 251-252
siting and location, 77, 79-80, 82, 90, 94, 99, 267
staffing, 80, 82, 89, 93, 94
treatment referrals, 8, 81, 82, 89, 90, 131, 199, 208, 211, 216, 232, 237, 249, 268, 309, 310
see also Community concerns and responses; *under names of individual jurisdictions, for descriptions and studies of specific programs*
Needle sales and distribution, 151, 265
availability, *see* Community availability
deregulation of, 136, 147, 152-158, 273
from diabetics, 265
and disposal of needles, 124, 125, 154, 157-158, 273
laws restricting, 6, 8, 75-77, 78, 122, 144, 147, 152, 156-157, 158
from pharmacies, 123-126, 136, 150, 152-155, 265
renting, 25-26, 65, 219
scarcity, *see* Needle sharing. relation to needle scarcity
by secondary exchangers, 91-92, 206, 264-265
see also Needle exchange programs
Needle sharing, 2, 10, 24-26, 39-40, 44, 45, 65, 159n, 167-168, 186, 272
and Connecticut needle legalization, 154-155
factors in, 149, 150-151
impacts of exchange programs, 199, 206, 207, 211, 212, 218, 219, 220, 251, 302-304
indirect, 26-28, 44, 65, 169, 179, 186-187, 266, 267, 272
relation to needle scarcity, 10, 150-151
as ritual, 150
Needlestick injuries, 136, 216
of health care workers, 24-25
of law enforcement officers, 121, 122, 155, 237
Netherlands
exchange program, 2
needle sharing, 157
Newark, New Jersey
injection drug use estimates, 59
intranasal heroin use, 68
New Hampshire, laws, 147
New Haven, Connecticut, exchange programs, 84, 86, 205, 226-234, 302
New Jersey
AIDS cases, 31
laws, 147
New Orleans, Louisiana, pharmacy sales, 124

New York City
 AIDS and HIV prevalence, 10, 31-
 32, 38, 39, 223
 bleach distribution program, 177-178
 exchange programs, 84, 86, 89-90,
 91, 92-93, 120, 121, 136, 218-
 220, 223-224
 injection drug use studies, 59, 60,
 175, 187
 intranasal heroin use, 68
 public opinion, 108, 110, 111, 113
 women at risk, 41
New York State
 AIDS cases, 31
 laws, 77, 147
North Dakota, laws, 147
Northeastern region
 AIDS and HIV cases, 32, 34, 37, 38,
 39
 condom use, 42
 injection drug use rates, 10, 59, 60

O

Observational epidemiologic studies,
 274, 275
Occupational Safety and Health
 Administration (OSHA), 125, 155
Office of National Drug Control Policy,
 105, 144
One-for-one exchange programs, 80,
 90, 156, 216, 235, 268, 302
Ordinary least squares (OLS) method,
 300, 301

M

Paraphernalia laws, 7, 75, 76, 121, 136,
 144-147, 156-157
 Baltimore, 265
 constitutionality, 147
 federal, 145
 impacts on needle sharing, 6, 123,
 150, 151, 158
 as tool for arresting dealers, 122-123
Pediatric cases, 31, 36, 37

Pennsylvania, laws, 147
Pentazocine, 67
Perinatal transmission, 29-30, 31, 46n
 and injection drug use, 2, 10, 29, 31,
 43-44
Pharmacists and pharmacies, 104, 123-
 126, 135, 136, 156, 273
 and Connecticut needle sale law,
 123, 152-155
 drug-user incidents and problems,
 124, 125, 153-154
 education of, 155, 156
 foreign studies, 124
Phenmetrazine, 67
Philadelphia, Pennsylvania
 injection drug use estimates, 59
 seroprevalence study, 39
Plausibility, 203-204
Population characteristics, *see*
 Demographic characteristics
Portland, Oregon, exchange programs,
 84, 86, 216, 220, 226
Pregnancy, *see* Perinatal transmission
Prescription laws, 6, 8, 75-77, 78, 121,
 122, 123, 144, 145-147, 152, 156,
 157, 158, 265
 constitutionality, 147-148
 federal, 143-144
 as tool for arresting dealers, 122-123
Prevention Point program, 282
Prisons and prisoners
 bleach distribution participants, 96
 injection drug use estimates, 64, 65
 Montréal study, 286-287, 288-289
 prevention research, 274
Professional associations, 127-130, 307-
 312
Programmatic research, 268
Promotion and increase of drug use, 4,
 105, 122, 126, 127, 132-133, 200,
 214-216, 217, 224-226, 251-252
Proportionalist approach, 105-106
Prospective studies, 202
 community-based, 265
 Connecticut needle deregulation,
 152-154

Prostitution, 41, 42, 43, 222
  for drugs, 41-42
*Public Health Impact of Needle
    Exchange Programs in the United
    States and Abroad, see* University
    of California (Lurie) report
Public Health Service (PHS)
  HIV infection estimates, 32
  injection drug use estimates, 58
  Tuskegee Syphilis Study, 107
Public opinion polls, 4, 104, 106-107,
    108-115, 133, 136
Puerto Rico
  HIV infection, 34
  injection drug use rates, 10
Pure Food and Drug Act, 143

Q

Quality assurance programs, 268

R

Race and ethnicity
  AIDS and HIV seroprevalence, 31,
    34, 36, 37, 40, 271
  and ancillary services, 268
  bleach distribution participants, 96
  exchange program participation, 83,
    99
  homosexual transmission, 34
  injection drug transmission, 10, 36
  injection drug use estimates, 62
  women with AIDS, 36
  see also African Americans; Asian
    Americans, exchange program
    participation; Latino/Hispanic
    population; White population
Randomized trials, 201, 202, 203, 274-
    275
Rangel, Charles, 117, 118-119
Reagan administration, 144
Recall and response bias, 201, 265
Recruitment and retention, 75, 268
Regional differences, *see* Geographic
    variation

Registering, 25
Relapse, 130, 131, 132
Rhode Island
  exchange programs, 74
  laws, 147
Rinse water, 26-27, 65, 169, 176, 186
Risk knowledge and perception, 149,
    150-151
Riverside, California, injection drug use
    estimates, 59
Roving vans, 77, 79
Running partners, 65
Rural areas, 69n

S

San Diego, California, injection drug
    use, 67
San Francisco, California
  AIDS cases, 31
  bleach distribution program, 97,
    175-176, 177, 187, 188, 217-218
  condom use, 42
  exchange programs, 84, 121, 219,
    223, 226, 281-285
  injection drug use estimates, 59,
    175, 215
  young program participants, 83
San Juan, Puerto Rico, injection drug
    use, 59, 60
School-distance zoning, 90
Screening and counseling services, 75,
    81, 82, 90, 91, 97, 179-180, 236-
    237
Secondary and surrogate exchangers,
    81, 236, 264-265
Selection and sampling bias, 39, 64,
    221, 246, 247-248, 283, 284-285,
    288, 291
Sepsis, 27
Seroconversion, *see* HIV
    seroconversion
Serrano, Yolanda, 120, 121
Sex, *see* Gender; Men; Prostitution;
    Sexual transmission; Women

Sexually transmitted diseases, 29, 45,
    75, 81, 82, 272, 274
Sexual transmission, 1, 9-10, 24, 28-29,
    31, 32, 34-36, 40-43, 182, 184
    and crack use, 41-42
    homosexual, 1, 9, 28, 32, 34, 36, 40,
        218
    and injection drug use, 2, 28, 36, 40-
        43, 44, 96, 218, 266-267
    prevention of, 45, 46, 82, 211, 213,
        218, 220
    social networks, 272
    women at risk, 28, 34-35, 40-43
    see also Condoms; Prostitution
Shooting galleries, 25-26, 40, 149, 179,
    218
Single-time users, 264
Siting and location, 77, 79-80, 82, 90,
    94, 99, 267
Situational factors, 149
Snorting, 60, 68
Social desirability effects, 246
Social networks, 65-66, 149, 269-270,
    271, 272, 276
    and bleach distribution programs,
        180, 181
Social services, 7, 13, 75, 81-82, 94,
    99, 254, 268
Socioeconomic status, 268
Sodium hypochlorite, see Bleach and
    bleaching methods
South Carolina, laws, 147
Southern region
    AIDS and HIV cases, 35, 37-38
    injection drug use rates, 60
Speedball, 65
Staffing, 80, 82, 89, 93, 94
Starter needles, 80, 216
State and local laws, 75-77, 144-147,
    see also under names of
        individual jurisdictions
    challenges to, 147-149
    constitutionality, 147-148
    deregulation and repeal, 147, 152-
        155, 156, 157, 158, 275
    drug-free zones, 77, 90
    impacts on needle sharing, 150-151

pharmacy sales, 124, 125-126, 152-
    155
precedence of public health laws,
    148
prostitution, 77
Stationary vans, 77, 79
Statistical sensitivity, 201, 207-208
Sterilization, 169-170
Stimulants, 67
Storefronts, 77, 79
Street sites, 77, 79
Subpopulations, see Demographic
    characteristics
Substance Abuse and Mental Health
    Services Administration
    (SAMHSA), 60. See also Center
    for Substance Abuse
Supreme Court, 147
Surgeon General, 2, 7, 11, 253
Surrogates, see Secondary and
    surrogate exchangers
Surveillance and monitoring
    at community and local level, 7, 38-
        39, 66-68, 69, 255, 268-269, 271
    of injection drug use, 7, 10, 57-69
    see also Epidemiologic data
Surveys and studies, see Case-control
    studies; Community-based
    studies; Comparison and cross-
    sectional studies; Epidemiologic
    data; Ethnographic research;
    General Accounting Office
    review; Mathematical models;
    Methodological problems and
    limitations; Monitoring the Future
    Survey; National AIDS
    Demonstration Research (NADR)
    studies; National Household
    Survey on Drug Abuse;
    Prospective studies; Public
    opinion polls; Randomized trials;
    Surveillance and monitoring;
    University of California (Lurie)
    report; Washington DC
    Metropolitan Area Drug Study;
    Youth Risk Behavior Survey
Syphilis, 27, 29, 42, 107

Syringes, *see* Bleach and bleaching methods; Bleach distribution programs; *under terms beginning* Needle *in this index*
Systematic measurement error, 292, 301

T

Tacoma, Washington, 69*n*
  exchange programs, 82, 84, 86, 205, 234-250
Tacoma Pharmacy Exchange, 86
Tagged syringes, 92-93
Texas
  condom use, 42
  injection drug use estimates, 59
The Works, 82
Time and temporal variation, 64, 266, 284
  of injection equipment availability, 149, 157
Track marks, 81
Transient populations, 60, 61
Transmission mechanisms, *see* Injection drug use; Needle sharing; Perinatal transmission; Sexual transmission
Treatment, *see* Addiction treatment services
Trend analysis, 68
Tripelennamine, 67
Ts and blues, 67
Tuberculosis, 75, 81, 82, 90, 91, 237
Tuskegee Syphilis Study, 107
Two-stage least-squares (2SLS) procedure, 299, 300-301

U

Underground exchanges, *see* Illegal exchange operations
Unemployment, injection drug use estimates, 65
Uniform Controlled Substances Act, 145
Uniform Crime Reports (UCR), 216

University of California (Lurie) report, 13, 74, 75, 86, 124, 201, 208-217, 275
Urinalysis data, 67, 216
User-friendliness, 91-93, 94, 95, 99, 268
Utah, public opinion, 108, 113

V

Vans, 77, 79
Volunteers, 80, 82, 93

W

Walk routes, 77, 79
Washington, D.C.
  exchange programs, 84, 90-91, 136
  injection drug use estimates, 59
  laws, 147
Washington DC Metropolitan Area Drug Study (DC*MADS), 61-63, 70*n*
Washington State
  exchange programs, 148
  public opinion, 108-111
Western region
  AIDS and HIV cases, 35, 37, 38
  injection drug use rates, 10, 59
White population
  AIDS and HIV seroprevalence, 36, 38, 182
  bleach distribution participants, 96, 182
  exchange program participation, 83, 84, 233
  injection drug use, 62, 65, 67
  women with AIDS, 36
Wishart Drug Problems Centre, 89
Women
  AIDS and HIV seroprevalence, 1, 31, 34-36, 37-38, 40
  bleach distribution participants, 96
  and crack, 34, 41-42
  exchange program participation, 8, 83, 84, 254

injection drug use estimates, 62, 65
sexual transmission risk, 28, 34-35,
   40-43
see also Perinatal transmission

Y

Youth and adolescents
   AIDS and HIV seroprevalence, 31,
      34, 38, 40, 83

exchange program participation, 8,
   81, 83, 215, 254, 272
homosexual transmission, 34
injection drug use, 61, 63, 215, 272
Youth Risk Behavior Survey, 63

Z

Zidovudine (AZT), 30